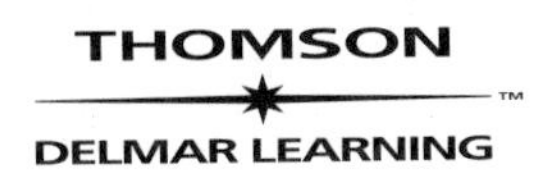

Legal Aspects of Health Information Management, Second Edition
Dana C. McWay, JD, RHIA

Executive Director Health Care Business Unit:
William Brottmiller

Executive Editor:
Cathy L. Esperti

Acquisitions Editor:
Rhonda Dearborn

Developmental Editor:
Marah Bellegarde

Editorial Assistant:
Jill O'Brien

Executive Marketing Manager:
Dawn F. Gerrain

Channel Manager:
Jennifer McAvey

Production Editor:
James Zayicek

Printed in the United States of America
5 XXX 06 05 04

For more information contact Delmar,
5 Maxwell Dr. PO Box 8007,
Clifton Park, NY 12065-8007

Or find us on the World Wide Web at
http://www.delmarhealthcare.com

Library of Congress Cataloging-in-Publication Data

McWay, Dana C.
Legal aspects of health information management / Dana C. McWay.—2nd ed.
p. cm. — (The health information management series)
Includes index.
ISBN 0-7668-2520-5
1. Medical records—Law and legislation—United States. I. Title. II. Series.

KF3827.R4 M395 2002
344.73′041—dc21 2002019401

NOTICE TO THE READER

Publisher does not warrant or guarantee any of the products described herein or perform any independent analysis in connection with any of the product information contained herein. Publisher does not assume, and expressly disclaims, any obligation to obtain and include information other than that provided to it by the manufacturer.

The reader is expressly warned to consider and adopt all safety precautions that might be indicated by the activities described herein and to avoid all potential hazards. By following the instructions contained herein, the reader willingly assumes all risks in connection with such instructions.

The publisher makes no representations or warranties of any kind, including but not limited to, the warranties of fitness for particular purpose or merchantability, nor are any such representations implied with respect to the material set forth herein, and the Publisher takes no responsibility with respect to such material. The Publisher shall not be liable for any special, consequential or exemplary damages resulting, in whole or in part, from the readers' use of, or reliance upon, this material.

Legal Aspects of Health Information Management

Second Edition

The Health Information Management Series

Dana C. McWay, JD, RHIA

THOMSON
DELMAR LEARNING

Australia Canada Mexico Singapore Spain United Kingdom United States

Contents

Preface ix

About the Author xii

About Legal Citations xiv

About Legal Research xvi

Chapter 1 Workings of the American Legal System 1

Public and Private Law 2
- *Private Law* 2
- *Public Law* 4

Sources of Law 5
- *Constitutions* 5
- *Statutes* 8
- *Administrative Decisions and Regulations* 8
- *Judicial Decisions* 10

Branches of Government 13
- *Legislative Branch* 14
- *Executive Branch* 15
- *Judicial Branch* 15

Quasi-Legal Requirements 16

Chapter 2 Court Systems and Legal Procedures 19

Court Systems 20
- *Jurisdiction* 20

Court Structure 22
Legal Process 24
Beginning the Lawsuit 25
Discovery 26
Pretrial Conference 29
Trial 30
Appeal 32
Satisfying the Judgment 32
Alternative Dispute Resolution 33

Chapter 3 Principles of Liability 37

Health-Care Relationships 39
Physician–Patient Relationships 39
Hospital–Patient Relationships 40
Hospital–Physician Relationships 42
Theories of Liability 43
Nonintentional Torts 43
Intentional Torts 52
Breach of Contract 55
Defenses and Limitations on Liability 55
Statutes of Limitations 55
Charitable Immunity 57
Governmental Immunity 57
Good Samaritan Statutes 58
Contributory and Comparative Negligence 59
Assumption of Risk 60

Chapter 4 Patient Record Requirements 63

Function and Use of the Medical Record 65
Legal Requirements for Medical Record Content 67
Content of the Medical Record 67
Timely and Complete Medical Records 70
Retention Requirements 75

Statutes and Regulations 76
Other External Forces 77
Bases for Decision 78
Record Destruction 78
Destruction in Ordinary Course 78
Destruction Due to Closure 80

Chapter 5 Access to Health Information 87

Ownership of Health Information 89
Notice of Use and Disclosure 90
Access by or on Behalf of the Patient 96
General Principles of Disclosure Information 96
By the Patient 100
To Third Parties 101
Reasonable Fees 102
Access by the Researcher 103
Access by the Business Associate 104
Access Pursuant to Reporting Laws 106
Access to Adoption Records 107

Chapter 6 Confidentiality and Informed Consent 115

Confidentiality 116
Constitutional Basis 119
Statutory Basis 120
Common Law Basis 121
Informed Consent 121
Historical Development 122
Scope of Informed Consent Doctrine 122

Chapter 7 Judicial Process of Health Information *133*

Medical Records as Evidence 135
Hearsay 135
Privilege 137

Responses to Legal Process 138
- *Subpoenas* 139
- *Court Orders* 142
- *Response Methods* 143

Chapter 8 Specialized Patient Records 149

Drug and Alcohol Abuse 151
- *Confidentiality* 152
- *Release of Information* 153
- *Miscellaneous Issues* 161

Mental Health and Developmental Disability Care 163
- *Content Requirements* 163
- *Privacy Restrictions* 165

Home Health Care 167

Genetic Information 168

Chapter 9 Risk Management and Quality Management 175

Risk Management 176
- *General Principles* 176
- *Patient Record Requirements* 178
- *Incident Reports* 181

Quality Management 184
- *Peer Review Privileges* 185
- *National Practitioner Data Bank* 187

Chapter 10 HIV Information 195

Testing 196
- *Background Information about HIV/AIDS* 196
- *Voluntary Testing* 197
- *Mandatory Testing* 198
- *Anonymous Testing* 199

Patient Confidentiality 200

Legal Challenges 201
- *Employment Challenges* 201
- *Improper Disclosure Challenges* 203

Chapter 11 Computerized Patient Records 209

Accreditation and Licensure Issues 212
- *Creation and Storage 213*
- *Authentication 214*

Liability Issues 215
- *Admissible Evidence 216*
- *Security Issues 218*

Electronic Health Issues 224
- *Internet 224*
- *Electronic Mail 226*
- *Digital Imaging 227*
- *Telemedicine 228*

Chapter 12 Health-Care Fraud and Abuse 237

Fraud and Abuse 238
- *Major Laws Addressing Fraud and Abuse 239*
- *Law Enforcement Agencies 243*

Compliance Programs 244

Appendix 251

Case Studies: Things to Consider 253
Table of Cases 265
List of Common Acronyms 271
A Patient's Bill of Rights 277
Principles of Medical Record Documentation 281
Durable Power of Attorney for Health Care and Health Care Directive (Sample Form) 287
Sample Living Will 293
Patient Self-Determination Act 297
Health Care Quality Improvement Act 307

Glossary 325

Index 341

Dedicated to
Patrick, Conor, William, and Ryan

Preface

Whether taking the form of a paper medical record, a computerized medical record, or an abstract of patient-specific information, the health information contained in these formats plays a primary role in the delivery of health care. In addition to its role in direct patient care, health information maintained in these formats serves as the health-care provider's legal record of patient care. As such, it is subject to stringent legal requirements. Therefore, managers of this health information have a professional stake in understanding the legal requirements governing policies designed to safeguard this information.

Unfortunately for students and managers of health information, many of the books currently available do not have as their focus the numerous legal issues present in the unique area of health information management. Rather, the available books generally fall into one of two areas: either they focus on legal issues but are geared to a far broader audience and therefore do not address concerns specific to health information managers, or if geared to health information managers, the legal issues covered are not comprehensive and comprise only a very small portion of the book. For that reason, this book is directed toward assisting students and managers in the health information field, and others involved in health-care activities, with understanding the legal principles that govern this particular area of health care. The knowledge gained in this study is not designed as a substitute for appropriate consultation with legal counsel; rather, it is designed as a guide to the recognition of legal problems. Nor is it designed as a substitute for the broader teachings of health information management, such as those dealing with ethics and quality improvement.

To achieve this goal, this book is organized into three main areas: (1) a study of the law in general, including the American legal system, legal procedures, and principles of liability; (2) control and use of patient-specific health information, including confidentiality and release of information; and (3) specialized areas of concern in health information management. Additionally, each chapter includes a case study. The case study is designed so that the learner may use both critical thinking skills and the knowledge gained in the chapter to formulate an answer. The case studies are designed to approximate real life situations and, as in real-life, no one "right" answer exists.

New to This Edition

The second edition of *Legal Aspects of Health Information Management* has been carefully designed to enhance the study of health information management. Much is new in this edition:

- The Health Insurance Portability and Accountability Act (HIPAA) and its implementing regulations are covered extensively in Chapter 5 and in other chapters where appropriate.
- Updates in electronic technology, such as the use of the Internet, electronic mail, digital imaging, and telemedicine, are included in an extensive revision of Chapter 11 on electronic health issues.
- An emerging area in health information management, health-care fraud and abuse, is covered in Chapter 12, new to this edition. An understanding of this area is important because the health information management professional manages risk areas critical to an allegation of health-care fraud and abuse, such as accurate documentation, coding, and billing. This understanding can assist the health-care organization in preventing the submission of false or inaccurate claims to the government or private payors.
- Review questions that test the comprehension of concepts have been added to every chapter. Enrichment activities that offer activity suggestions to the reader that will reinforce the material presented in the chapter and help the reader develop and hone critical thinking skills can be found in each chapter.
- One comprehensive glossary has been added to the back of the book to make looking up terms easier.

- The Table of Cases has been reordered by chapter, as well as in alphabetical order, to make locating cases by subject matter easier. All cases have been indexed.

Following publication of the first edition of this book, the American Health Information Management Association (AHIMA) recognized *Legal Aspects of Health Information Management* for offering "practical guidance to legal principles of information management." AHIMA awarded the Legacy Award for 1997 to me in recognition of the book's "contribution to the HIM profession."

Acknowledgments

This preface would not be complete without acknowledging the assistance and support of the many people who have made this book possible. I am most thankful to my family, whose patience has encouraged and sustained me in so many ways. In particular, to my husband and three sons, I owe my unending gratitude. Additionally, the research assistance provided by Jill Shipley, a former student at St. Louis University Law School, has proved invaluable. My editors for the second edition, Maureen Muncaster and Marah Bellegarde, guided me through the revision process and encouraged me with every effort. Thank you to the reviewers of my manuscript. Your comments were invaluable. The reviewers were:

Sue Ellen Bice, MS, RHIA
HIT/MR and Allied Health Programs
Mohawk Valley Community College
Utica, NY

Nancy Coffman-Kadish, MS, RHIA
Health Information Technology Program
Indiana University, Northwest
Gary, IN

Thomas J. Falen, MA, RRA, LHCRM
Health Information Management
University of Central Florida
Orlando, FL

Maribeth Schneider, RHIA
Health Information Management
Northwest Iowa Community College
Sheldon, IA

Julie Wolter, MA, RRA
Health Information Management
Saint Louis University
St. Louis, MO

D.C.M.

About the Author

Dana C. McWay, JD, RRA, is a lawyer working as the Clerk of Court for the U.S. Bankruptcy Court for the Eastern District of Missouri. She is responsible for all executive and administrative matters of the court. Prior to this position, she worked in court administration with the U.S. Court of Appeals for the Eighth Circuit. Before taking this position, Ms. McWay was associated with the law firm of Peper, Martin, Jensen, Maichel & Hetlage, a multispecialty firm located in St. Louis, Missouri. Ms. McWay's legal practice encompassed a variety of health law topics, including contracts, medical records, and physician practice issues. Before entering private practice, she worked as a judicial clerk to the Honorable Myron H. Bright of the U.S. Court of Appeals for the Eighth Circuit. She is admitted to practice in both Illinois and Missouri.

Prior to her legal career, Ms. McWay worked in health information management as both a director and assistant director of medical records at a large teaching hospital and a for-profit psychiatric and substance abuse facility. She has served as a member of the Legislative Committee of the Missouri Health Information Management Association and, with the Peper, Martin law firm, revised *The Legal Manual to Medical Record Practice in Missouri* in 1991. Between 1993 and 1996, she served as a member of the Committee for Professional Development of the American Health Information Management Association.

Other activities include service as a member of the Advisory Board of the Health Information Management program at St. Louis University from 1990 to 1991 and as a member of the Institutional Review Board at Washington University Medical School from 1991 to present. She has received national recognition from the National Bar Foundation, a component of the American Bar Association, for creating the "Kids in Court Program," now operated by the Bar Association of Metropolitan St. Louis, which was cited as one of the five most outstanding children's legal education programs for 1995.

Ms. McWay is a magna cum laude graduate of the St. Louis University School of Allied Health Professions with a degree in medical record administration and a cum laude graduate of the St. Louis University Law School. While in law school, Ms. McWay served as the health law editor of the *St. Louis University Law Journal.*

About Legal Citations

A legal citation identifies a legal authority or reference work, such as a constitution, statute, court decision, administrative rule, or treatise. Legal citations are used throughout this work to (1) identify the source of a quotation, (2) identify an authority referred to in the text, or (3) support the propositions stated. Legal citations are found in both the body of the text and the endnotes.

The learner may be interested in legal citations for more than one reason: to identify legal authority that is binding on the health-care provider or to learn how to obtain full copies of a citation to read as a supplement to the text. For most citations other than statutory provisions and court decisions, the legal citation is self-explanatory. Some explanation is warranted for understanding how to read citations of statutes and court decisions.

Both federal and state statutes are published in either official or unofficial codes. For federal statutes, the official code is the *United States Code* (U.S.C.); unofficial codes include the *United States Code Annotated* (U.S.C.A.) and the *United States Code Service* (U.S.C.S.). Every effort has been made in this book to cite federal statutes published in the official code. A typical federal statutory citation cites first to the title number, next to the abbreviation of the official code, third to the numbered section or paragraph, and finally to the year that appears on the spine of the volume cited. Where statutory material can be found in a supplement to the official code, it is identified as a supplement with the year of the supplement identified. For example, the citation 42 U.S.C. § 11101 (1988 & Supp. V 1993) shows that the particular statute may be found in title 42 of the *United States Code* as section number 11101 in both the volume published in 1988 and the fifth supplement to that volume published in 1993.

Similarly, state statutes are published in either official or unofficial codes and generally follow the same practice as federal statutes. For example, the citation FLA. STAT. ANN. § 395.0197 (West 1993) shows that the particular statute may be found in the unofficial code *Florida Statutes Annotated* at section 395.0197 published by the West Publishing Company in 1993. Multiple state statutory citations are listed in alphabetical, rather than year, order, using standard abbreviations.

Court decisions are cited according to a similar approach. The name of the case and the numbers, letters, and years following it are referred to as the citation for the decision. For example, the citation *Warwick v. Bliss,* 195 N.W. 502 (S.D. 1923) shows that the case involving those named parties may be found in volume 195 of the *NorthWestern Reporter* on page 502. The initials and year in parentheses refer to the identity of the court that issued the decision, in this case the Supreme Court of the State of South Dakota, and the year the decision was issued.

The same case may show more than one citation, indicating that a decision has been issued in the same case by different courts. If the first citation is followed by the abbreviations *aff'd, rev'd,* or *cert. denied,* the citation indicates the subsequent history of the case, namely, that a higher court has reviewed the decision of the lower court. For example, the citation *Johnson v. Misericordia Community Hospital,* 294 N.W.2d 501 (Wis. Ct. App. 1980) *aff'd,* 301 N.W.2d 156 (Wis. 1981) shows that the case involving those named parties appears in two different reporters. First, the case may be found in volume 294 of the *NorthWestern Reporter,* second series, on page 501, and was issued by the Wisconsin Court of Appeals in 1980. Second, the case was affirmed by the Wisconsin Supreme Court in 1981 and can be found in volume 301 of the *NorthWestern Reporter,* second series, on page 156.

The legal citations listed in this book are cited according to the standards of the book *A Uniform System of Citation, Fifteenth Edition,* commonly referred to as *The Blue Book,* a joint publication of the Columbia Law Review Association, the Harvard Law Review Association, the University of Pennsylvania Law Review, and the Yale Law Journal.

About Legal Research

To the uninitiated, legal research can be bewildering, overwhelming, or intimidating. Entire books have been devoted to the subject, making the topic difficult to summarize easily. Nonetheless, a basic review of legal research methods is provided so that the learner may research an area of law covered in this book or to review the exact wording of a constitutional provision, statute, or administrative regulation.

Before beginning any research project, the learner must first obtain an understanding of the sources of law in order to know where to look. The sources of law are explained in detail in Chapter 1, and a brief description is provided here. The sources of law are divided into two categories: primary sources and secondary sources. Primary sources are *the law themselves*, including constitutions, statutes, court decisions, and administrative decisions and regulations. They are located in official and unofficial codes in the case of constitutions, statutes, and administrative regulations, and in case digests when looking for court cases or administrative decisions. Case digests are grouped by cases issued by federal courts, state courts, or courts found in a particular region of the United States. Citations to these primary sources are explained in the "About Legal Citations" discussions previously. Secondary sources are the writings or commentaries *about the law*, including legal encyclopedias, articles found in professional journals, and legal treatises. This book is an example of a secondary source.

With so many sources to choose from, how does the learner find the answer? There are several techniques to choose from, all of which apply to the traditional method of using books for research or through the newer method of using computer-based legal databases. The learner should choose from the following techniques when beginning legal research:

1. *Generalized approach.* This approach is most applicable when the learner has little or no general knowledge about the problem or area that is the subject of research. It begins with a review of secondary source materials, such as legal encyclopedias or articles in professional journals. These materials often have a table of contents or indexes to guide further research, leading to review of topics of interest. Many of these topics of interest list citations, footnotes, or references to primary source material, which will further aid the learner's research.
2. *Known authority approach.* This approach is most applicable when the learner knows the citation to the constitutional provision, statute, case, or administrative decision or regulation (the "authority"). It begins with a review of primary source materials to locate the citation of the authority in question and follows with a review of that authority.
3. *Descriptive word or fact word approach.* This approach is most applicable when the learner knows general information about the subject matter but does not have a specific citation to the relevant primary authority. After choosing a descriptive or fact word, the learner should look in the index to a set of official or unofficial codes to find constitutions, statutes, and administrative regulations or to the applicable case digest to find a court case or administrative decision.
4. *Known topic approach.* This approach is most applicable when the learner knows the area of law involved but not the specific legal authority. For constitutions, statutes, and administrative regulations, the learner should look to the subject matter grouping within the official and unofficial codes. For court cases or administrative decisions, look to the topic and subtopic sections of the applicable case digest.

Once the learner has found the authority being researched, the research activity is not over. Rather, the learner must continue the research to check the current status (i.e., validity) of the authority. The easiest, most thorough, and complete method to check the status of the authority in question is through the use of a computer-based legal database. A search begins for references to the citation by typing the authority's citation into the database. The learner should review the listed references to evaluate their effect, if any, on the citation in question.

Alternatively, nonelectronic methods of checking the current status of an authority are available. Many hardbound volumes contain so-called pocket parts, which are paperbound pamphlets inserted into a slot in the cover of the hardbound volume. The pocket parts follow the same format as the hardbound volume to which they correspond and report any additions or decision to the main text. Supplements to hardbound volumes follow the same principles. The learner should review the references to the citation to evaluate their effect, if any, on the citation in question.

Another method is to trace the subsequent work of a legal authority through a citator publication; the best known is *Shepard's Citations*. The entries contained in *Shepard's* list authorities (e.g., other cases, journal articles, and attorney general opinions) that have cited the legal authority that is the subject of the research. Detailed instruction on the use of a citator publication such as *Shepard's* is beyond the scope of this book.

Chapter 1

Workings of the American Legal System

Learning Objectives

After reading this chapter, the learner should be able to:

1. Differentiate between public and private law.
2. Compose a scenario that illustrates the difference between the substantive and procedural aspects of criminal law.
3. Identify and explain the differences between various sources of law.
4. Describe the branches of government and their roles in creating, administering, and enforcing law.
5. Explain the process of how a bill becomes a law.
6. List and describe quasi-legal requirements to which health-care organizations are subject.

Key Concepts

Common law
Constitution
Contract law
Felony
Misdemeanor
Private law
Procedural law
Public law
Res judicata
Stare decisis
Statutes
Substantive law
Tort law

Introduction

As health care becomes more complex, the interplay between the law and health care increases. Government regulation of the health-care field continues almost without pause while lawsuits against health-care providers appear to increase. The interplay of these forces significantly affects the health information manager's ability to manage patient-specific health information. Thus, the health information manager must possess a fundamental understanding of the law. This chapter provides that understanding through a discussion of the differences between public law and private law, the sources of law, the branches of government and their respective roles, and quasi-legal requirements to which health-care organizations are subject.

Public and Private Law

In the most general sense, law is defined as a system of principles and processes devised by organized society to deal with disputes and problems without resorting to the use of force. Law establishes certain standards for human behavior. When those standards are not met, conflict emerges. Individuals and governments then look to the law to resolve the conflicts and enforce the established standards.

Conflicts between private parties constitute **private law**; by contrast, conflicts between the government and private parties constitute **public law**. It is not always easy to make a distinction between these two types of law because in certain instances behavior that deviates from the established standard violates both public and private law. For example, an assault and battery violates both private and public law. Although no clear distinction is possible, understanding the differences between public and private law will assist the health information manager in understanding the American legal system. The distinctions between public and private law are illustrated in Figure 1-1.

Private Law

Private law consists of the body of rules and principles that governs the rights and duties between private parties. Private law is sometimes referred

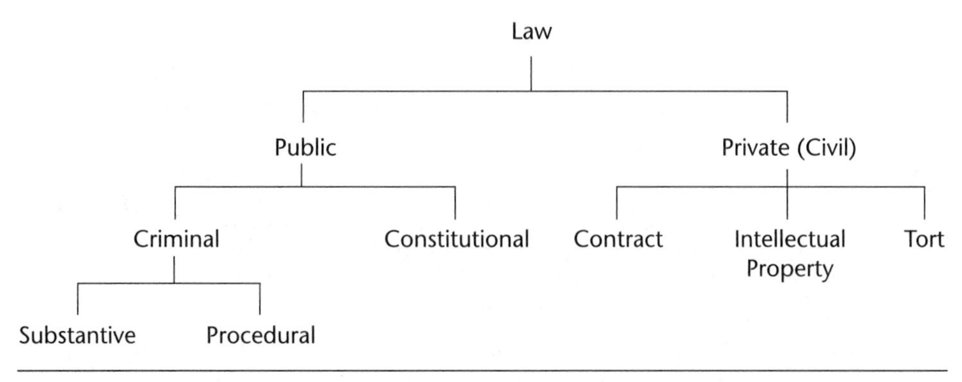

Figure 1-1. Distinctions between Public Law and Private Law

to as civil law because it is concerned with private rights and remedies. Civil law is more properly defined, however, as that part of the law that does not include criminal law.

Generally, lawsuits brought between private parties fall into one of two categories: contract law or tort law. **Contract law** is concerned with an agreement between two or more parties that creates some type of obligation to act (do something) or refrain from acting (not do something). When a party fails to fulfill the terms of the contractural agreement, a breach of contract occurs and the aggrieved party may sue to force performance of the terms of the contract or seek compensation.

An example of a lawsuit involving breach of contract is *Mordecai v. Blue Cross/Blue Shield of Alabama.*[1] In *Mordecai,* the patient sued her insurance company after it denied payment for the majority of her claim for medical expenses. The court held that the patient could proceed against the insurance company for breach of contract on the issue of whether the insurer correctly determined that the patient's care was not medically necessary.

Claims of breach of contract were also at the heart of *Prevost v. Coffee County Hospital Authority.*[2] In *Prevost,* the hospital sued a doctor for breach of contract, seeking to recover a loan it made to induce the doctor to open a medical practice at the hospital. The doctor counterclaimed, asserting that the hospital failed to comply with the terms of the contract by not purchasing certain medical equipment to facilitate his practice or reimbursing him for expenses in renovating his office space. A jury found that each side breached the contract and awarded damages to each. Other examples of activities covered by contract law include the sale of goods, the employment of others, the furnishing of services, and the loaning of money.

Tort law encompasses the rights and duties that exist between parties that are independent of a contract. When one party claims that the wrongful conduct of the other party has caused harm, the aggrieved party may seek compensation. An example of a lawsuit involving tort law is *John Roe v. Jane Doe.*[3] In *Roe,* the court held a physician liable for negligence and breach of confidentiality after the physician improperly disclosed her patient's HIV status. Other examples of activities covered by tort law include medical malpractice, defamation, and invasion of privacy.

While most legal issues in the health-care field involve either contract or tort law, one emerging area of law is that of intellectual property. Ordinarily associated with patents and trademarks, intellectual property law involves the question of legal rights to processes and products of technology, in particular, the concrete application of a principle or idea. Intellectual property law is used in the health information management field as the basis for the legal rights to the software used to control and store information in the computerized patient record.

Public Law

Public law is the body of rules and principles that governs the rights and duties between government and a private party, or between two parts or agencies of government. Public law defines appropriate behavior between citizens, organizations, and government.

One very large segment of public law is criminal law. The essence of criminal law is to declare certain conduct injurious to the public order and provide specified punishment for those found to have engaged in such conduct. Criminal law can be divided into two subcategories: **substantive law** and **procedural law.** Substantive criminal law defines the specific offenses, the general principles of liability, and the specific punishment. Examples of specific offenses are **felonies**, crimes of a grave or serious nature punishable by a term of imprisonment exceeding one year, and **misdemeanors**, crimes of a less serious nature punishable by fine or a term of imprisonment of less than one year. Criminal procedure focuses on the steps through which a criminal case passes, from the initial investigation of a crime through trial and sentence, and the eventual release of the criminal offender.

A second large segment of public law consists of constitutional provisions, statutes, and regulations that govern society by requiring governmental entities and private parties to follow certain courses of action. Although some government regulations contain criminal penalties, their purpose is not to punish offenders but to secure compliance with the goals of the law.

To further understand the contrast between private and public law, their sources must be examined. The primary source of private law is decisions of the courts, which may be subsequently modified by statute or regulation. The primary sources of public law are written constitutions, statutes, regulations, and decisions from both judicial and administrative bodies. The interplay of these sources within private and public law provides the starting basis for understanding the legal aspects of health information.

Sources of Law

Because private and public law originate from a variety of sources, there is no one document or place to turn to find the rules governing health information. Even if such a document or place existed, its value would be questionable because law is not constant; rather, it is constantly changing. Accordingly, it is important to understand that all of the following sources of law may affect the management of health information.

Constitution

A **constitution** is the fundamental law of a nation or state and may be written or unwritten.[4] A constitution establishes the basic principles to which the nation or state must conform, organizes the branches of government, and limits the functions of its different departments.

A constitution familiar to most Americans is the Constitution of the United States, which has as its basic premise the ensuring of each person's rights to life, liberty, and religious freedom. As illustrated in Figure 1-2, the main body of the U.S. Constitution establishes and defines the three branches of government: (1) the legislative branch, (2) the executive branch, and (3) the judicial branch. Following the main body of the Constitution are twenty-six amendments that have been ratified by at least three-fourths of the states in existence at the time of their ratification. The first ten amendments are referred to as the Bill of Rights and include the rights to freedom of speech and religion, freedom from unreasonable search and seizure, freedom to bear arms, freedom to be protected against self-incrimination, freedom to demand a jury trial, and freedom to be afforded due process of law. A listing of the Bill of Rights is contained in Table 1-1.

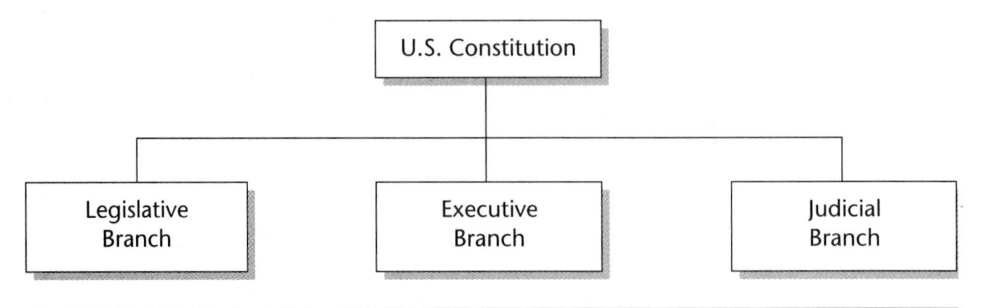

Figure 1-2. Branches of the Federal Government

Table 1-1. The Bill of Rights

Amendment I

Congress shall make no law respecting an establishment of religion, or prohibiting the free exercise thereof; or abridging the freedom of speech, or of the press; or the right of the people peaceably to assemble, and to petition the Government for a redress of grievances.

Amendment II

A well regulated militia, being necessary to the security of a free State, the right of the people to keep and bear arms, shall not be infringed.

Amendment III

No Soldier shall, in time of peace be quartered in any house, without the consent of the owner, nor in time of war, but in a manner to be prescribed by law.

Amendment IV

The right of the people to be secure in their persons, houses, papers, and effects, against unreasonable searches and seizures, shall not be violated, and no warrants shall issue, but upon probable cause, supported by oath or affirmation, and particularly describing the place to be searched, and the persons or things to be seized.

Amendment V

No person shall be held to answer for a capital, or otherwise infamous crime, unless on a presentment or indictment of a Grand Jury, except in cases arising in the land or naval forces, or in the militia, when in actual service in time of war or public danger; nor shall any person be subject for the same offense to be twice put in jeopardy of life or limb; nor shall be compelled in any criminal case to be a witness against himself, nor be deprived of life, liberty, or property, without due

Table 1-1. *(continued)*

process of law; nor shall private property be taken for public use, without just compensation.

Amendment VI

In all criminal prosecutions, the accused shall enjoy the right to a speedy and public trial, by an impartial jury of the State and district wherein the crime shall have been committed, which district shall have been previously ascertained by law, and to be informed of the nature and cause of the accusation; to be confronted with the witnesses against him; to have compulsory process for obtaining witnesses in his favor, and to have the assistance of counsel for his defense.

Amendment VII

In Suits at common law, where the value in controversy shall exceed twenty dollars, the right of a trial by jury shall be preserved, and no fact tried by a jury, shall be otherwise reexamined in any Court of the United States, than according to the rules of the common law.

Amendment VIII

Excessive bail shall not be required, nor excessive fines imposed, nor cruel and unusual punishments inflicted.

Amendment IX

The enumeration in the Constitution, of certain rights, shall not be construed to deny or disparage others retained by the people.

Amendment X

The powers not delegated to the United States by the Constitution, nor prohibited by it to the States, are reserved to the States respectively, or to the people.

In addition to the U.S. Constitution, each state has its own constitution. These state constitutions provide the fundamental laws for each state but are subordinate to the U.S. Constitution. A state constitution typically contains language similar to the U.S. Constitution but also language that is unique to that state. Sometimes, state constitutions provide even broader rights and protections than the U.S. Constitution. For example, one state's courts have interpreted its state's constitutional provision guaranteeing the right to privacy to include a patient's right to die and right to refuse treatment—matters that the U.S. Constitution does not expressly address.[5]

Statutes

A second source of law flows from federal and state legislatures. The laws written by these legislatures are called **statutes** and become effective after being signed by the president, in the case of federal statutes, or by the governor, in the case of state statutes. As a general rule, statutes passed at the federal level address matters of national concern; statutes passed at the state level address matters of particular interest to the individual state.

Statutes written in one state can differ greatly from statutes written in other states on the same topic. For example, one state's statute may directly address a patient's access to his or her own medical record, whereas the neighboring state's statute governing access to patient records may be silent on the issue of direct patient access. For more information concerning the patient's right of access to health information, see Chapter 5.

Similarly, one state's response to a perceived problem may result in statutes that are imitated by other states. For example, several states have responded to allegations of high photocopy charges for copies of medical records by passing statutes that place caps on the amount the health-care provider may charge for these copies. Other states have followed suit and adopted statutes that vary in detail (i.e., the cap amount) but address similar results (i.e., need for a cap). More information concerning the reasonableness of photocopying fees is provided in Chapter 5.

In addition to these legislative bodies, legislatures on the local level, such as city councils or boards of aldermen, may pass laws regulating matters not already covered by federal or state law. City councils or boards of aldermen may also pass laws to supplement federal or state laws. Frequently, laws passed at the local level are called ordinances. Areas typically not governed by federal or state law but by ordinances include zoning, building, or public safety. Areas where ordinances supplement federal or state law include content requirements for medical records.

Administrative Decisions and Regulations

A third source of law comes from the decisions and regulations of administrative agencies. Common at both the federal and state levels, administrative agencies are governmental bodies charged by the legislature with administering and implementing particular legislation. The legislature delegates to the agency the power to promulgate rules, adopt regulations, and decide how the statutes, rules, and regulations apply to particular situations.

When promulgating rules, adopting regulations, and making decisions, agencies must follow certain procedures contained in administrative procedure acts. Administrative procedure acts exist on both the federal and state levels. Under these acts, agencies may not make certain decisions until after they (1) have given advance notice, (2) allowed affected parties an opportunity to present arguments for or against the proposed action, and (3) provided a public record for their action.

The second part of the process is commonly known as providing a notice and comment period. Proposed rules and regulations on the federal level are first published in the *Federal Register.* After the time for notice and comment has expired, the agency determines what comments it will incorporate in its final rules and regulations. These final rules and regulations are then published in the *Code of Federal Regulations,* commonly referred to as the *CFR,* and have the force of law.

A recent example of a federal agency following the requirements of an administrative procedure act is the final privacy rule issued pursuant to the Health Insurance Portability and Accountability Act (HIPAA). HIPAA required the Congress to take action to establish privacy standards within a prescribed time frame; if it did not take action the U.S. Department of Health and Human Services (HHS) was required to establish privacy standards. After Congress failed to act within the requisite time period, HHS published a proposed rule in the *Federal Register* concerning privacy standards and received widespread commentary. After determining what comments to incorporate, HHS issued the revised rule in the *Federal Register*. This rule would have become effective in the ordinary course with publication in the *CFR*, but because a new presidential administration was taking office, the effective date of the rule was delayed by several months. Eventually, the rule was incorporated into the *CFR*, meaning that it received the force of law.

In addition to these federal publications, many states issue comparable publications. For example, the state of Missouri initially publishes proposed rules and regulations in the *Missouri Register.* After the expiration of the notice and comment period, the final rules and regulations are published in that state's *Code of State Regulations* or *CSR* In addition, Missouri's *CSR* includes references to cases that have interpreted the individual rule or regulation. These case references are termed annotations.

Administrative rules and regulations are valid only to the extent that they fall within the scope of the authority granted to the agency by the legislature. Legislatures are limited by both the U.S. and state constitutions in delegating authority to governmental agencies; they cannot abdicate their responsibilities and delegate too extensively. To accommodate those limits, legislatures generally identify the specialized subject matter and empower the agency to develop rules and regulations within that specialized subject matter.

In addition to rule-making authority, legislatures on both the federal and state levels often grant agencies quasi-judicial powers. These powers include the authority to make decisions concerning certain defined matters and provide hearings for parties dissatisfied with the agency's decision. For example, the Centers for Medicare and Medicaid Services (CMS), formerly known as the Health Care Financing Administration (HCFA), of the Department of Health and Human Services administers the Medicare program for the federal government. CMS determines the amount of reimbursement to be paid to health-care providers who participate in the Medicare program. Dissatisfied providers may request a hearing before the Provider Reimbursement Review Board. If still dissatisfied, the provider can pursue an appeal of the board's decision within the Department of Health and Human Services. Then, if the provider is dissatisfied with the agency's final decision, the provider can request judicial review—that is, review of the final agency decision by a U.S. district court. Decisions of administrative agencies, such as those of the Department of Health and Human Services, are published chronologically in sets of administrative reports.

Judicial Decisions

A fourth source of law is the decisions of courts, sometimes referred to as common law. **Common law** is formed when a court, attempting to resolve a dispute, renders a decision. In reaching this decision, courts may interpret relevant constitutional provisions, federal or state statutes, regulations, and/or previous court decisions. The resulting court decision establishes a precedent that may be relied on in future court cases involving similar issues. This reliance on precedent is referred to as ***stare decisis.***

Stare decisis applies to all courts within the same geographic area and within the same jurisdiction. *Stare decisis* operates in a pyramid-type fashion. Courts at the top of the pyramid issue decisions on particular topics. All lower courts within the pyramid that have the same geographic area and jurisdiction are then bound to follow the decisions issued by the court above it in the pyramid.

An example of this pyramid structure would be the federal court system. At the top of the pyramid is the U.S. Supreme Court, the highest court in the land. Immediately below are the U.S. Courts of Appeal. These courts of appeal, called circuit courts of appeal, are divided into geographic areas and are numbered 1 through 11, except for one named court of appeal, the U.S. Court of Appeals for the District of Columbia. Additionally, one court of appeal is not defined by its geography but by the type of cases it can hear. This court is the U.S. Court of Appeals for the Federal Circuit, which hears, among other subjects, cases involving patent appeals from all over the United States. The geographic breakdown of the thirteen circuit courts of appeal is illustrated in Figure 1-3.

Finally, the lower level of the pyramid includes the trial courts, called U.S. District Courts. Each state has at least one federal trial court, and depending on the size and population of the state, may have more.

Under *stare decisis,* U.S. District Courts are bound by decisions of both the U.S. Supreme Court and the U.S. Court of Appeal that is located in their geographic area. However, the doctrine of *stare decisis* does not operate in the reverse direction. For example, the courts of appeal are not bound by trial court decisions, only by decisions of the U.S. Supreme Court and prior decisions of that particular court of appeal. In turn, the U.S. Supreme Court is not bound by decisions of either the trial court or the court of appeal, only by its own previous decisions. If certain circumstances exist, such as significantly changed conditions, the U.S. Supreme Court may decide to overrule its precedent and not follow the doctrine of *stare decisis.*

In addition to *stare decisis,* courts are also subject to the doctrine of ***res judicata,*** which literally means a thing or matter settled by judgment. Whenever a court with jurisdiction over the lawsuit renders a final decision on the merits, the parties to the lawsuit are forever barred from bringing a subsequent action raising the same claim or demand. *Res judicata* applies only after all avenues of appeal have been exhausted. It differs from *stare decisis* in that *res judicata* applies only to the parties and issues involved in a particular lawsuit; by contrast, *stare decisis* applies to future decisions involving different parties with similar issues.

Unlike constitutions and statutes, many court decisions are not made available to the general public for review. Cases settled either before or during trial generally do not involve published decisions; many times a written trial court decision is made available only to the parties involved in the case. If one of the parties later appeals the trial court's decision, the

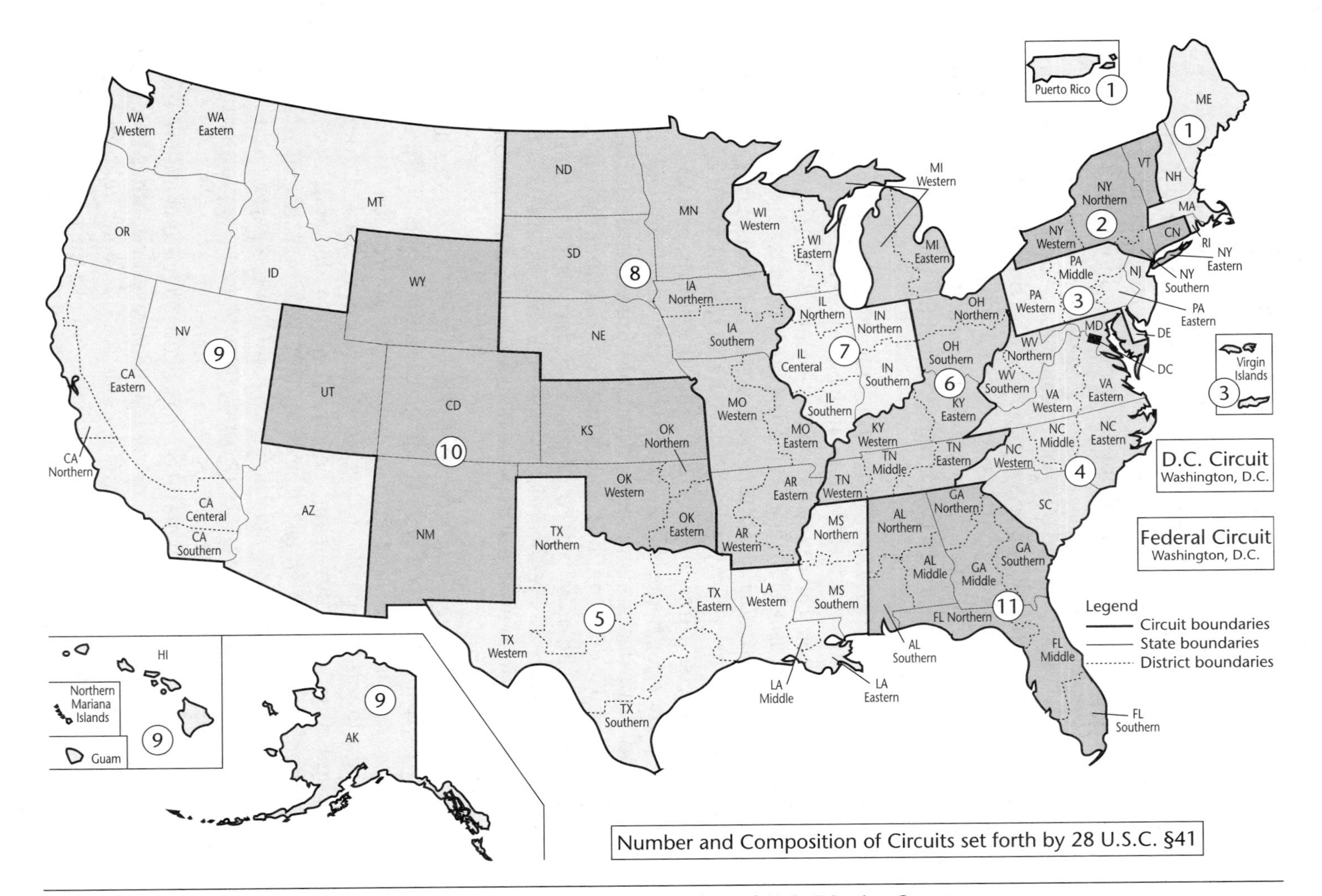

Figure 1-3. Geographical Boundaries of U.S. Courts of Appeals and U.S. District Courts

appellate court may publish its decision, therefore making it available for review.

Despite the fact that not all court decisions are published, numerous cases are available for study. By reviewing cases with similar circumstances, an idea can be obtained of how a court may view a new controversy involving similar circumstances. In making this determination, it is important to remember that the doctrine of *stare decisis* applies at both the state and federal levels. In the state systems, *stare decisis* applies so that the decisions in one particular state have binding precedence only over future decisions of courts in that same state; decisions of other states regarding similar circumstances have only persuasive value. For this reason, cases involving similar circumstances but involving courts in different states may result in opposite conclusions.

Branches of Government

In the federal and state systems, the powers of government are described in the system's respective constitution. These powers are divided into three distinct branches: legislative, executive, and judicial (Figure 1-4). As their names indicate, the legislative branch enacts the laws, the executive branch enforces and administers the laws, and the judicial branch interprets the laws. Each branch exercises those powers that belong to its branch and refrains from exercising those powers that properly belong to the other branches, except in instances in which the constitution expressly directs or permits. This division of power was designed so that no one

	Legislative Branch	***Executive Branch***	***Judicial Branch***
Government of the United States (federal government)	United States Congress	President of the United States	Federal courts
State governments	State legislatures	Governors	State courts

Figure 1-4. The Division of Governmental Power

branch of government would dominate over the other two. This system of checks and balances is referred to as the separation of powers.

Although the three branches of government maintain a separation of powers, they do interact in certain areas. For example, the president of the United States may see the need for particular legislation to advance his agenda and may therefore ask a member of Congress to act as sponsor of the particular bill the president has drafted. Additionally, the names of individuals nominated by the president for appointment to the federal judiciary must be submitted to the Senate for its approval (the advise and consent process). And while Congress and the president may not change any decision reached by the U.S. Supreme Court in a specific controversy, the Congress may pass new or revised legislation to replace the law previously held unconstitutional. In addition, the amendment process to the constitution can serve as a mechanism to offset or override a U.S. Supreme Court decision.

Legislative Branch

The legislative branch functions to enact laws. The legislature determines the need for new laws and for changes in existing laws. At the federal level and in almost all states, the legislature is bicameral, consisting of two houses: one upper house (called the Senate) and one lower house (called the House of Representatives or Assembly). At the federal level, the Senate and the House of Representatives are collectively referred to as the Congress.

Legislative proposals are called bills. Bills are shepherded through the legislature by means of a committee system. When a particular bill is introduced into one of the houses, it is assigned or referred for study to a committee with prescribed areas of concern or interest. To assist their study of a bill, committees may conduct investigations and hold hearings, inviting interested persons to present their views. Some bills "die in committee," meaning they never reach the full legislative body. If a bill does emerge from committee, it is subject to further consideration and debate, and eventually approved or rejected by one of the houses.

Before a bill can be sent to the chief executive for signature, both houses must pass identical versions of the bill or resolve their differences by way of a joint conference committee. If the joint conference committee approach is used, the bill must be resubmitted to both houses for vote before being forwarded to the chief executive for signature.

Executive Branch

The executive branch functions to enforce and administer the laws. The executive branch is organized on a departmental basis, with each department assigned a particular responsibility. The departments are subdivided into administrative agencies, each with defined powers to administer and implement particular legislation.

Health-care providers deal most frequently with the executive branch. Although each agency by definition is assigned a particular area of responsibility, health-care organizations are subject to the rules and regulations of multiple agencies on both the federal and state levels. For example, at the federal level, the Department of Health and Human Services regulates Medicare payments to health-care providers and the Department of Labor regulates the hours and wages of employees of these same providers. At the state level, various licensing boards issue licenses to practice medicine, nursing, and pharmacy and to operate hospitals and nursing homes.

The role of the executive branch is not limited to the action of administrative agencies; the chief executive plays a large role in this branch of government. For instance, it is only after the chief executive approves a particular bill by signing it that the bill becomes law. If, however, this chief executive disapproves of the bill, he or she may veto the bill, effectively killing the legislation unless the legislature successfully overrides the veto through the voting process.

Moreover, the chief executive can issue executive orders. These orders interpret, implement, or give administrative effect to a provision of the constitution or law. Executive orders have the effect of law after being published in the *Federal Register,* in the case of the federal system, or in a comparable publication on the state level.

Judicial Branch

The judicial branch functions to interpret the law through the adjudication and resolution of disputes. In situations where the parties cannot resolve their dispute among themselves, they may resort to a lawsuit, asking the court to resolve their dispute.

In order to resolve a particular dispute, a court looks to the relevant statutes, constitutional provisions, and administrative rules and regulations, and applies them where appropriate to the facts of the case. The court also applies the doctrines of *stare decisis* and *res judicata* where necessary.

Where the circumstances of the case warrant, a court will examine the specific law or regulation to determine if it conforms to or violates the U.S. Constitution. Where the law violates the terms of the U.S. Constitution, the court will declare that law, or portion thereof, invalid. The power of the courts to pass on the constitutionality of an act of Congress was decided in the landmark U.S. Supreme Court case of *Marbury v. Madison*.[6] The configuration of the judicial branch is explained in detail in Chapter 2.

Quasi-Legal Requirements

In addition to the many requirements imposed directly by law, health-care organizations are subject to a multitude of additional requirements: ethical, accreditation, and licensure. To add a further layer of requirements, health-care institutions frequently develop their own policies, procedures, and medical staff bylaws in response to state licensing requirements, accrediting standards, and/or the recommendations of professional associations. While these additional requirements are not laws in and of themselves, they greatly influence the running of health-care organizations. Furthermore, health-care organizations can be held responsible for failing to meet these requirements. For these reasons, they are referred to as quasi-legal requirements.

In the legal context, quasi-legal requirements are most often used to establish the standard of care in a medical malpractice lawsuit or a licensing hearing. As discussed in Chapter 3, if the standard of care established under the quasi-legal requirements is higher than the minimally acceptable standard found in a statute, it is the higher standard against which the health-care organization will be measured.

Conclusion

In large measure, the sources of law define the government's authority to control the activities of individuals and organizations. By understanding these sources of law and the separate branches of government, the health information manager should be better equipped to deal with the government's regulation of the health-care industry. And as the branches of government pose even further regulation, the health information manager may be able to influence the direction of this further regulation.

Case Study

You are the director of health information services for a medium-sized health-care facility. Like many of your peers, you have contracted with an outside copying service to handle all requests for release of patient health information at your facility. You have learned that a lobbying organization for trial attorneys in your state is promoting legislation to place a cap on photocopying costs, which is significantly below the actual cost incurred as part of the contract. Discuss the roles each branch of government will play in considering this legislation and how you and your professional organization may act to influence this process.

Review Questions

1. Why should a health information manager possess a fundamental understanding of the law?
2. Does a single document or source of law exist where an individual can find all of the rules governing health information? Why or why not?
3. How does the content of state constitutions compare with the content of the federal constitution?
4. Statutes governing health information are found at what three levels?
5. Explain the concepts of *stare decisis* and *res judicata.*
6. When does an executive order have the effect of law?
7. What is the function of the judicial branch of government?

Enrichment Activity

Through the use of the Internet, identify bills pending in your state legislature that deal with health-care issues. Contact by written mail, e-mail or telephone the office of the sponsoring state legislator of one of the bills. Identify yourself as a student, indicate your course of study, and request to interview the legislator about the sponsored bill. Ask about the origins of the bill, the amount of support or opposition the bill has garnered, and the chances for successful passage and signature by the governor. Report your results to your instructor, and/or discuss the results with your classmates.

Notes

1. 474 So.2d 95 (Ala. 1985).
2. 453 S.E.2d 760 (Ga. Ct. App. 1995).
3. 599 N.Y.S.2d 350 (N.Y. App. Div. 1993).
4. In the United States, constitutions on the federal and state levels are written. By contrast, Great Britain's constitution is unwritten.
5. *See, Bartling v. Superior Court,* 163 Cal. App. 3d 186, 195 (1984).
6. 5 U.S. 137 (1803).

Chapter 2

Court Systems and Legal Procedures

Learning Objectives

After reading this chapter, the learner should be able to:

1. Compare and contrast subject matter jurisdiction between the federal and state court systems.
2. Differentiate between subject matter jurisdiction and personal jurisdiction.
3. Explain the basic differences between a trial and an appeal.
4. Identify the steps in a civil lawsuit.
5. Distinguish among the different forms of discovery.
6. Describe the roles of the judge and the jury during a trial.
7. Compare and contrast an order of garnishment and writ of execution.
8. Differentiate the types of alternative dispute resolution.

Key Concepts

Alternative dispute resolution
Appeal
Arbitration
Complaint
Court structure
Defendant
Discovery
Diversity jurisdiction
Federal question jurisdiction
Jurisdiction
Legal process
Mediation
Negotiation and settlement
Plaintiff
Satisfying the judgment
Subpoena duces tecum
Trial

Introduction

It is truly an American phenomenon that a primary method of resolving disputes in the United States is through the court system. Although alternative methods of dispute resolution increasingly are being used, filing a lawsuit has become the way many Americans deal with resolving their disputes. Understanding the court systems and the legal procedures employed to process cases through these systems will assist the health information manager in understanding the use of health information in a legal action.

Court Systems

Federal and state courts are similar in certain respects but differ in other respects. Both the federal and state court systems employ a multitier structure: trial courts, intermediate courts of appeal, and a supreme court. They differ, however, on what matters can be brought before them.

Jurisdiction

Jurisdiction is the authority by which courts and judicial officers may hear and decide a case. Jurisdiction encompasses authority not only over the parties involved, called personal jurisdiction, but also authority over the question at issue, called subject matter jurisdiction. This distinction is illustrated in Figure 2-1. The scope and extent of subject matter jurisdiction vary between federal and state courts, with subject matter jurisdiction in the fed-

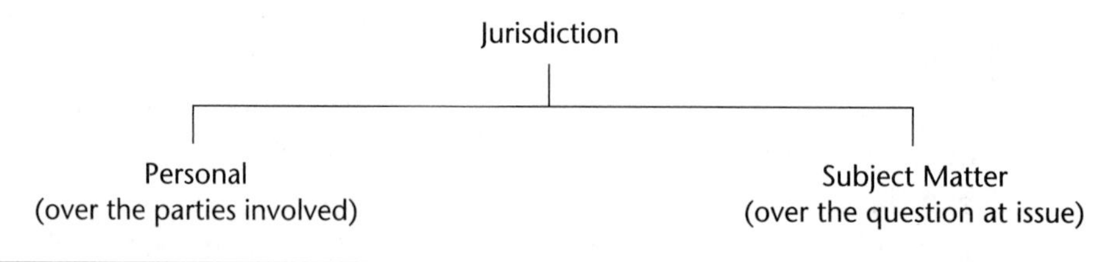

Figure 2-1. Types of Jurisdictions

eral courts being more limited in nature than subject matter jurisdiction in state courts. The contrast between jurisdictions is illustrated in Figure 2-2.

Subject matter jurisdiction in federal court is limited by both the U.S. Constitution and statute. As a general rule, cases may be brought to federal court if they meet the requirement of either federal question jurisdiction or diversity jurisdiction. **Federal question jurisdiction** refers to cases that call into question or involve a U.S. constitutional principle, treaty, federal statute, or federal rule or regulation. It also involves those cases that would traditionally be considered state cases but occur on federal land. For example, negligence occurring at a military base hospital or theft of property at a national park would fall within federal question jurisdiction.

Additional cases may be brought to federal court under the theory of **diversity jurisdiction**: the case in question involves parties who are citizens of different states and the amount in controversy is over $50,000. Both points must exist in order to meet the requirements of diversity jurisdiction. In diversity cases, the federal courts apply the substantive law of the particular state in which the federal court is located to resolve the dispute. Procedural matters in diversity cases are governed by federal common law and the pertinent rules of court, such as the Federal Rules of Civil Procedure.

By contrast, state courts usually maintain courts of general jurisdiction, meaning that the subject matter is not limited. Within a particular state system, the state courts may be subdivided into special courts dealing with limited subjects, such as probate court, juvenile court, or small claims

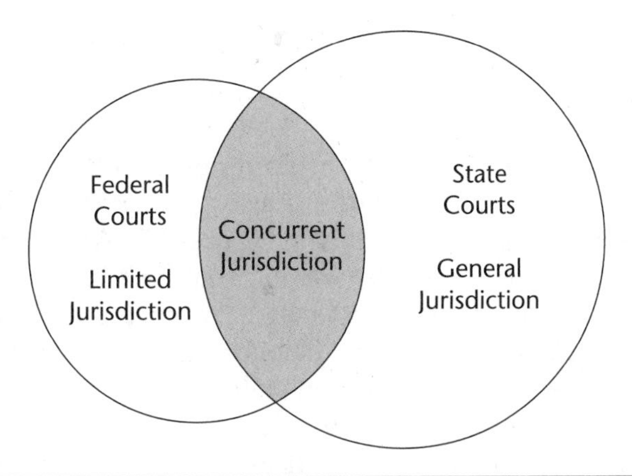

Figure 2-2. Jurisdictional Contrasts between Courts

court. Lawsuits that cannot be brought before the state's specialized courts will be brought in the court of general jurisdiction.

In some instances, federal courts have exclusive jurisdiction over a certain subject matter; therefore, a lawsuit covering that subject matter may be brought only in federal court. For example, judicial review of a decision by the Provider Reimbursement Review Board can occur only in a U.S. District Court.

In other instances, jurisdiction is concurrent between the federal and state courts. Where concurrent jurisdiction exists, the party bringing the lawsuit may go to either federal or state court and thus must choose between the two court systems. For example, a medical malpractice action involving a citizen of one state (the patient) and a citizen of a second state (the health-care provider) could be brought in either a federal court using diversity jurisdiction, if the jurisdictional amount is also met, or in a state court of general jurisdiction. The decision over which court to choose rests on many factors, including how long it will take before obtaining a trial date in a certain court and whether certain procedural rules are more advantageous to one side over another.

In addition to subject matter jurisdiction, courts must have personal jurisdiction in order to issue a valid judgment. Personal jurisdiction refers to the authority of a court over the person as opposed to authority over the person's property. When a plaintiff files a lawsuit, the plaintiff voluntarily submits to the personal jurisdiction of the court. Personal jurisdiction over the defendant depends on a number of factors, mainly whether the defendant was properly served with the summons and complaint.

Court Structure

As stated in Chapter 1, both the federal and state court systems operate within a multitier structure. An organizational chart illustrating these **court structures** is included in Figure 2-3. At the bottom tier is the trial court. Above trial courts are intermediate courts of appeal and above these courts are the highest courts, supreme courts. In the federal court system, all three levels exist. Each of the fifty states has at least a trial court and a supreme court. In some states, however, no intermediate courts of appeal exist; therefore, cases moving through the court system in those states may go directly from a trial court to the supreme court of the state.

Trial courts conduct trials in civil and criminal matters and supervise the discovery process that occurs before trial. In a trial, the judge and jury

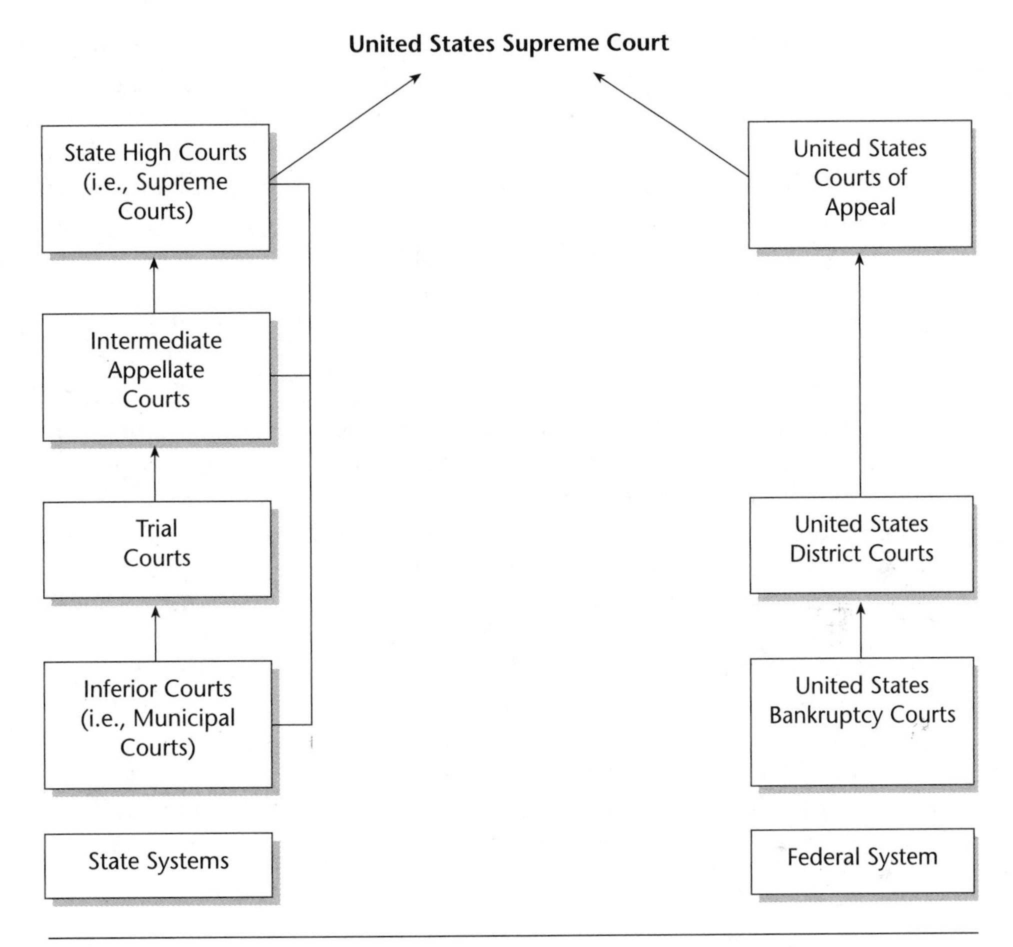

Figure 2-3. Structure of Court Systems

listen to the testimony of witnesses and view exhibits in an attempt to reach a verdict. The names of trial courts vary within the fifty states; trial courts in the federal system are called district courts.

It is the nature of a trial that one party must lose, either in whole or in part. The losing party at trial may then decide to appeal. If so, the lawsuit moves to the intermediate appellate court.

Appellate courts differ dramatically from trial courts in that the appellate court looks to the record of events at trial to determine if error in law or procedure occurred, which would warrant reversal or modification of the result reached at trial. In an appellate court, there is no testimony of witnesses or introduction of exhibits. In short, there is not another trial. Cases proceed on the basis of the parties' written briefs; the only "live" portion of an appeal consists of the oral argument the parties present to the court after the briefs are filed. Appellate courts in the state systems are generally referred to as courts of appeal for that particular state, for example, the Missouri Court of Appeals. Appellate courts in the federal system are divided by geographic region and are referred to as circuit courts of appeal (see Chapter 1).

The highest level of court is the supreme court. Each of the fifty states and the federal government has a court of last resort called a supreme court, with one exception. In New York State, the court of last resort is called the court of appeals, whereas the trial court is termed the supreme court.

These supreme courts, except in New York State, hear appeals from the intermediate appellate courts. Under very limited exceptions, a case may be brought directly in the supreme court without first having been heard in a trial or intermediate appellate court.

The U.S. Supreme Court hears appeals brought from the various federal circuit courts of appeal and the highest state courts in cases involving the U.S. Constitution, federal statutes, treaties, or rules and regulations. The U.S. Supreme Court decides which cases to hear by granting a writ of certiorari. Each year, litigants in thousands of cases apply for writs of certiorari; the U.S. Supreme Court grants only approximately 150 of these writs per year. Similarly, state supreme courts maintain guidelines concerning the type and number of cases they can decide per year.

Legal Process

As stated in Chapter 1, the law is divided into two general areas: criminal law and civil law. The stages through which a lawsuit passes are referred to as **legal process.** Because the civil lawsuit has traditionally played a large role in health care, its steps are described in this section and are illustrated in Figure 2-4.

The characteristics of a civil lawsuit vary somewhat from state to state because of the differences in each state's procedural rules. The following description is modeled on the Federal Rules of Civil Procedure, which is the pattern more than half of the states have used to develop their own procedural rules. For simplicity, all references are made to persons and not organizations or corporations.

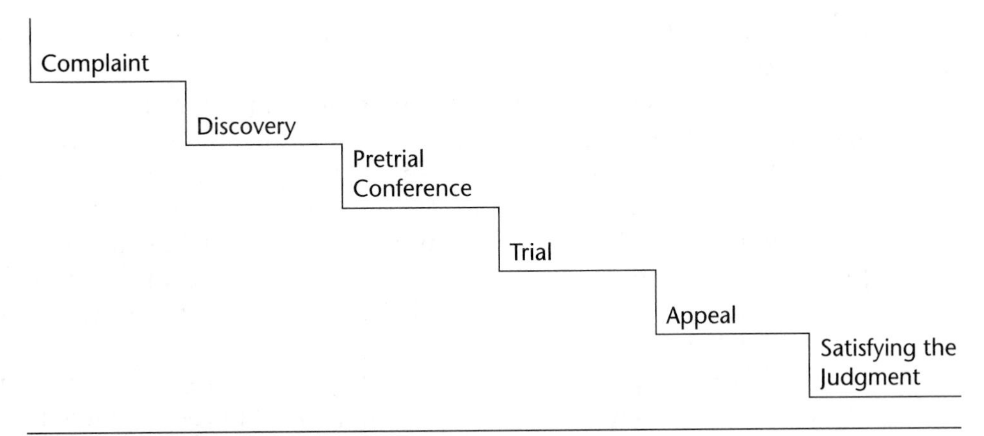

Figure 2-4. Steps in a Civil Lawsuit

Beginning the Lawsuit

The person who initiates the lawsuit is called the **plaintiff**. The person sued by the plaintiff is called the **defendant**. Additional parties may also be present, depending on the complexity of the lawsuit. Where appropriate, these additional parties are identified in this discussion. They are also identified in Figure 2-5.

The first step of every lawsuit is the filing of the plaintiff's complaint. The **complaint** is a written document that describes (1) the grounds of jurisdiction of the court, (2) the plaintiff's claim in a short and plain statement, and (3) the demand for relief to which the plaintiff feels he or she is entitled, for example, damages. After filing the complaint with the court clerk, the plaintiff or his or her attorney receives a summons from the clerk that must be personally delivered to the defendant along with a copy of

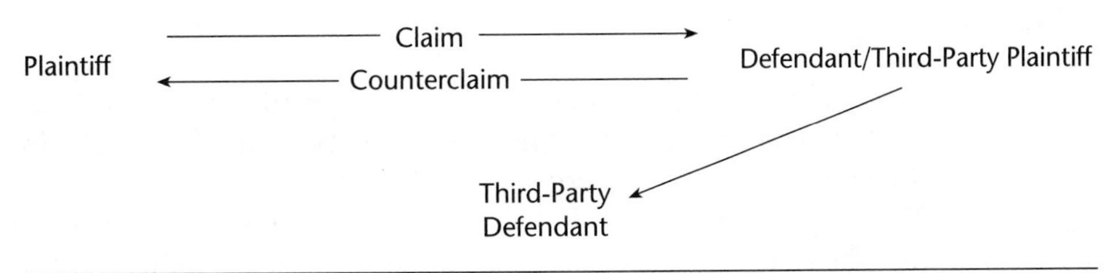

Figure 2-5. Parties to a Lawsuit

the complaint. The delivery of the summons and complaint is referred to as service of process.

After receiving the complaint, the defendant must file a written response, called an answer. In the answer, the defendant admits or denies the contents of the complaint and raises any affirmative defenses, such as contributory negligence. The defendant may also include in the answer a counterclaim, which is a claim presented by the defendant against the plaintiff. For example, a physician sued in a medical malpractice action may decide to raise as a counterclaim against his or her former patient a claim of malicious prosecution.

Furthermore, the defendant may decide to pursue a claim against someone who was not originally part of the lawsuit but is liable for all or part of the plaintiff's claim. In that case, the defendant is referred to as a third-party plaintiff in addition to being the defendant. In this situation, the person being sued by the defendant is called a third-party defendant.

The defendant has only a limited time frame in which to file an answer, generally twenty days after service of process. If the defendant fails to file an answer, the court may decide the case against the defendant by entering a default judgment. The rules on answering the complaint also apply to third-party defendants who must file an answer or risk a default judgment.

In addition to the answer, a defendant may also file any of a number of motions in the hope that the case can be decided without going to trial. For example, the plaintiff can file a motion to dismiss the case or a motion for summary judgment, citing specific reasons such as failure to state a claim or that no disputed facts exist and no reasonable jury could find in the plaintiff's favor. If the motion is granted, the lawsuit in the trial court stops, and the only action the losing party can then take is to pursue an appeal.

Discovery

The delay between the commencement of a lawsuit and a trial date is usually explained by the quantity and complexity of the discovery in a case and the volume of cases before the court.

Discovery can be defined as those devices or tools used by one side to obtain facts and information about the case from the other side in order to prepare for trial. Types of discovery include depositions, written inter-

Method	***Defined***
Deposition	Testimony given under oath outside the courtroom pursuant to a subpoena
Interrogatories	Written questions presented to a party or witness designed to gather information
Production of documents and things	Inspection and/or copying of documents or other physical evidence upon written request
Physical/mental examination	Ordered by the court upon a party's request with good cause shown
Requests for admissions	Written questions presented to a party designed to obtain admission of a certain fact

Figure 2-6. Methods of Discovery

rogatories, production of documents or things, physical and mental examinations, and requests for admissions (Figure 2-6). The parties may use any or all of these forms of discovery.

Depositions

A deposition is a discovery device in which one party subpoenas a witness to appear at a given time and place to testify under oath. The person answering the questions is called the deponent. Depositions take place outside the courtroom, frequently in a lawyer's office, in the presence of counsel for both sides and a court reporter who administers the oath and transcribes the testimony word for word. Depositions can include both written and oral questions, with the questions presented in the same manner as during trial, with direct examination and cross-examination of the deponent. Counsel can object to any of the questions asked of the deponent. Although depositions are relatively expensive, they are considered by many to be the most effective way of obtaining a hostile individual's knowledge of the facts.

The main purpose of a deposition is to uncover details of the case. Depositions are also submitted as evidence at trial if the deponent is unavailable, or to contradict a deponent's testimony if an inconsistent statement was given.

Written Interrogatories

Written interrogatories are a far less expensive method to uncover details of a case. This discovery device consists of one party submitting written questions about the case to another party or witness. The questions are answered separately in writing, with the person answering the questions signing a sworn statement that the answers are true. The party or witness may object to answering the question, stating the reason for the objection in writing. The party must answer the interrogatories generally within thirty days from the time they are sent.

Production of Documents and Things

This discovery device permits one side to inspect and copy documents and things that are not already in that side's physical possession. In this instance, a written request is served on the other side, identifying the item and category along with a reasonable time, place, and manner in which to inspect and copy the document or thing. A party receiving the request must respond in writing, generally within thirty days, either stating that inspection and copying will be permitted as requested or that the party has an objection to the request.

This discovery tool is subject to wide variation. In some cases, a written request for documents may only require the respondent to photocopy documents and send them to the requestor. A complete and valid release of information submitted to a health-care provider asking for photocopies of a medical record would be an example of this type of request. By contrast, a request accompanied by a **subpoena duces tecum**, a formal request to produce a record, would require a person who possesses the document in question to produce the document at a certain time and place pursuant to the authority of the court supervising the lawsuit, unless the subpoena duces tecum indicates that personal delivery is not required and mailing of the document will suffice.

Physical or Mental Examination

When the physical or mental condition of the plaintiff is at issue in the case, the defendant may ask the court to order the plaintiff to submit to a physical or mental examination by a physician. The request must be supported by a demonstration of good cause to order the examination. A notice is given to the person to be examined of the time, place, manner, conditions, and scope of the examination, along with the name of the physician who will conduct the examination. The physician then prepares a detailed written report of his or her findings, the results of all tests, diagnoses, and conclusions. The report is made available to the party examined at that party's request.

Requests for Admission

Requests for admission are similar to written interrogatories in that one party asks the other side a series of written questions. They differ from written interrogatories in that these questions are not designed to gather information; rather, the questions are designed so that the other side will admit certain facts. A party must respond in writing to a request for admission within thirty days or else the subject matter of the request for admission will be deemed admitted.

Many routine and mundane matters are the subject of requests for admission, for example, the date, day of the week, and time of occurrence of a particular event. Conversely, disputed matters may be the subject of a request for admission. In those instances, the party responding to the request may object to the question or deny the fact that is central to the question. Any matter that is admitted pursuant to a request for admission is conclusively established for purposes of that lawsuit only. Under certain circumstances, the trial court may later permit withdrawal or amendment of the admission.

Once admitted, the parties do not need to resort to presenting unnecessary proof at trial concerning the subject matter of the admission. Admissions save each side both time and expenses.

Pretrial Conference

Many trial courts have local rules that require the parties to meet with the trial judge before a trial date is set and discuss the status and issues of the case. At the pretrial conference, the trial judge rules on any outstanding motions, resolves certain discovery disputes, helps the parties further define the issues, and discusses the possibility of settlement. If the case is not settled at that time, the trial judge sets the court date and enters a pretrial order that controls the course of the trial.

Trial

A **trial** is a hearing or determination by a court of the issues existing between the parties to an action. Cases that proceed to trial will be decided by either the trial judge or the jury. Certain categories of cases are not entitled to jury trials, for example, divorce and adoption proceedings. In those instances, the trial judge will make decisions about the disputed facts in the case. Where the case is tried before a jury, the jury will decide the disputed facts in the case.

After choosing a jury, each side's counsel presents an opening statement to the jury. The opening statement is an outline or summary of the case and the evidence that each side anticipates will be presented to the jury during the course of the trial. The opening statement gives a general picture of the facts so that the jury will be able to understand the evidence as it is presented. The plaintiff's attorney presents her opening statement first. The defendant's attorney immediately follows unless she defers until after the plaintiff rests her case.

The next step is the presentation of the plaintiff's case. The plaintiff's lawyer may call witnesses to explain the facts of the case. The plaintiff's lawyer engages the witness in a question and answer dialogue, which is called direct examination. After direct examination is completed, the defendant's lawyer has the right to question the same witness. This is referred to as cross-examination.

During either direct or cross-examination, the lawyer who is not questioning the witness may choose to object to a question asked or the answer given if the lawyer believes that either is outside the bounds of admissible evidence. The lawyer voices the objection to the trial judge, giving reasons that the question or answer is improper. The trial judge allows the opposing counsel to respond to the objection. The trial judge then decides whether to allow the evidence to be considered by the jury. This decision is based on many factors, including trustworthiness of the witness, relevance of the evidence, and prior appellate decisions concerning that particular form of evidence. The trial judge announces his or her decision by saying that the objection is sustained or is overruled, and the case proceeds.

After the plaintiff has called all witnesses and introduced the remaining evidence, such as exhibits, she rests her case. At that time, the defendant can ask the court to rule in the defendant's favor because the plaintiff has failed to prove her case. This request is called a motion for directed verdict. If the trial judge grants the motion, the lawsuit stops; if denied, the trial proceeds with the defendant presenting his case. The same procedures used in the plaintiff's case, direct and cross-examination, are followed in the defendant's case for each of the defendant's witnesses.

After both sides have "rested," either side may renew the request for a directed verdict. If granted, the lawsuit is over; if denied, the case is ready for closing statements. Similar to opening statements, a closing statement summarizes the evidence that has been presented during the trial and highlights the weaknesses of the other side's case. As a general rule, the plaintiff first presents the closing statement; the defendant then replies with a closing statement, with the plaintiff being allowed to rebut the defendant's closing statement. This scenario may differ, however, if any party elects not to present a closing statement.

Closing statements often include references to a witness's credibility. The lawyer will explain to the jury why a particular witness should be believed and another witness not believed. Decisions concerning credibility are among the most difficult decisions a jury must make. Credibility decisions call into play the jury's understanding of the witness's intelligence, knowledge of the circumstances in question, reputation for telling the truth, and impartiality to the matter at issue in the case.

Following closing statements, the trial judge will provide directions to the jury concerning the law that applies to the case. These directions are called jury instructions. The jury uses these instructions to reach its ultimate decision in the case, which is called the verdict.

After the jury returns the verdict, the losing party can ask the trial judge to overturn the verdict by filing a motion for judgment notwithstanding the jury's verdict. The losing party can also seek a new trial by submitting a list of errors to the trial judge that the party believes caused her to lose. The trial judge may grant either of these posttrial motions if the jury verdict is against the weight of the evidence submitted at trial. Whatever the trial court's decision on these posttrial motions, the trial court eventually enters a judgment indicating who won and lost in the case.

As this discussion illustrates, distinct roles exist for both the trial judge and the jury. The trial judge determines the admissibility of the evidence, instructs the jury on the applicable law, and can remove a case from the jury by granting a directed verdict, a motion notwithstanding the verdict, or a motion for new trial. It is the role of the jury to decide the facts in the case and reach the ultimate decision of whether the plaintiff has proved her case. Simply stated, it is the trial judge who decides questions of law and the jury that decides questions of fact.

Appeal

Once all posttrial motions are decided and judgment is entered, the losing party in the trial court may pursue an appeal. On **appeal,** a case may be affirmed, modified, or reversed. Furthermore, a new trial may be ordered. The written opinion issued by the appellate court provides reasons for the decision made by that court. Any party losing on appeal from a decision of an intermediate appellate court may then choose to pursue an appeal with that state's court of last resort or with the U.S. Supreme Court, as discussed earlier in this chapter.

On appeal, the order of each party's name may be reversed from how they were listed in the trial court. For example, the title of the case at trial may have been *Mary Smith v. John Doe,* with the plaintiff being Mary Smith and the defendant being John Doe. If John Doe loses and takes the appeal, the order of the parties is frequently switched to show who is the party initiating the appeal, for example, *John Doe v. Mary Smith.* If Mary Smith loses and takes the appeal, the order of the names will usually remain the same. Although this is a fairly minor point, it can cause some confusion.

Satisfying the Judgment

After all appeals have been exhausted, the winning party must still collect the amount of the judgment if a money award has been made. This process is frequently referred to as **satisfying the judgment.**

Among the most common ways to satisfy a judgment is to obtain a writ of execution or an order of garnishment. A writ of execution, the most common method used in the federal court system, is a written document that orders the sheriff or other local official to take the property of the losing party and sell it to satisfy the judgment. An order of garnishment is an order directed to a third person to whom the losing party is indebted that orders payment of the debt directly to the winning party in the lawsuit. Garnishment is frequently used to obtain a portion of the losing party's wages. In this situation, the employer of the losing party is directed to pay a certain percentage of the losing party's wages to the winning party.

Alternative Dispute Resolution

Alternative methods of dispute resolution are increasing in popularity in the United States. Commonly referred to as **alternative dispute resolution** or ADR, these methods seek to resolve conflicts and disagreements to the satisfaction of all parties without using the court system. ADR arose as a result of dissatisfaction with the existing legal system and its costs to litigants in terms of time, stress, and fees. ADR has steadily grown in popularity because it involves decision making in an expedited and economically feasible manner. Although most often used in the business world, ADR is now seen more frequently in the health-care field.

The most frequently used form of ADR in the United States is mediation. In **mediation,** a neutral third party assists both sides of a dispute in resolving their differences and reducing their resolution to writing. Unlike a court decision imposed on the parties to a lawsuit, mediation allows the parties themselves to reach a decision that binds all sides to the controversy. After learning the positions of the respective sides, the third-party mediator tries to reach some form of common ground. That common ground is then agreed to by both sides, and the mediator reduces the agreement to writing. Because the mediator is seeking the active involvement of the parties in reaching common ground, it is not necessary that the mediator be an expert in the field in which the dispute arises. Mediation is popular because it allows the parties to remain in control of their destiny; the mediator cannot force a decision upon the parties. Its popularity also stems from the fact that it is generally voluntary, not mandatory, and is a private process with no documents filed in the public record.

A second form of ADR is arbitration. Like mediation, **arbitration** uses a neutral third party to hear both sides of a dispute and render a written decision, called an award. The neutral third party is called an arbitrator. Unlike mediation, the arbitrator's award is not based on the parties' agreement;

rather, the arbitrator's award is imposed on the parties after consideration of each side's position. Depending on the situation, the arbitrator's award may be binding on the parties. A party unhappy with the arbitrator's award may seek to appeal it by bringing a lawsuit in a court of general jurisdiction to overturn the award.

One advantage to the use of arbitration is the arbitrator is frequently an expert or at least knowledgeable about the field in which the dispute arises. This knowledge often give confidence to the parties that the decision to be reached is solidly grounded not only on the facts but on the business practices in the field in which the dispute arises. Parties may agree to keep the written arbitration award confidential. If, however, a party wanted to warn others of the danger posed by whatever is the subject of the arbitration, a confidential award will not suffice. Additionally, it can be hard to predict the outcome of an arbitration award, leaving parties with a feeling of uncertainty until an award is reached.

A third method of ADR is negotiation and settlement. Like arbitration and mediation, negotiation and settlement seeks to resolve a dispute. **Negotiation and settlement** differs in that no neutral third party is used. The parties (or their representative) must work with each other (the negotiation) in order to succeed in reaching resolution of the dispute (the settlement). A written document memorializing the settlement is then drafted and signed by all the parties involved. Settlement agreements often contain a release of claims, meaning that the parties agree to give up any rights to otherwise pursue the claims listed in the release.

Negotiation and settlement is frequently used where there is minimum animosity between the parties. It is also pursued as an avenue to defray costs, as no neutral third party is involved who must be paid by the parties for the time expended in the mediation or arbitration. Negotiation and settlement is also attractive because the parties themselves control the process.

All three forms of ADR are used throughout the United States. Depending on the situation, more than one form of ADR may be used if the first form of ADR does not result in a successful outcome. For example, the parties may try negotiation and settlement but reach a stalemate. They may then proceed with either mediation or arbitration to resolve their differences. These forms of ADR may be used even after the parties have resorted to a lawsuit to resolve their differences.

Conclusion

Each lawsuit filed in the United States differs in some respect from every other lawsuit. These lawsuits may vary not only by the type of law involved and the facts underlying the case, but also by the jurisdiction of the court in which they are filed and by the types of discovery devices used. Furthermore, Americans are increasingly using alternative forms of dispute resolution to address their legal issues. A thorough understanding of these variations will assist health information managers in complying with the requirements of the legal process.

Case Study

You are the in-house counsel at General Hospital. You have been contacted by an attorney for a former patient of the hospital whose inpatient hospitalization resulted in some harm to the patient. That harm was memorialized in an incident report prepared by hospital staff. Your review of the incident report indicates that the harm described by the attorney is consistent with the harm described in the incident report. Based on your conversations with the attorney, you believe a lawsuit is imminent. Because you believe it is in the best interests of all concerned to avoid the cost of litigation, you wish to consider methods of alternative dispute resolution. Discuss the relative advantages and disadvantages of each method.

Review Questions

1. Why should a health information manager need to understand the court system and legal procedures?
2. Name examples of federal question jurisdiction and diversity jurisdiction.
3. Does each state have trial courts, intermediate courts of appeal, and supreme courts?
4. What is meant by the term *legal process*?
5. What are the elements of a complaint?

6. What are the similarities and differences between opening and closing statements at trial?
7. How did alternative dispute resolution become a popular alternative to litigation?

Enrichment Activity

Contact the Clerk of Court's Office of your local trial court or court of appeals to learn the date of a scheduled trial or scheduled oral argument on appeal. Attend and observe the trial or oral argument. Discuss your observations with your class and/or instructor.

Chapter **3**

Principles of Liability

Learning Objectives

After reading this chapter, the learner should be able to:

1. Describe each of the following relationships: physician–patient, hospital–patient, and hospital–physician.
2. Define medical malpractice and negligence.
3. Identify the elements of a negligence claim.
4. Define the meaning of standard of care and explain its role in medical malpractice cases.
5. List the methods a plaintiff may use to establish the standard of care in a medical malpractice case.
6. Distinguish among the three types of damages.
7. Analyze the difference between negligence and *res ipsa loquitur.*
8. Compare and contrast vicarious liability and corporate negligence.
9. Explain the difference between assault and battery.
10. Describe each of the following intentional torts: defamation, invasion of privacy, and medical abandonment.
11. Explain the difference between a claim for nonperformance and improper performance.
12. Identify the defenses commonly raised in lawsuits involving health-care providers.
13. Differentiate between contributory and comparative negligence.

Key Concepts

- Assault
- Assumption of risk
- Battery
- Breach of contract
- Breach of duty of care
- Causation
- Charitable immunity
- Comparative negligence
- Contributory negligence
- Corporate negligence
- Damages
- Defamation
- Duty of care
- Failure to warn
- Good Samaritan statutes
- Governmental immunity
- Health-care relationships
- Hospital–patient relationship
- Hospital–physician relationship
- Intentional torts
- Invasion of privacy
- Malpractice
- Medical abandonment
- Medical malpractice
- Medical staff privileges
- Negligence
- Nonintentional torts
- Physician–patient relationship
- *Res ipsa loquitur*
- Statute of limitation
- Vicarious liability

Introduction

Liability for injury is feared by many health-care providers. Injury may encompass not only physical damage but also damage to a party's rights, reputation, or property. Improper disclosure of health information is an injury for which a party is entitled to bring a lawsuit. Accordingly, individuals engaged in protecting health information must understand the principles of liability.

To understand the principles of liability, the nature of the relationships from which liability can arise must be understood. The legal theories underlying lawsuits in the health-care field and the type of defenses raised in many of these lawsuits can then be studied.

Health-Care Relationships

Before an individual can bring a lawsuit to establish some form of liability against a health-care provider, the individual must have established a relationship with that provider. Without this relationship, the parties to a lawsuit are basically strangers who have no obligation to each other that could serve as the basis for a malpractice lawsuit.[1] Although many variations of **health-care relationships** exist between provider and patient, this section addresses those relationships most common to a lawsuit in the health-care field as illustrated in Figure 3-1. Furthermore, this section addresses a relationship that does not directly involve patient care, the physician–hospital relationship, because this relationship increasingly serves as the subject of lawsuits.

Physician–Patient Relationships

Physician–patient relationships have traditionally served as the cornerstone of health care in the United States. As other health-care providers assume a larger role in the health care of tomorrow, new questions of liability may arise. Many of the basic principles of the physician–patient relationship apply not only to physicians but also by analogy to other types of health-care providers, such as nurses and physical therapists. An understanding of the basic principles of the physician–patient relationship will assist the student in making these analogies to situations involving other health-care providers.

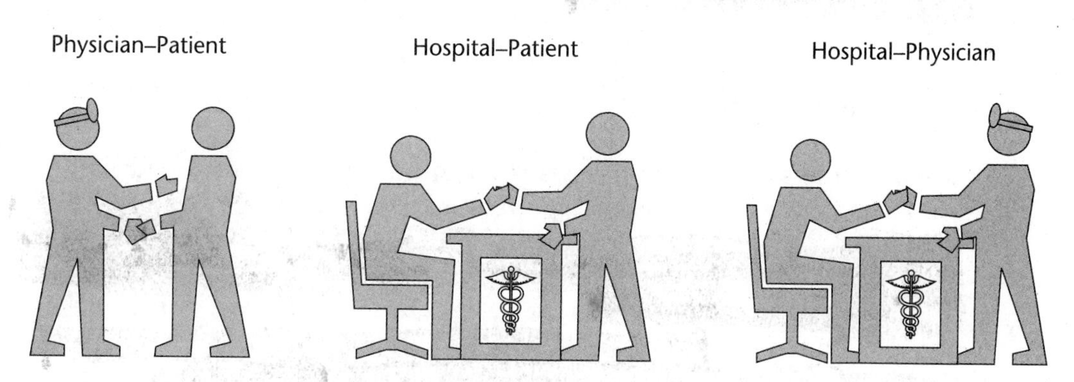

Figure 3-1. Health-Care Relationships

The **physician–patient relationship** begins when the patient requests treatment and the physician agrees to render that treatment. This relationship is a contractual one because it involves both an offer (the request for treatment) and an acceptance (the agreement to render the treatment). This contractual relationship can exist as either an express contract or an implied contract.

In an express contract, the terms, rights, and responsibilities of the parties are agreed on either orally or in writing. For example, an express contract is established when a physician and a patient agree, in advance of any treatment, on the amount the patient must pay and what treatment or result the physician will render for that payment. By contrast, an implied contract exists when the conduct of the parties and the circumstances of the situation create a tacit understanding that an agreement has been reached. In this instance, details of the contract are not reached in advance of treatment. For example, an implied contract is created when a physician treats the patient prior to an agreement on the terms for payment and treatment.

Once the physician–patient relationship is established, it continues until such time that it has been properly terminated or the patient no longer requires treatment. Terminating this relationship can be accomplished in a number of ways: (1) the physician may withdraw from the contract, (2) the patient may dismiss the physician, or (3) the physician and patient may mutually agree to end the relationship. If the physician decides to withdraw from the contract, he or she must give the patient reasonable notice so that the patient may obtain alternative treatment. Most often, termination is due to the fact that the patient is either cured or has died. The relationship may also terminate as a result of the patient's failure to comply with the physician's orders.

Hospital–Patient Relationships

Many of the same concepts addressed in the physician–patient relationship also apply to the **hospital–patient relationship**. The relationship begins when the patient is voluntarily admitted to the hospital. At the time of admission, the patient signs certain forms, agreeing to pay for the treatment that will be rendered. This act establishes an express contract to receive health care. The hospital–patient relationship ends when the patient is discharged or leaves the hospital against medical advice.

As a general rule, a hospital does not have a responsibility to treat every patient who arrives at its door. The exception to this rule is an emergency-care situation. Under various provisions of federal and state law, along with the Joint Commission on Accreditation of Healthcare Organizations (JCAHO) standards, the general rule has been modified so that hospitals must have, at minimum, a procedure for assessing whether an ill or injured person who appears at the hospital's door can be treated at that hospital or transferred to another facility for treatment.

Under the Emergency Medical Treatment and Active Labor Act (EMTALA)[2] of the Consolidated Omnibus Budget Reconciliation Act of 1985, hospitals and physicians who participate in the Medicare program must follow certain guidelines for the treatment and transfer of all patients, regardless of whether a particular patient who appears for care is eligible for Medicare. Commonly referred to as the "antidumping law," EMTALA requires a hospital or physician to treat a patient who is in active labor or in an emergency medical condition until the condition is stabilized. Once the condition is stabilized, the hospital and physician have three choices: (1) continue to treat the patient, (2) transfer the patient, or (3) discharge the patient.

An example of a physician's failure to comply with EMTALA is illustrated in *Burditt v. U.S. Department of Health and Human Services*.[3] In *Burditt*, a pregnant woman in active labor with dangerously high blood pressure presented at the hospital's emergency room. The patient had not received prenatal care and did not have the means for payment of her medical treatment. The on-call obstetrician initially refused to treat her, but when pressured by the hospital staff, arranged for her transfer to a hospital 170 miles away. Despite repeated attempts by hospital staff to challenge the obstetrician's transfer order, the patient began transfer by ambulance to the designated facility. Within forty miles of the original hospital, the patient delivered her child. When the nurse accompanying the patient in the ambulance notified the obstetrician of the birth, he ordered her to continue the transfer to the second hospital. The nurse instead returned the patient to the original hospital, where the obstetrician directed the patient's discharge. At that point, the hospital arranged for the patient's treatment with a second obstetrician. The court held that the obstetrician's conduct in ordering the patient's transfer violated EMTALA and supported imposition of a $20,000 fine.

The requirement under EMTALA and similar state laws to treat emergency-care patients necessarily influences the hospital's ability to decide whether to create a hospital–patient relationship. As these laws illustrate, the law may create a duty to treat the patient, which in turn forms the basis for the hospital–patient relationship. A branch of this duty implicates the possibility of liability.

Hospital–Physician Relationships

Unlike the relationships previously discussed, this relationship is not based on direct patient care. Rather, it is based on the contract between hospital and physician that allows the physician to bring patients to the hospital to receive health care. In this relationship, the hospital furnishes and coordinates patient care along with the physician.

The **hospital–physician relationship** begins with the credentialing process. Merely being licensed as a physician is not sufficient to become a member of a hospital's medical staff. The credentialing process involves examination by the hospital's governing board of the physician's background, experience, and licensure against established criteria. If the established criteria are met, the physician is admitted to the medical staff.

Once admitted to the medical staff, the governing board determines the scope and limit—that is, **medical staff privileges**—of the physician's practice in the hospital. In determining medical staff privileges, the board again reviews the physician's background, experience, and licensure against criteria established by the medical departments or specialties of the hospital. The physician then may exercise only those privileges that have been granted or be subject to a charge of practicing beyond the scope of his or her privileges.

Medical staff admission and privileges may be curtailed or terminated for a variety of reasons, among them the failure to meet applicable quality of care standards or misconduct by the physician. Depending on the circumstances, the physician may have a right to a formal hearing to challenge the action taken against him or her. The Health Care Quality Improvement Act of 1986 allows hospitals to summarily suspend or restrict medical privileges to avoid imminent danger to patients, provided that the procedures specified by the act are followed. Further discussion of the act is provided in Chapter 9.

In sum, hospitals have a duty to ensure that their medical staffs are competent. Failure to perform this duty may result in a finding of direct liability to the patient. Such liability is discussed later in this chapter under the section on corporate negligence.

Theories of Liability

The theories of liability underlying lawsuits in the health-care field can be divided into three areas: breach of contract, intentional torts, and nonintentional torts. **Intentional torts** are torts committed by persons with the intent to do something wrong. **Nonintentional torts,** by contrast, are torts committed by persons who lack the intent to do something wrong. Table 3-1 lists the theories of liability of intentional and nonintentional torts. A fuller description of contract and tort law is provided in Chapter 1. The majority of medical malpractice lawsuits filed in the United States involve nonintentional torts.

Nonintentional Torts

Negligence and Medical Malpractice

Because of its frequent use in medical malpractice lawsuits, negligence has become almost synonymous with medical malpractice, although they are separate legal terms. Negligence is the most frequently used theory of liability, but it is only one of many theories that may support a medical malpractice claim.

Table 3-1. Theories of Liability

Intentional Torts	***Nonintentional Torts***
Assault and battery	Negligence
Defamation	*Res ipsa loquitur*
Invasion of privacy	Vicarious liability
Medical abandonment	Corporate negligence
	Failure to warn

Negligence refers to someone failing to do something that a reasonably prudent person would do in a similar situation or, alternatively, doing something that a reasonably prudent person would *not* do in a similar situation. **Malpractice,** on the other hand, refers to professional misconduct. This misconduct involves a professional who fails to follow a standard of care prevalent for his or her profession that results in harm to another person. In **medical malpractice,** this misconduct generally involves the failing of a physician to follow a standard of care, which results in harm to the patient.

Medical malpractice actions are not limited to physicians and may also be brought against other health-care providers and institutions. Underlying any medical malpractice action is, of course, the existence of a relationship between the patient and the health-care provider or institution.

To succeed in a negligence claim for medical malpractice, the plaintiff (the patient) must prove the following four elements; (1) a duty of care is owed to the patient; (2) a breach of this duty of care; (3) a causal connection between the breach of duty and the patient's injury; and (4) damages. If all four elements are not proved, the plaintiff will lose the case. Figure 3-2 illustrates this interrelationship. The following discussion defines each of these elements and describes how they fit in a medical malpractice lawsuit.

Duty of care

A **duty of care** is an obligation, to which the law gives recognition and effect, to conform to a particular standard of conduct toward another. That is, this duty of care requires a person to behave in a particular way, with

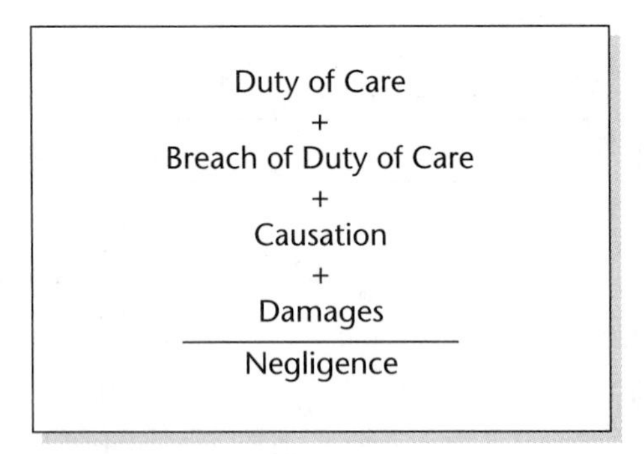

Figure 3-2. Elements of a Negligence Claim

the risk that if he or she does not do so, he or she will become subject to liability for any harm sustained by another because of his or her actions. For example, an automobile driver has a duty to drive in a safe manner and will become liable for damages resulting from an accident if he fails to do what a reasonably prudent automobile driver would do.

As the example illustrates, the duty of care is measured under the reasonably prudent person standard. The mythical reasonably prudent person is someone with average intelligence and experience. This standard is applied when negligence is alleged against someone who is not a professional. Where negligence is alleged against the professional, however, a different standard of care is involved: that of a reasonably prudent professional.

Breach of duty of care

The basis of every negligence claim in a medical malpractice case is the allegation of a **breach of duty of care,** meaning that the medical professional failed to maintain a certain standard of care. This standard of care is the level of care a reasonably prudent professional would have rendered in the same or similar circumstances. Like the reasonably prudent person, the reasonably prudent professional is someone with average intelligence and comparable training and experience.

During a medical malpractice trial, the plaintiff attempts to show that the defendant, the medical professional, deviated from the appropriate standard of care. To do this, the plaintiff must first establish what standards were appropriate at the time the care was received. This procedure can be accomplished in several ways.

First, the plaintiff may introduce into evidence the general standards contained in state laws and regulations governing the pertinent profession, such as nursing practice acts. If the state law and/or regulation was designed to protect a class of persons from certain types of harm and the law was violated, a court and jury will find the medical professional liable.

Second, general standards of care can be found in written materials from various sources. For example, a professional association or accrediting organization may have published general standards for the profession or the institution it accredits. Furthermore, certain textbooks provide guidelines that illustrate the appropriate standard of care.

A health-care facility's internal policies and procedures, including medical staff bylaws and manuals, are a third way to establish the standard of care. As a general rule, an institution's policies and procedures are more specific than the standards found in textbooks. In some instances, an institution's policies and procedures may establish a higher standard of care than the minimally acceptable standard found in textbooks. If a higher standard is established by an institution's policies and/or procedures, it is the higher standard of care against which the institution will be measured.

Fourth, a plaintiff uses expert testimony to establish a breach of the standard of care. Under this scenario, the plaintiff contacts a medical professional who is proficient in the same area of practice as the defendant. After reviewing the facts of the plaintiff's case, the medical professional, referred to as the expert witness, testifies in court, describing what he or she believes to be the appropriate standard of care and comparing that standard to the care the defendant provided to the plaintiff.

When trying to establish the standard of care, the plaintiff is not limited to using only one of these methods. And, of course, courts and juries may use ordinary common sense when establishing an appropriate standard of care. If the very nature of the act committed by the medical professional indicates improper treatment and malpractice, such as amputating the wrong limb, expert testimony would not be necessary and the court and jury could rely on ordinary experience and knowledge to determine the standard of care. For example, the patient was not required to use the testimony of an expert in *Larrimore v. Homeopathic Hospital Association,*[4] to establish a failure to meet the standard of care. In *Larrimore,* a nurse injected the patient with a medication rather than administer it orally, despite the patient's protest that the physician had prescribed oral administration of the medicine in question. The court held the jury could rely on their own common sense to conclude that the nurse's failure to follow the doctor's written instructions constituted a breach of the standard of care.

At one time, courts looked to the locality where the care was rendered to determine the standard of care. Commonly referred to as the locality rule, the standard of care under this rule is measured in a given situation solely against the practice of other medical professionals in the same locality. The locality rule was formulated at a time of great variance between the knowledge and skill of medical professionals in rural and urban areas. Due to improved transportation and communication systems, the trend since the 1970s has been away from a locality-based standard of care toward a national standard of care that exists in every state in the country. Whether the state in which a lawsuit is brought uses the locality rule or a national standard of care is determined by that state's rules of evidence and its case law.

Causation

Once the patient has demonstrated that the medical professional breached the standard of care owed him, he must then establish that it was this breach that caused the injury. The breach of duty must constitute the proximate cause of his injury, meaning the primary or moving cause without which the injury would not have occurred.

Proving the causal connection, sometimes referred to as **causation,** can be difficult. In some cases, all or part of an injury is not the direct result of the medical professional's negligence, but is the indirect result of an intervening force. Under these circumstances, the test to determine proximate cause is foreseeability: if the reasonably prudent medical professional had anticipated that the intervening force would occur, then the injury is considered foreseeable and the medical professional will be held liable.

Damages

After establishing the causal link between the breach of duty and the injury, the patient is entitled to damages. **Damages** may be of three types: (1) nominal, (2) actual, or (3) punitive.

Nominal damages are awarded for the vindication of a right in which minimal injury can be proved. These damages constitute a *very small* amount of money, for example, $1, and are awarded as a recognition of a technical invasion of a person's rights. Where other types of damages are proved, nominal damages are not awarded. An example in which nominal damages can be awarded is discussed in the section dealing with assault and battery.

Actual damages, sometimes referred to as compensatory damages, are awarded to "make the plaintiff whole" and restore him to his position before the injury. These damages compensate for actual loss and include, but are not limited to, the value of past and future medical expenses and past and future loss of income.

Punitive damages, sometimes referred to as exemplary damages, are awarded above and beyond actual damages. These damages are awarded when there is proof of outrageous, malicious, or intentional conduct. The theory behind punitive damages is a public policy consideration: by punishing wrongdoers or making an example of them, others will be deterred from future outrageous, malicious, or intentional conduct. Punitive damages are not often awarded in medical malpractice cases because most of these cases are based on a negligence theory involving deviation from the standard of care, as opposed to intentional tort theories involving conduct that is outrageous, malicious, or intentional.

Res Ipsa Loquitur

In addition to the traditional negligence theory just described, a second negligence theory, ***res ipsa loquitur,*** can serve as the basis for a medical malpractice action. In the most fundamental sense, *res ipsa loquitur* means "the thing speaks for itself."[5] This theory is not widely used and applies only when a plaintiff cannot prove negligence with the direct evidence available.

Using this theory, the patient attempts to convince the jury that the injury would not have happened except as a consequence of negligence, therefore creating a presumption of negligence that the medical professional must rebut. Underlying this theory is the belief that the medical professional has better access to evidence of what happened than does the patient.

To succeed on this claim, the patient must prove the following elements: (1) the injury is of such a character that it would not ordinarily occur without someone's negligence; (2) the medical professional had exclusive control and management over the instrument or cause of the accident; and (3) the injury could not have occurred as a result of any action by the patient. In some states, the patient must also prove that the medical professional had superior knowledge of the course of the accident.

The doctrine of *res ipsa loquitur,* by its definition, can apply in only limited situations. For example, the doctrine may be used in instances in which the patient is undergoing surgery and emerges from the anesthetic with a foreign object inside his body, for example, a sponge. Applying the elements listed previously, the patient would be able to prove his claim because (1) the foreign object would not ordinarily be present in the patient following surgery but for the medical professional's negligence; (2) the medical professional had exclusive control and management over the operation; and (3) the patient did not contribute in any way to leaving a foreign object inside his body.

At one time, *res ipsa loquitur* could not be applied in a lawsuit if the patient sued more than one defendant. The case of *Ybarra v. Spangard*[6] changed this rule. In *Ybarra,* the court reasoned that any one of the medical professionals involved in the surgery to remove the appendix (i.e., the surgeon, the anesthesiologist, the consulting physician, and hospital employees) could have been responsible for the patient's subsequent paralysis in his right shoulder. The court ruled that the patient was not required to show which medical professional was responsible for his injury because the patient did not have access to direct evidence proving which medical professional was responsible. The court allowed the patient to use *res ipsa loquitur* to create a presumption of negligence that any of the medical professionals involved in the surgery could have been responsible for the injury, and then allowed the medical professionals the opportunity to rebut the presumption and individually prove their innocence.

Vicarious Liability

The doctrine of **vicarious liability,** also referred to as *respondeat superior,* makes a health-care organization, such as a hospital, responsible for the negligent acts of its employees committed within the course and scope of their employment. Underlying the doctrine is the common law concept that a master is subject to liability for the torts of his servants if the servants were acting within the scope of their duties. Moreover, the reasoning holds that if an individual will be held responsible for the consequences of his own actions, so should employers be held responsible for the consequences of the acts of their agents and employees who act within the scope of their employment.

Vicarious liability is a derivative concept. If a jury determines that the employee is not liable, liability cannot be imposed on the employer under this theory. That is to say that the employer can be found liable under other theories, but the vicarious liability theory will not apply.

Whether an employment relationship exists may vary from case to case. To determine the existence of this relationship, courts look to a number of factors, including (1) who selected the employee, (2) who pays the employee, (3) who has power to fire the employee, and (4) who has power to control the details of the employee's work.

Among these factors, control is the most important. If the employer has control over the employee's work, an employment relationship will generally be found. In the health-care field, hospitals have generally been found vicariously liable for the negligent conduct of nurses, interns, residents, and technicians due to the level of control hospitals generally have over these employees. For example, the hospital in *Bernardi v. Community Hospital Association,*[7] was found negligent under the doctrine of *respondeat superior* when a nurse improperly injected a patient with medication, causing the patient to lose normal use of her right foot. The court ruled that the nurse was acting within the scope of her employment of the hospital, and therefore the hospital was responsible for her negligent acts.

By contrast, hospitals have generally not been found vicariously liable for the negligent conduct of physicians because the physicians are typically classified as independent contractors. Courts frequently classify the physician as an independent contractor because of the high degree of skill, learning, and judgment the physician exhibits, which the hospital is incapable of controlling. If, however, the physician is an employee of the hospital, the classification of independent contractor generally does not apply, and vicarious liability can be used.

Corporate Negligence

Unlike vicarious liability, **corporate negligence** recognizes that a healthcare organization, such as a hospital, owes a duty directly to a patient with regard to care and treatment. The doctrine has been defined as "the failure of a hospital, entrusted with the task of providing the accommodations necessary to carry out its purpose, to follow the established standard of conduct to which it should conform."[8] This duty cannot be delegated, and because it is not centered on the physician–hospital relationship, it is separate and distinct from the doctrine of vicarious liability.

The doctrine of corporate negligence was first applied in the landmark case of *Darling v. Charleston Community Memorial Hospital.*[9] In *Darling,* a college football player broke his leg during a game and was treated at the emergency room of the hospital. The on-call doctor, who had no orthopedic training, improperly applied a cast to the leg, which impaired blood circulation. Despite the patient's complaints, the cast remained on for fourteen days. After the patient was transferred to another hospital, his new physician removed the cast, discovered accumulated dead tissue, and subsequently amputated the leg.

In the player's lawsuit against the first hospital, the court found the first hospital liable under the theory of corporate negligence, reasoning that the hospital had a duty to require that the patient be examined by members of the hospital staff who were skilled in the particular treatment required under the circumstances. The hospital's failure to provide this examination, along with its failure to review the treatment the patient received, as well as not requiring consultants to be called in, was a breach of its direct duty to the patient.

The doctrine of corporate negligence also encompasses the hospital's duty to adhere to its own bylaws and the applicable state statute governing the credentials process. In *Johnson v. Misericordia Community Hospital,*[10] the hospital failed to investigate the qualifications of the physician who was accused of negligence. By granting staff privileges without doing this investigation, the court determined that the hospital created a foreseeable and unreasonable risk that unqualified physicians might be appointed and harm to patients would result. For that reason, the doctrine of corporate negligence applied.

Failure to Warn

Failure to warn, sometimes referred to as failure to protect, is a negligence theory that applies to a psychotherapist's failure to take steps to protect an innocent third party from a dangerous patient. First developed in the case of *Tarasoff v. Regents of University of California,*[11] the theory holds that when a psychotherapist determines that his patient presents a serious danger of violence to a third person, he incurs a duty to use reasonable care to protect the third person from this danger.

After determining that such a danger exists, the psychotherapist must then determine what steps to take to protect the intended victim. These steps may include warning the victim directly, warning others who can apprise the victim of the danger, notifying the police, or taking other steps that are reasonable under the circumstances.

In addition to being a legal duty, the duty to warn is an ethical duty. For example, the ethics code of the American Psychological Association provides that despite the general duty of confidentiality, a psychologist may reveal patient confidences if not doing so would pose a clear danger to the patient or others.[12] This provision illustrates how a professional association's own guidelines and requirements can be used to establish a standard of care.

Failure to warn is only one of a variety of possible theories that could support a lawsuit involving a patient's danger to a third party. Among other theories are the failure to adequately diagnose the patient, the failure to treat the patient so that the patient's violent tendencies could be brought under control, or the failure to commit the individual to a mental institution for care.

Intentional Torts

Assault and Battery

Although frequently referred to in connection with each other, assault and battery are two separate torts. An **assault** occurs when an individual is placed in reasonable anticipation of being touched in such a way that is insulting, provoking, or will cause the individual physical harm. An assault is a threat that does not involve physical contact. By contrast, a **battery** consists of physical contact involving injury or offense. In assault and battery, the individual does not give permission or authority for either act.

In addition to being considered a tort, assault and battery is considered a crime, punishable under the criminal law. A medical professional, like any other person, may be accused of the crime of assault and battery. It is infrequent, however, that a medical professional is accused of assault and battery in a civil matter. When that occurs, it is usually an accusation of technical battery.

Technical battery occurs when a medical professional, in the course of treatment, exceeds the consent given by the patient. In so doing, the medical professional does not necessarily intend a wrongful act and most likely sincerely hopes to aid the patient. Nonetheless, the medical professional does not have the patient's permission to act beyond that to which the patient originally consented. Unless an emergency is present, the patient may recover damages for the technical battery. If, however, the patient benefited from the technical battery, the patient may recover only nominal damages.

For example, a claim of battery succeeded in a case where the patient consented to exploratory surgery but instead received a mastectomy.[13] Similarly, a battery claim has succeeded where there has been an obvious mistake, such as operating on the wrong ear.[14]

Defamation

Defamation consists of the wrongful injuring of another person's reputation. Defamation may expose the other person to ridicule, contempt, or hatred and tends to diminish the esteem, respect, goodwill, or confidence in which the other person is held.

Defamation expressed in print, writing, pictures, or signs is referred to as libel; defamation expressed by oral expressions or transitory gestures is referred to as slander. In both libel and slander, the defamatory statement must be "published," meaning that the defamatory statement must be made to a third party and not just to the patient.

As a general rule, truth of the statement at issue is an absolute defense in a defamation lawsuit. This defense can be applied in cases against health-care institutions alleging wrongful release of medical records because the contents of a medical record are generally considered true.

Where the defense of truth does not apply, because some or all of the statement at issue is false, health-care providers may be able to use the defenses of absolute privilege and qualified privilege. Under absolute privilege, publications made as part of judicial, legislative, and/or administrative proceedings are protected in a subsequent defamation lawsuit. For example, a health-care provider who releases information pursuant to lawful judicial process, for example, a lawful subpoena, and then is sued for defamation, is protected from liability.

Similarly, qualified privilege may be used as a defense if the statement was made in good faith, without malice, under a reasonable belief to be true, by someone with an interest or legal duty to disclose the statement to another with a corresponding duty or interest. For example, a health-care provider who possesses a duty to inform another of her possibility of contracting a contagious disease from the physician's patient, and does so in good faith, without malice and reasonably believing the diagnosis to be true, can avail himself of the defense even if he later learns he was mistaken concerning the contagious disease.

Invasion of Privacy

Invasion of privacy involves the dissemination of information about another person's private, personal matters. To charge invasion of privacy, the plaintiff must show any one of the following: (1) an unwarranted appropriation or exploitation of an individual's personality; (2) a publication of an individual's private affairs, which would cause embarrassment; (3) a wrongful intrusion upon an individual's private concerns or activities; or (4) some form of publicity that paints the individual in a false light.

Invasion of privacy lawsuits in the health-care field can arise in a number of ways, including using a patient's likeness for commercial purposes without the patient's consent. For example, using "before" and "after" photographs of a surgery patient for purposes of medical instruction would constitute an invasion of privacy if the patient had not given consent.

Similarly, a charge of invasion of privacy can be brought if there has been improper disclosure of a patient's health information given in the course of treatment. For further information discussing this topic, see Chapter 5.

Medical Abandonment

Medical abandonment generally means the unilateral severing, by the physician, of the physician–patient relationship without giving the patient reasonable notice at a time when there is a necessity for continuing care. To prove medical abandonment, the patient must establish the following elements: (1) the existence of a physician–patient relationship and (2) that the abandonment is the proximate cause of the injury for which the patient is suing. Unless the injury is an obvious result of the abandonment, the patient must use an expert witness to establish proximate cause between the abandonment and the injury. If there is abandonment but no injury, the physician will not be held liable.

Courts have found physicians liable for abandonment in a number of instances: for intentionally leaving their patients alone at a critical time[15] and for failing to be available because of the needs of other patients,[16] vacation,[17] or the physician's erroneous belief that the patient had recovered and no longer needed treatment.[18] Conversely, courts have found physicians not liable for abandonment in cases in which the patient does not need immediate treatment and the physician gives the patient a list of qualified substitute physicians. Courts have been split concerning whether a physician can be liable for failing to be available because of personal illness.[19]

Although the tort of medical abandonment is nearly one hundred years old, changes in the economics of health care provide new opportunities for its use. With the advent of health maintenance organizations, preferred provider organizations, and Medicare's Prospective Payment System, critics have charged that economic issues and pressures, rather than medical reasons, have caused the premature discharge of patients. These critics charge that hospitals and physicians may succumb to the temptation to discharge a patient prematurely, rather than extend the hospital stay or transfer the patient to another institution, in order to obtain full diagnostic-related group (DRG) reimbursement. This premature discharge raises the possibility of a medical abandonment claim if there is not adequate follow-up treatment for the patient.

Breach of Contract

Breach of contract claims generally involve express contracts and the failure to perform these contracts. In express contracts, the parties have agreed in advance upon a specific treatment, or the physician may have guaranteed a certain cure or result. If the physician fails to perform the particular act promised, the patient may sue under the theory of nonperformance.

Physicians who fail to perform as specifically promised have been found liable in court. For example, the physician in *Brooks v. Robinson*[20] expressly agreed to treat the patient for tuberculosis but took no action whatsoever. Similarly, in *Foran v. Carangelo*,[21] the physician agreed to perform a hysterectomy but did not do so. In both instances, the basis of the patient's successful lawsuit was nonperformance.

A claim for nonperformance should not be confused with a claim for improper performance. In a lawsuit for improper performance, the physician begins to take whatever action he and the patient agreed on, but performs it improperly. For example, the physician in *Horowitz v. Bogart*[22] agreed to remove the patient's ulcer but instead removed the patient's appendix. In such an instance, the lawsuit is not for breach of contract but for negligence or battery.

Defenses and Limitations on Liability

In virtually every lawsuit, the defendant must decide which defenses to present to the charges leveled against him. In addition to disputing the merits of the lawsuit, the defendant may choose to raise defenses that shield him from liability or reduce his level of liability, regardless of whether the defenses address the merits of the lawsuit. Defenses commonly raised in lawsuits involving health-care providers are addressed in the following sections.

Statutes of Limitations

A **statute of limitation** is a law that sets forth a fixed time period in which a lawsuit must be brought. If a lawsuit is not brought within the time frame specified in the applicable statute of limitations, the lawsuit is barred, and the court must dismiss the case.

Statutes of limitations are designed for two purposes: (1) to force those persons considering a lawsuit to bring the lawsuit at a time when memories are intact and evidence is available and, therefore, not "sit on their rights" and (2) to allow potential defendants a time frame from which to know that a lawsuit can no longer be maintained against them.

Statutes of limitations are technical in nature, as illustrated by the fact that the time period of each statute of limitations varies between the type of lawsuit—that is, contract or tort—and between each state's laws. Statutes in virtually every state provide a fixed time frame in which to bring medical malpractice lawsuits and other personal injury lawsuits.

In certain instances, specific statutes or court decisions have extended the time period of the general statute of limitation. For example, the time frame in which to bring a lawsuit is generally measured from the time the injury occurred. If, however, the injury involves a foreign object left in the body following surgery, the limitations period begins to run when the injured person discovers or should have discovered the injury.

Extensions of the statute of limitations period also apply to minors or persons under some type of legal disability. The extension of the statute of limitations period in these instances is referred to as tolling the statute of limitations. For example, a particular state's law may extend the period of time to a certain number of years after the minor reaches the age of majority to bring a lawsuit. This extension is granted so that the minor is not penalized for the failure of his parent to bring a lawsuit on his behalf.

For a variety of reasons, parents do not bring lawsuits on behalf of their injured children, including reasons of unwillingness or financial inability. For public policy considerations, the law allows children whose rights were not vindicated by their parents to bring lawsuits to vindicate their rights once they reach the age of majority. For this same reason, this extension concept applies to an injured person who is under some form of legal disability, such as being adjudged insane. Once the period of legal disability is removed, the time period of the statute of limitations begins to run.

Illinois law provides a perfect illustration of these concepts. The statute of limitation governing malpractice actions against physicians, dentists, registered nurses, or hospitals in Illinois provides a two-year time period in which to bring a breach of contract or tort lawsuit.[23] The two-year time period is measured from the time of injury or death, or the time the patient should have known or received notice of the injury or death, whichever occurred first. The statute provides that in no event can a lawsuit be brought more than four years from the date of injury or death at issue.

If, however, the person entitled to bring the lawsuit is a minor at the time of the injury, the statute provides an eight-year period to bring the lawsuit, measured from the date of injury. The statute further provides that in no event can the lawsuit be brought after the minor reaches twenty-two years old. Furthermore, if the person entitled to bring the lawsuit is under a legal disability, the time period does not begin to run until the disability is removed.

Charitable Immunity

At one time, a majority of the states permitted the use of the **charitable immunity** defense. In this defense, a charitable institution such as a hospital could be shielded from liability for any torts committed on its property or by its employees. The defense was permitted so that assets intended for charitable purposes would not be used for "improper" reasons, such as paying damage awards. The doctrine originated in England and was adopted in the United States in the late nineteenth century.[24]

The doctrine of charitable immunity was followed until the case of *Bing v. Thunig*.[25] In *Bing*, New York's highest court expressly overruled applying the doctrine to shield charitable hospitals from liability and proceeded to apply the doctrine of respondeat superior. The court in *Bing* reasoned that charitable institutions should be forced to compensate persons for the injuries the institutions caused, just as any other business organization would be required to compensate for injuries caused by the business organization. After the *Bing* case, virtually every state either limited or abolished the doctrine of charitable immunity.

Governmental Immunity

Governmental immunity precludes a plaintiff from asserting a meritorious lawsuit against a governmental entity unless the governmental entity consents to the lawsuit. The doctrine has its origin in the English common law concept that the king could do no wrong; therefore, he and his subordinates could not be sued. As developed in the United States, federal and state governments were immune from lawsuits arising out of the negligence of their officers, agents, and employees, *unless* the federal or state government expressly consented to the lawsuit.

Most jurisdictions have abandoned this doctrine in favor of permitting tort lawsuit with certain limitations and restrictions. For example, the government of the United States may not be sued without its consent. With the passage of the Federal Tort Claims Act in 1946, the U.S. government's immunity from tort liability was largely abolished and certain conditions for suits and claims against the U.S. government were established.

Among those conditions was the requirement that the government employee being sued had to be acting within the scope of her employment. Whether a government employee, such as an employee of a veterans' hospital, is acting within the scope of her employment depends on the facts of the particular case.

Conversely, certain restrictions on lawsuits against the United States do remain. The U.S. government is protected from liability for the traditional category of intentional torts and from claims brought against employees who exercise due care in executing a statute or regulation. Finally, the U.S. government is protected from claims brought against its employees based on the performance, or failure to perform, a discretionary duty. States that have passed laws abandoning the doctrine of governmental immunity have done so with similar conditions and restrictions.

Good Samaritan Statutes

Several states, seeking to encourage physicians and other rescuers to provide emergency treatment, have passed what are referred to as **Good Samaritan statutes.** As a general rule, these statutes protect physicians and other rescuers from civil liability as a result of their acts or omissions in rendering emergency care.[26] If, however, the rescuer acts in a willful, wanton, or reckless manner in providing emergency treatment, he cannot avail himself of the Good Samaritan statute as a defense.

Generally, the statutes are not designed to protect health-care providers who routinely treat patients in immediate need of emergency care, such as emergency room physicians. Rather, the statutes address those health-care providers who render emergency care in a nontraditional setting, such as at an automobile accident on the side of the road. If the nontraditional setting is present, the health-care provider may raise the Good Samaritan defense.

Contributory and Comparative Negligence

Contributory negligence and comparative negligence, although often used interchangeably, are separate legal concepts used to limit a defendant's liability. **Contributory negligence** means conduct of the plaintiff that contributes in part to the injury the plaintiff received. In some states, a finding of contributory negligence on the plaintiff's part is sufficient to bar any form of recovery. Therefore, even if the plaintiff proves every element of a negligence claim against a defendant, she still will lose if the defendant proves that the plaintiff contributed to her own injuries.

Comparative negligence, on the other hand, builds on the concept of contributory negligence, but is not as harsh in the result. Rather than bar recovery, proof that the plaintiff contributed to her own injuries only serves to reduce the amount of damages the plaintiff can recover.

Under comparative negligence principles, negligence is measured in terms of percentages. The percentage that can be attributed to the plaintiff will then be reduced proportionally from the overall award of damages. In some states, if the plaintiff's percentage of fault outweighs the defendant's percentage of fault, the plaintiff can recover nothing. The same situation in another state, however, may merely reduce the damage award. Similarly, some states permit recovery when the plaintiff and defendant are equally at fault; other states do not permit any form of recovery in such a situation.

Under both contributory and comparative negligence theories, the negligence of the defendant is not in doubt; it has already been proved by the plaintiff. The basic difference between the two concepts is that comparative negligence attempts to compensate the plaintiff for some portion of her injury, no matter how small, whereas contributory negligence serves to bar completely a damage award for injury.

In the health-care setting, documentation in the medical record may be the only successful way to support either of these defenses. For example, nurses' notes documenting the instructions given to a patient and the patient's multiple refusals to follow those instructions would support a defense that the patient's own actions caused, or contributed to, her complications.

Such documentation was used in *Seymour v. Victory Memorial Hospital*[27] to support a contributory negligence defense. In *Seymour,* the patient was instructed not to smoke unless someone was with her and to call the nurses' station when she wanted to smoke. The patient bought cigarettes from a volunteer cart, smoked alone, dropped a match, and burned herself.

She then sued the hospital, raising claims of both negligence and *res ipsa loquitur*. The court ruled that the hospital was not liable because the patient knew the smoking procedures and was aware of the danger if she did not follow the procedures. The patient's action in obtaining the cigarette without calling the nurse amounted to contributory negligence.

Assumption of Risk

Assumption of risk, like contributory and comparative negligence, is a method used to limit liability either completely or in part. Under this doctrine, a plaintiff who voluntarily exposes himself to a known and appreciated danger may not recover damages caused by incurring that risk. In order to prevail in this defense, the defendant must prove that the plaintiff knew of the risk, assumed the risk voluntarily, and was not coerced. If all elements are proved, the defendant cannot be held liable for negligence.

Conclusion

In order to manage health information wisely, the differences and similarities between the principles listed in this chapter must be understood. Each main section builds on its predecessor: understanding health-care relationships provides the basis for understanding the types of lawsuits that may be brought and the defenses that may be raised. Understanding these principles should assist the health information manager in recognizing potential legal situations.

Furthermore, those involved with managing health information must be aware that the principles of liability differ depending on which jurisdiction applies to a particular case. Learning the particular statutory, common law, and administrative requirements of that jurisdiction in order to make prudent decisions concerning health information is extremely important.

Finally, adopting a constant learning approach to the principles of liability is essential because the law is constantly changing. Keeping abreast of changes in the law at all levels, particularly statutory and common law changes, must be a goal of health information managers.

Case Study

A surgeon performs elective surgery on John Smith. Smith later complains to his surgeon about pain resulting from the surgery. His surgeon dismisses his complaints as not credible and eventually withdraws from the case. Smith is then treated by another surgeon, who determines that Smith developed complications from surgery and that the delay in treatment has made the complications worse. Smith sees an attorney about a possible lawsuit against the first surgeon. Describe the theories that could support a lawsuit under these circumstances.

Review Questions

1. How do the principles of liability influence the health information manager's role in protecting health information?
2. What are the requirements of the Emergency Medical Treatment and Active Labor Act that hospitals must meet?
3. What are medical staff privileges, and how are they determined?
4. Compare and contrast negligence and medical malpractice.
5. What are the different methods one can use to establish the standard of care?
6. What is the role of an expert witness in a negligence claim?
7. What is the failure-to-warn theory, and how may it be exercised in the context of a dangerous patient?
8. Compare and contrast the defenses commonly raised in lawsuits involving health-care providers.

Enrichment Activity

Construct a series of flowcharts. Each flowchart should illustate a health-care relationship, a type of lawsuit, and a defense that may be raised. Compare the differences between the flowcharts, and determine whether any of the elements in your flowcharts can be interchanged with another element.

Notes

1. LOUIS GOLDSTEIN & MILES ZAREMSKI, MEDICAL AND HOSPITAL NEGLIGENCE, Volume 1, § 6:01 (1990 & Supp. 1992).
2. 42 U.S.C. §§ 1395 et seq. (2000).
3. 934 F.2d 1362 (5th Cir. 1991).
4. 181 A.2d 573 (Del. 1952).
5. BLACK'S LAW DICTIONARY 1173 (5th ed. 1979).
6. 154 P.2d 687 (Cal. 1944).
7. 443 P.2d 708 (Colo. 1968).
8. *Johnson v. Misericordia Community Hospital,* 294 N.W.2d 501, 506 (Wis. Ct. App. 1980), *aff'd,* 301 N.W.2d 156 (Wis. 1981).
9. 211 N.E.2d 253 (Ill. 1965).
10. *Supra* note 8.
11. 529 P.2d 553 (Cal. 1974), *reargued,* 551 P.2d 334 (Cal. 1976).
12. AMERICAN PSYCHOLOGICAL ASSOCIATION, ETHICAL PRINCIPLES OF PSYCHOLOGISTS, Preamble to Principle 5 (1981).
13. *Corn v. French,* 289 P.2d 173 (Nev. 1955).
14. *Mohr v. Williams,* 104 N.W. 12 (Minn. 1905).
15. *Johnson v. Vaughn,* 370 S.W.2d 591 (Ky. Ct. App. 1963).
16. *Katsetos v. Nolan,* 368 A.2d 172 (Conn. 1976).
17. *Vann v. Harden,* 47 S.E.2d 314 (Va. 1948).
18. *Mucci v. Houghton,* 57 N.W. 305 (Iowa 1894).
19. *Dashiell v. Griffith,* 35 A. 1094 (Md. 1896) (finding the physician liable); *Warwick v. Bliss,* 195 N.W. 502 (S.D. 1923) (finding the physician not liable).
20. 163 So.2d 186 (La. Ct. App. 1964).
21. 216 A.2d 638 (Conn. 1966).
22. 217 N.Y.S. 881 (N.Y. 1926).
23. 735 ILCS § 5/13-212 (2000).
24. *McDonald v. Massachusetts General Hosp.,* 120 Mass. 432 (Mass. 1876).
25. 143 N.E.2d 3 (N.Y. 1957).
26. *See, e.g.,* CONN. GEN. STAT. § 52-557b (2000); FLA. STAT. ANN. § 768.13 (2000); MISS. CODE ANN. § 73-25-37 (1999); MONT. CODE ANN. § 41-1-405 (2000).
27. 376 N.E.2d 754 (Ill. 1978).

Chapter 4

Patient Record Requirements

Learning Objectives

After reading this chapter, the learner should be able to:

1. Summarize the multiple functions and uses of a medical record.
2. Identify and explain how the sources of law influence the content of the medical record.
3. Distinguish between authorship and authentication.
4. Differentiate between proper and improper methods for a health provider to correct the medical record.
5. Compare and contrast the procedures used to comply with or refuse a patient's request to correct the record.
6. Identify the factors influencing a record retention policy.
7. Explain what role a statute of limitations plays in a record retention policy.
8. Compare and contrast record destruction done in the ordinary course with that done due to closure.
9. Identify the importance of keeping permanent evidence of a record's destruction in the ordinary course.
10. Identify the special procedures involved with the destruction of alcohol and drug abuse records upon a program's closure.

Key Concepts

- Authentication
- Authorship
- Corrections to the record
- Medical record content
- Record destruction policies
- Record retention policies
- Statute of limitations

Introduction

The health information contained in a paper medical record, a computerized medical record, an abstract of patient-specific information, or some other format plays a primary role in the delivery of health care. In addition to its role in direct patient care, health information maintained in these formats serves as the health-care provider's legal record of patient care. As such, it is subject to stringent legal requirements.

While technology has advanced quite rapidly, advances in the law concerning technology have not been as rapid. Despite new methods of storing health information, legal requirements governing such information often reference only one format, the paper medical record. For purposes of simplicity, this chapter refers to the traditional concept of a medical record in explaining the legal requirements governing the content, retention, and destruction of health information. Despite this approach, many of the concepts addressed in this chapter may apply by analogy to the other formats. Where appropriate, other record formats are addressed.

To understand the legal requirements governing the medical record, the health information manager should first recognize its function and uses. Functions and uses, in turn, are affected by statutory, regulatory, accrediting, and institutional requirements. By understanding these concepts, effective policies governing **medical record content** (the characteristics essential to constitute an adequate medical record), retention, and destruction can be created.

Function and Use of the Medical Record

The multiple **functions and uses** of the medical record have resulted in various names such as health record, hospital chart, outpatient record, clinical record, electronic medical record, computerized patient record, and other such descriptors for the basic medical record. Generally defined, a medical record is a document that contains a complete and accurate description of a patient's history, condition, diagnostic and therapeutic treatment, and the results of treatment. The medical record includes detailed personal, medical, financial, and social data about the patient.[1] Figure 4-1 categorizes these data by their sensitivity and need for confidentiality. Because extensive literature already exists that addresses these types of data, more detail will not be given here.

The medical record serves both clinical and nonclinical uses, as shown in Figure 4-2. In the most basic sense, the medical record serves as the chronological document of clinical care rendered to the patient. Created contemporaneously with the clinical care rendered, it provides a method for various medical disciplines to communicate about the patient's illness and course of treatment during a particular episode of care. Further, it supplies information to caregivers involved in a patient's subsequent episode of care.

In addition to direct patient care, medical records serve other clinical purposes. Through concurrent and retrospective analysis, medical records are relied on by the medical, nursing, and scientific communities as a primary source of information for research. By identifying specific incidences of disease, medical records assist the public health community's efforts to

Least Sensitive
Personal and
Financial Data
More Sensitive
Social Data
Most Sensitive
Medical Data

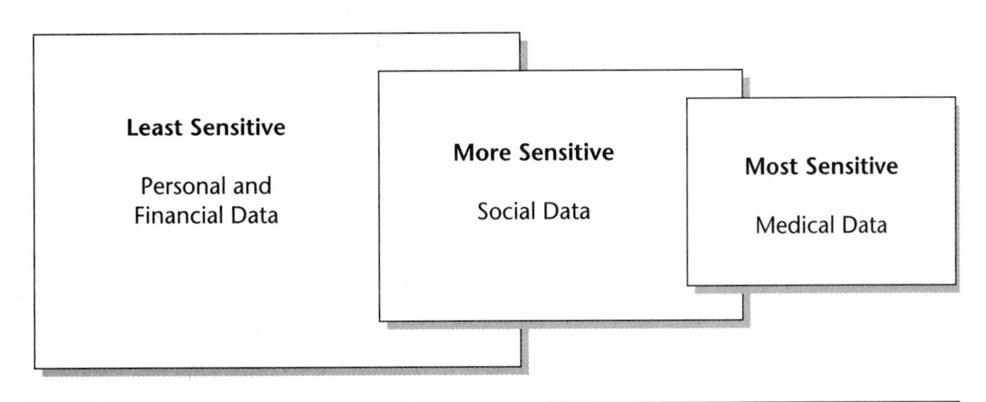

Figure 4-1. Patient Data Categories

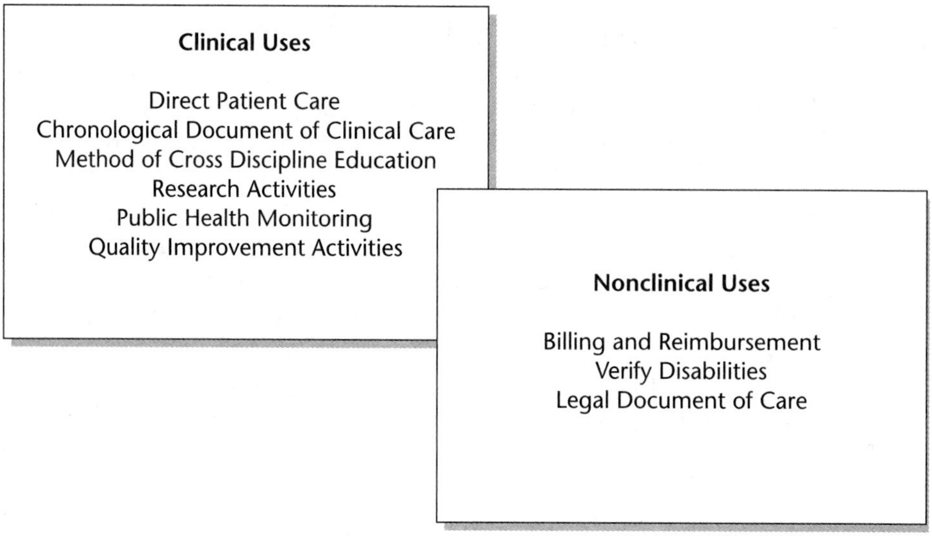

Clinical Uses

Direct Patient Care
Chronological Document of Clinical Care
Method of Cross Discipline Education
Research Activities
Public Health Monitoring
Quality Improvement Activities

Nonclinical Uses

Billing and Reimbursement
Verify Disabilities
Legal Document of Care

Figure 4-2 Uses of Medical Records

control disease and monitor the overall health status of a population. Furthermore, medical records assist in quality improvement activities because they provide a source from which to evaluate the adequacy and appropriateness of patient care.

In addition to clinical uses, medical records serve other secondary purposes. Health-care providers rely on medical records to support the billing of insurance and benefits claims of individual patients to whom they have provided care. Third-party payors rely on medical records to make payments on claims to health-care providers and to monitor the appropriateness of care and services rendered to the patient. Employers rely on medical records to document the extent of an employee's disability.

Finally, medical records serve as legal documents: the record of a particular episode of a patient's care. The backbone of virtually every professional liability action, medical records are used to prove what did or did not happen in a particular case and to establish whether the applicable standard of care was met. Because memories fade and persons who participated in direct patient care are not always available at the time of trial, the medical record serves as the most frequently used method to reconstruct an episode of patient care.

Legal Requirements for Medical Record Content

In the light of the many uses of medical records, it is incumbent on health information managers to design and manage systems that ensure accurate and complete medical records. Before doing so, health information managers must become aware of the legal requirements governing the content of a medical record.

Content of the Medical Record

Unfortunately, no one source of law definitely addresses the legal requirements governing the content of medical records. Rather, a myriad of sources supply these requirements: statutory, regulatory, accrediting, institutional, and professional guidelines. Although each source is separate, they must all be reviewed together to obtain an understanding of the legal requirements governing medical records. See Figure 4-3.

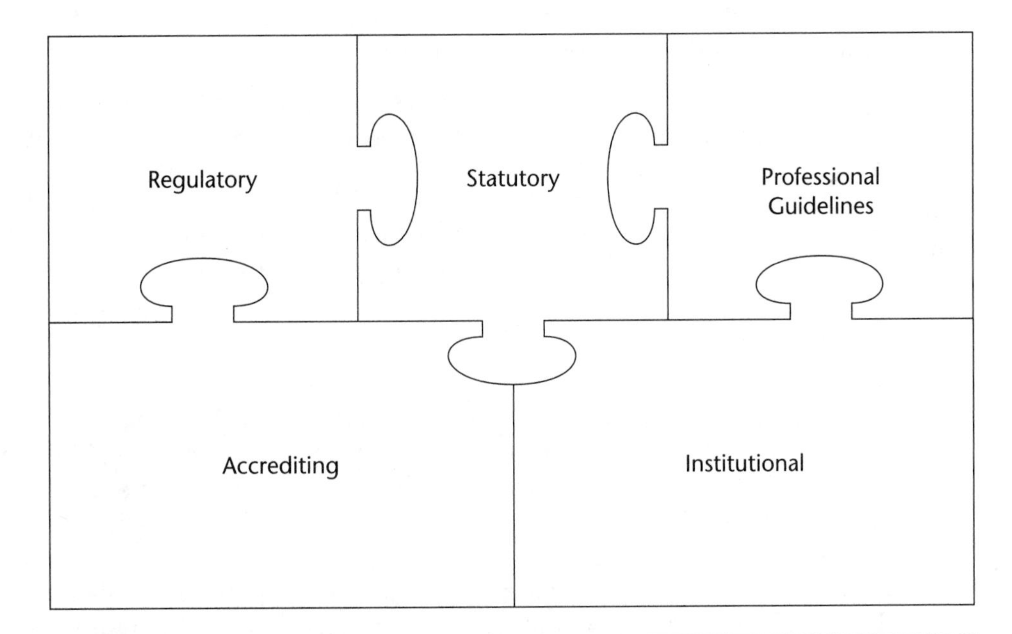

Figure 4-3. Interrelationship of Legal Requirements Governing Content of the Medical Record

Statutory Provisions

First and foremost in any review of the legal requirements governing medical records are statutory provisions. Although very few statutes address the contents of medical records specifically, statutory provisions should be reviewed first because of the critical role they play in the legal system.

As explained in Chapter 1, statutory provisions can be federal or state laws or municipal codes. Unfortunately, no one federal law addresses the legal requirements governing all patient records. Rather, a small patchwork of federal and state laws on this subject exists. For example, the section of federal law that establishes the Conditions of Participation in federal reimbursement programs such as Medicare defines a hospital, in part, as an institution that "maintains clinical records on all patients."[2] That same section does not, however, define what a clinical record must contain.

Similarly, states that have passed statutes referring to medical records generally limit the statute to the requirement that the health-care provider merely create a medical record.[3] If the content of the medical record is defined by statute, the definition is often provided in the context of hospital licensing. For example, a portion of the Tennessee law that licenses health facilities, referred to as the Medical Records Act of 1974, defines the content of a medical record. It provides:

> (5) (A) "Hospital records" means those medical histories, records, reports, summaries, diagnoses, prognoses, records of treatment and medication ordered and given, entries, X rays, radiology interpretations, and other written, electronic, or graphic data prepared, kept, made or maintained in hospitals that pertain to hospital confinements or hospital services rendered to patients admitted to hospitals or receiving emergency room or outpatient care.[4]

Regulations

Closely related to statutory provisions are regulations promulgated by executive agencies. Frequently, statutory provisions delegate certain powers to the executive agency responsible for licensing a health-care facility, such as the power to promulgate and enforce rules and regulations governing the health-care facility's medical records.

Found on both the federal and state levels, these regulations vary between (1) general statements that a medical record be maintained, (2) broad listings of content requirements, and (3) specific, detailed provisions governing content.

An example of specific, detailed provisions on the federal level include a regulation promulgated by the Department of Health and Human Services as a Condition of Participation in the Medicare program. This regulation states:

> (b) Standard: Content. The clinical record contains sufficient information to identify the patient clearly, to justify the diagnosis(es) and treatment, and to document the results accurately. All clinical records contain the following general categories of data:
>
> (1) Documented evidence of the assessment of the needs of the patient, of an appropriate plan of care, and of the care and services provided,
>
> (2) Identification data and consent forms,
>
> (3) Medical history,
>
> (4) Report of physical examinations, if any,
>
> (5) Observations and progress notes,
>
> (6) Reports of treatments and clinical findings, and
>
> (7) Discharge summary including final diagnosis(es) and prognosis.[5]

In place of specific regulations, some states have adopted as their own all or portions of the requirements of the Medicare Conditions of Participation.[6] Finally, at least two states have adopted the Accreditation Standards of the Joint Commission on Accreditation of Healthcare Organizations (JCAHO) as the governing regulations.[7]

Accrediting Standards

Although accrediting standards do not have the force of law standing alone, they are frequently used to establish the standard of care in negligence actions against health-care providers. As stated previously, at least two states have adopted accrediting standards as their governing regulations. Thus, health-care providers must pay close attention to these standards of accreditation. For further information concerning the standard of care in negligence actions, see Chapter 3.

The primary source for accrediting standards in health care is the JCAHO. JCAHO standards require hospitals to maintain medical records for each patient and describe in detail the contents of the medical record.[8]

Institutional Standards

Where no specific statute or regulation specifically addresses the existence or content of a medical record, health-care institutions may wish to create their own standards or adopt the standards issued by an accrediting agency. These institutional standards may be either broad statements or detailed listings or fall somewhere in between. They serve as a guide to medical record content for that institution.

Similar to accrediting standards, institutional standards do not carry the force of law. Nevertheless, they are useful to establishing the standard of care in a negligence action. And, as indicated in Chapter 3, if the institutional standards are higher than the minimally acceptable standard found in a statute or textbook, it is the higher standard against which the institution will be measured.

Professional Guidelines

In addition to the sources listed previously, allied health professional organizations publish guidelines that address the existence and content of medical records. For example, the American Health Information Management Association, in conjunction with a number of health-care associations, has published a brochure entitled *Principles of Medical Record Documentation*.[9] (This brochure is reproduced in the appendix of this book.) Similarly, health-care associations publish position statements on issues related to medical records. Although these health-care associations are not providing legal advice when publishing these guidelines and position statements, the documents address sensitive legal issues related to medical records. As such, they assist health information managers to ensure accurate and complete medical records.

Timely and Complete Medical Records

As described earlier, a medical record serves multiple functions and uses. It is axiomatic that a timely and complete medical record is essential to achieving these purposes.

Authentication and Timeliness

All entries in the medical record must be authored and authenticated. **Authorship** identifies the health-care provider who has made the entry, either in writing, by dictation, keyboard, or keyless data entry. **Authentication** confirms the content of the entry, either by written signature, initials, or computer-generated signature code. This confirmation implies that the entry as recorded is accurate.

In some localities, the licensing authority may consider authentication to include the use of a rubber stamp signature by the medical staff member the signature represents. In such an instance, the licensing authority may require the health-care institution to maintain in its administrative offices a signed statement that the medical staff member whose signature stamp is involved is the only one who has the stamp and is the only one authorized to use it. Duplication and delegation of the stamp by others would be strictly prohibited[10] and, if allowed, would defeat the concept of verifying the accuracy of the entry in the medical record.

Because accuracy of the medical record is paramount, authentication principles dictate that only the author of the entry may authenticate the entry. For example, it would not be legally sound for a physician within a group practice to sign for another physician within that same practice unless specific accreditation standards or regulations allowed for this action. This is because the proper foundation for admitting medical records into evidence requires that the record be made by a person with knowledge of the acts, events, conditions, opinions, or diagnoses appearing within it. Presumably the physician who signs an entry she did not author cannot have the requisite knowledge of the acts, events, conditions, opinions, or diagnoses in question—in other words, the physician would not have firsthand knowledge of what transpired to support the entry in the medical record. Allowing a physician to sign for another physician therefore raises a question concerning the reliability and integrity of the medical record.

As an ordinary matter, health-care providers who make an entry in the medical record must do so contemporaneously with the actual occurrence of the event. This need for timeliness is not only critical to delivering quality patient care; it is required as a condition of both licensing and accreditation.[11]

Completeness

Completeness of a medical record is not only a matter addressed by state laws, federal and state regulations, and accrediting standards; it is a matter of common sense.[12] Without a complete medical record, the health-care provider's ability to render quality patient care and conduct research and education is impaired. In addition, the health-care provider's ability to present a defense in a lawsuit is called into question.

The impact of an incomplete record on a medical malpractice lawsuit is illustrated by *Ravenis v. Detroit General Hospital.*[13] In *Ravenis,* two patients who received cornea transplants from a cadaver subsequently developed ophthalmitis and eventually lost their sight. In the lawsuit the patients brought against the hospital, the evidence indicated that the results of lab tests that had been performed on the deceased and that revealed an acute infection were not made a part of the record at the time the decision to harvest the organs was made. Because the hospital failed to maintain complete records showing the medical history of the eye donor, the jury found the hospital liable for medical malpractice.

Completeness of a medical record is measured against the requirements governing medical record content examined earlier in this chapter. An incomplete record may be discovered during concurrent or postdischarge review by the health information management department. A health-care provider's immediate attention to the deficiencies identified in such a review support a conclusion that the health-care provider is documenting the actual treatment rendered rather than making belated entries to support a defense in a lawsuit.

For considerable time, courts have held the opinion that if an event or aspect of patient care was not recorded in the medical record, it is appropriate to conclude that it did not occur. This is sometimes phrased as: "If it wasn't charted, it didn't happen or "not documented, not done." The impact of the absence of proper documentation in the medical record on the health-care provider's defense in a negligence lawsuit is illustrated by *Collins v. Westlake Community Hospital.*[14]

In *Collins,* the plaintiff alleged that the nursing staff's failure to observe and record the condition of his leg while it was in a cast culminated in amputation of the leg. The court examined the plaintiff's medical record and noted that no entries were made in the nurses' notes during a critical seven-hour time period, despite a physician's order directing the nursing staff to "watch condition of toes." Testimony by the nurse on duty that a nurse does not always record her observations on the chart every time the patient is checked, and that she usually records only abnormal findings did not overcome the inference that no observations were actually made of the patient.

By contrast, the absence of documentation of patient care was overcome in the case of *Hurlock v. Park Lane Medical Center.*[15] In *Hurlock,* the attending physician had ordered the nursing staff to turn a paraplegic patient every two hours to avoid development of decubitus ulcers. The patient developed decubitus ulcers at multiple sites, which eventually contributed to amputation of her leg.

The medical record introduced at trial indicated that the nurses' notes contained only eighteen entries concerning turning the patient. Had the order to turn the patient been complied with and properly documented, the patient's medical record should have included 117 such entries in the nurses' notes. This absence of documentation allowed the jury to infer that the nurses had not turned the patient as ordered by the physician. The jury's verdict in the patient's favor was later overturned on appeal because the court determined that the patient had failed to prove definitively that the nurses were negligent.

Although both *Collins* and *Hurlock* resulted in different outcomes, they illustrate the necessity for a complete medical record reflecting the patient care rendered, even routine care.

Corrections to the Record

By the health-care provider

No matter how careful the health-care provider is, at times, details of patient care may be incorrectly recorded. Perhaps the patient information is recorded in the wrong patient's medical record or words are misspelled. When these mistakes occur, it is appropriate for the person who made the original entry to make **corrections to the record.**

The proper method to correct the record is to draw a single line through the entry and write "error" next to it, along with the date, time, and initials of the person making the correction. The line should be drawn so that whatever was written can be read. Under no circumstances should the original entry be obliterated or covered with correction fluid. Where appropriate, the reason for the correction should be noted, for example, "wrong patient record." Finally, only the individual who made the mistaken entry should correct the entry.

The same principles apply to correction of information stored in a computerized patient record. The difference is in the method of making that correction. Typically, the correction is made by way of an addendum to the computerized record. Unlike the paper record, the original document in the computerized record is left in an unaltered state. A new document showing the correction is created and added to the computerized record, with a computer code attribute used to reference the original document to the addendum. An electronic signature is required to authenticate the addendum. Specific guidelines for the correction of computerized patient record entries have been issued by standards organizations.[16]

A case illustrating the wrong way to correct the record is *Ahrens v. Katz.*[17] In *Ahrens,* a portion of the nurses' notes had been covered up with correction fluid. To determine what was recorded under the correction fluid, the court allowed x-rays to be taken of notes in question. Testimony at trial indicated that the use of correction fluid to make corrections to the record was not in accordance with correct nursing practices.

A case illustrating the principle that the only individual who should correct the record is the one who made the mistaken entry is *Henry by Henry v. St. John's Hospital.*[18] In *Henry,* a child was born with cerebral palsy, allegedly because of the use of an inappropriate amount of anesthetic. At trial, it became clear that the physician who had administered the anesthetic had corrected the entries made by a nurse concerning the amount of anesthetic given. The court noted that a physician would not ordinarily write on, or correct, nursing notes. Because the physician had altered the entry of another health professional, it created an inference that she was attempting to conceal information and was therefore liable for negligence.

By the patient

Although health-care providers typically are the individuals who discover the need to correct the record, this is not always the case. For example, the patient who has received a copy of her medical record may discover some inaccuracy or incompleteness and may decide to correct the record accordingly. Such correction by the patient is a matter governed by both federal and state law.

Federal standards for the privacy of patient-specific health information issued pursuant to the Health Insurance Portability and Accountability Act, also known as the HIPAA final privacy rule, dictate that an individual possesses a right to have a covered entity[19] amend patient-specific health information or a record about the individual contained in a designated record set for as long as the patient-specific health information is maintained in that record set.[20] If the covered entity grants the amendment request in whole or in part, it must insert or provide a link to the amendment, inform the requestor it has accepted the amendment, and make reasonable efforts to inform other persons identified by the requestor as having previously received patient-specific health information. The covered entity may deny the request for amendment for a limited number of reasons, but in doing so must give written notice to the requestor.

The HIPAA final privacy rule sets a floor requirement for health-care providers to respond to patient requests to correct the record. Similar requirements exist at the state level. Where state law requirements are more stringent than those outlined under the federal standards, health-care providers must comply with both sets of requirements.

One state statute illustrating the proper method for the patient to correct the record is that of Washington State. Under Washington law, a patient who determines that her record is inaccurate or incomplete may request in writing that the health-care provider correct or amend the record.[21] The health-care provider then has a limited time frame in which to make the correction or amendment and inform the patient of the action. The procedure to make the correction or amendment involves adding the amending information to the record and marking the challenged entries as corrected or amended entries. The health-care provider then must indicate where in the record the corrected or amended information is located.

If the health-care provider refuses to make the requested correction or amendment, the health-care provider must inform the patient in writing of that decision and of the patient's right to add a statement of disagreement. Upon receipt of a concise statement of the correction or amendment requested and the reasons, the health-care provider must file the statement as part of the patient record, mark the challenged entry as inaccurate or incomplete according to the patient, and note where in the record the corrected information is located.

The health-care provider who fails to comply with these requirements may be subject to liability. The statute permits the patient to bring a lawsuit against the health-care provider or facility for noncompliance and receive actual damages along with attorney's fees and costs.[22] Such potential for liability should cause all health information managers to examine their policies governing patient correction to the medical record for compliance with their own state's laws.

Retention Requirements

Retention of health information has long been influenced by both external and internal forces. Certain statutes and regulations provide specific requirements on record retention. The ability of a health-care provider to meet the needs of continuing patient care, education, research, and defense of professional liability actions influences how long health information will be retained. Furthermore, storage constraints, new technology, and fiscal concerns play a role in reaching a decision on this issue. See Figure 4-4.

The health information manager must be able to reconcile these forces when creating effective **record retention policies.** Record retention policies are the general principles determining the length of time medical records must be maintained by the health-care provider. For example, should a health information manager choose a form of document imaging rather than retain records in their paper form? If so, what form is cost-effective? Or if computerized patient records are the norm, when should the health information manager consider transferring these records to an archival database? Whatever choice is made, that choice should be guided by a record retention policy that addresses legal requirements in addition to institutional needs.

Statutes and Regulations

Statutes on the state level and regulations on both the state and federal levels address retention requirements. For example, some state statutes establish specific time frames for which to retain the medical record following the death or discharge of a patient.[23] These time frames may differ if the patient is an adult or minor or has a mental disability.[24]

Statutory and Regulatory Requirements

Health-Care Provider's Ability to:
- Render continuing patient care
- Conduct education and research
- Defend a professional liability action

Storage Constraints

New Technology

Fiscal Concerns

Figure 4-4. Forces Influencing Retention of Health Information

More often, it is regulations rather than statutes that provide the specific time frames. On the federal level, the Conditions of Participation in the Medicare program require hospitals to maintain medical records for the period of the state's applicable **statute of limitations** or, if there is no applicable statute, for five years after discharge.[25] For more information concerning statutes of limitation, see Chapter 3.

Finally, statutes of limitation in contract and tort actions also influence retention decisions because the ability to defend a lawsuit successfully depends in part on the availability of the medical record. An example of the unavailability of a medical record to defend a lawsuit is illustrated by *Bondu v. Gurvich.*[26] In *Bondu,* Mrs. Bondu's husband died of a heart attack during the administration of anesthesia as part of heart surgery. When she sought copies of her husband's medical record as part of the evidence to support her medical malpractice lawsuit, she discovered that the hospital had either lost or destroyed it.

In addition to suing the hospital and the physicians for medical malpractice, Mrs. Bondu sued the hospital for negligent loss of records. Not only did the court find that state statutes required the hospital to maintain patient records, the court found that state regulations required the hospital to maintain medical and surgical treatment notes and reports as part of the content of the medical record. The hospital's inability to produce the records caused a shift in the burden of proof to the hospital to prove that it was not negligent. With this significant change in burden of proof, the court let both claims proceed to trial.

Other External Forces

Beyond these strictly legal considerations, other external forces may guide health information managers in developing a retention policy. For example, the health information manager may look to professional organizations for guidance. Along this line, the American Health Information Management Association (AHIMA) recommends a ten-year retention period on adult patient records, measured from the date of the patient's last encounter.[27] Furthermore, AHIMA recognizes that records of minor patients pose special concerns and therefore recommends retaining records until the patient reaches the age of majority plus the statute of limitations period governing medical malpractice lawsuits.

Similarly, the American Hospital Association (AHA) suggests a ten-year retention period for clinical records, again measured from the date of the patient's last encounter.[28] The AHA's policy permits storage of inactive records, either in the hospital or off-site if permitted by law or the appropriate licensing body.

Another external force that should be considered in a retention discussion is new technology. In the near future, the push toward a computerized patient record will become a reality. One of the many advantages to a computerized patient record is the physical space savings it offers. The previously discussed factors pertaining to the retention of health information stored in a traditional medical record format should also be considered when retaining health information stored in a computerized format. For more information concerning computerized health information, review Chapter 11.

Bases for Decision

As this discussion demonstrates, there is no answer to the question of how long medical records should be retained. Under the reasoning of the *Bondu* case, it is clear that institutions should strive to retain their records for at minimum the period specified under statute and regulation. Retaining medical records beyond that period should be decided based on medical and administrative needs, along with fiscal, technological, and storage constraints.

Record Destruction

Each institution that retains medical records faces the prospect of destroying those records at some future date. When that time arrives, the institution should have in place a policy governing destruction. Destruction of medical records occurs in either of two instances as outlined in Figure 4-5 and as described in the following paragraphs.

Destruction in Ordinary Course

Record destruction policies should address, at minimum, the controlling statute and/or regulation. These controlling statutes and regulations may

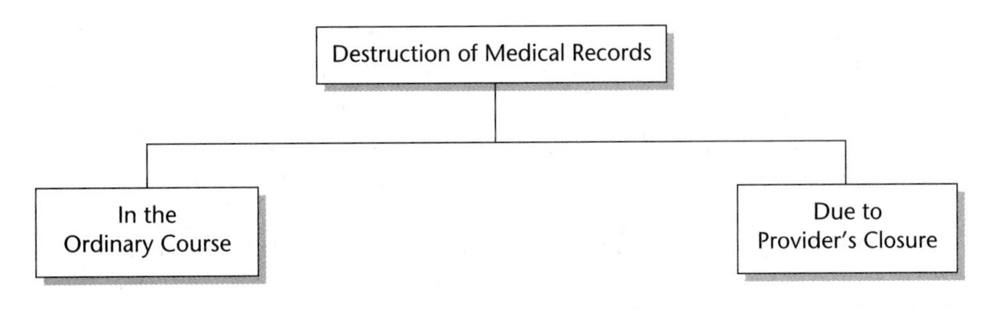

Figure 4-5. Instances of Destruction of Medical Records

specify or recommend the method of destruction, for example, shredding, burning, or recycling.[29] Some laws may also require the hospital to create an abstract of patient data before destroying the patient's record.[30] Other state laws may require the facility to notify the patient or the licensing authority before destroying the patient's record.[31]

No matter what method is selected, the paramount concern should be one of keeping the contents of the record confidential. Institutions may attempt to protect this confidentiality by destroying the records internally or by using a commercial contractor that is subject to stringent restrictions. If a commercial contractor is involved, the institution should include restrictions in the written contract that specify the method of destruction, the safeguards to be employed, the indemnification provided in the event of an unauthorized disclosure, and the certification procedure indicating that the records received were properly destroyed.[32]

Whether destroyed internally or externally, the institution should retain permanent evidence of the record's destruction in the ordinary course of business. This permanent evidence would most likely be a dated certificate indicating destruction of a particular record. This certificate could subsequently be used to defend a health-care provider in an investigation before a governmental agency or in a medical malpractice lawsuit in which the absence of a medical record is an issue.

Failure to retain a certificate of destruction of medical records opens the health-care provider to a charge that an individual record was destroyed for suspicious reasons, such as to gain advantage in a lawsuit. Just such a claim was made in *Carr v. St. Paul Fire & Marine Insurance.*[33] In *Carr,* the hospital briefly treated the patient in the emergency department and then sent him home. Shortly after returning home from the emergency department, the patient died. Because the hospital could not produce the emergency department record upon request or show that it had been destroyed in the ordinary course of business, it was accused of destroying the patient's record contrary to acceptable hospital practice. This claim went to trial, and the jury was allowed to infer that the destroyed record may have shown evidence of a medical emergency necessitating further care than that provided by the hospital staff.

As the *Carr* case illustrates, destruction of records in other than the ordinary course of business may result in civil liability. Criminal liability may also apply if the destruction is for the purpose of concealing responsibility for a patient's illness, injury, or death.[34] Finally, health-care providers should not destroy records currently involved in litigation, audits, or investigations, even if the retention period would otherwise have ended, because of the possibility of civil or criminal penalties.

Destruction Due to Closure

Destruction of the medical record may be necessary after a health-care institution closes or a medical practice dissolves. Health-care providers generally are liable for accidental or incidental disclosure of health information at such a time.

State laws and regulations vary on how a health-care provider should handle this situation. Some states recommend that the health-care provider transfer medical records to another health-care provider, while other states recommend delivery of medical records to the state licensing authority for storage.[35] Some states require the health-care provider to notify the appropriate licensing authority before taking action.[36]

Additionally, if the health-care provider offered alcohol and/or drug abuse services, the health information manager should examine federal regulations governing these areas to determine how to proceed. These regulations require health-care providers to obtain the patient's written authorization before transferring records to an acquiring program or any other program named in the authorization. If transfer has not been authorized and records must be retained for a period specified by law, the records must be placed in a sealed envelope or other container and labeled as follows:

> Record of [insert name of program] required to be maintained under [insert citation to statute, regulation, court order or other legal authority requiring that records be kept] until a date not later than [insert appropriate date][37]

These sealed records must be held confidential under the procedures outlined in the regulations until the end of the retention period. At that time, the records may be destroyed. Further information concerning the special handling of alcohol/drug abuse records is in Chapter 9.

If the health-care provider closes due to filing for bankruptcy protection, the issue of disposal or destruction of medical records is unclear. Bankruptcy, while a creation of federal law and governed primarily by federal statute and rules, also incorporates state law, rule, and regulation in situations when federal law is silent. Currently, no federal statute or rule addresses the question of disposal or destruction of medical records when a health-care provider files for bankruptcy protection under Chapter 7 (Liquidation), Chapter 9 (Adjustment of Debts of a Municipality), or Chapter 11 (Reorganization).[38] For that reason, the bankruptcy court and the trustee appointed to administer the case would look to state law for guidance.

Conclusion

The legal requirements governing the content, retention, and destruction of health information most closely resemble a patchwork quilt: a variety of federal and state laws and regulations address issues central to these health information matters. No one reliable scheme exists that addresses the issues contained in this chapter.

Until one such scheme exists, health information managers must review and understand those legal requirements that apply to their particular situation. A review of the legal requirements should begin with the applicable statutes and regulations. The review should also include quasi-legal requirements such as accrediting and institutional standards and professional guidelines. Health information managers must then incorporate these legal and quasi-legal requirements into policy, balancing these factors against the functions and uses of health information and very practical concerns, such as storage constraints. Striking such a balance should lead to policies that are not only legally sound but realistic and practical.

Case Study

You are the director of health information at a large medical center that offers inpatient, outpatient, and emergency care at several sites in one state. Your medical center has announced that it will acquire a facility offering similar services in a neighboring state. The laws and regulations governing the retention and destruction of medical records differ between these states. Discuss how the lack of a consistent set of laws and regulations on these two matters affects the institution you serve, and outline the steps you will take to deal with the situation.

Review Questions

1. Compare and contrast the clinical uses of a medical record with the secondary purposes of a medical record.
2. How does a medical record serve as a legal document?
3. Is it legally proper for a physician in a group practice to sign medical entries made by another physician in the same practice? Why or why not?
4. How can a computerized patient record be corrected?
5. Explain the concept of an amendment to the record under the HIPAA final privacy rule.
6. What legal requirements apply to a record retention policy?
7. Will civil or criminal liability apply to a health-care institution that destroys a record in other than the ordinary course? Why or why not?

Enrichment Activities

1. Review the record retention requirements for the Medicare Conditions of Participation and the statutes and regulations for your state. Develop a record retention policy for a fictional hospital that complies with those requirements. With the applications of new technologies to health information management, can you see any inadequacies in those requirements?

2. Discuss with a fellow student the functions and uses of a medical record. With the permission of the administration of a local health-care facility, jointly survey members of the facility's staff to determine their awareness of the functions and uses of a medical record. Do not limit your survey to health information department staff. Categorize your results by department. Share those results with the facility's administration and health information department manager. Present recommendations, if survey results so indicate, to educate facility staff as to the functions and uses of the medical record. If it is impractical to survey a local health-care facility, arrange with the permission of your faculty advisor or department chair to survey other students at your educational institution to determine their awareness of the functions and uses of a medical record. Share those results with your instructor, and brainstorm what efforts you can make to raise awareness of the functions and uses of the medical record to the student population.

Notes

1. For example, Missouri regulations specify the contents of a medical record in the hospital context to include:

   a unique identifying record number, pertinent identifying and personal data, history of present illness or complaint, past history, family history, physical examination, provisional admitting diagnosis, medical staff orders, progress notes, nurses' notes, discharge summary, final diagnosis and evidence of appropriate informed consent. Where applicable medical records also shall contain reports such as clinical laboratory, X-ray, consultation, electrocardiogram, surgical procedures, therapy, anesthesia, pathology, autopsy and any other reports pertinent to the patient's care.

   MO. CODE REGS. tit. 19, § 30.20.021(2) (D) (1993).
2. 42 U.S.C. § 1395x(e) (2) (Supp. 1993).
3. *See, e.g.,* N.J. REV. STAT. ANN. § 26:8-5 (2001) (requiring institutions treating disease to "make a complete medical record covering the period of such person's confinement . . ."); N.Y. PUB. HEALTH LAW § 4165 (Consol. 2000) (requiring health-care providers to "make, at the time of their admittance, a record of all the personal and statistical particulars relative to the patients and inmates in their institutions . . .").
4. ARIZ. STAT. ANN. § 12-2291 (2000); TENN. CODE ANN. § 68-11-302 (2000).
5. 42 C.F.R. § 405.1722(b) (1992).

6. *See, e.g.,* Mass. Regs. Code tit. 105, § 130.200 (1987); Mont. Admin. R. 16.32.320 (1990).
7. Alaska Stat. § 18.20.080 (2000); N.H. Code Admin. R. He-P 802.12 (1990).
8. Joint Commission, Comprehensive Accreditation Manual for Hospitals, Management of Information, IM 7.2 (2001). These characteristics include not only those items specified in the Medicare Conditions of Participation, but also include items such as evidence of known advance directives, the patient's legal status if the patient receives mental health services, and details of emergency, operative, and anesthetic care.
9. Developed by representatives from American Health Information Management Association, American Hospital Association, American Managed Care and Review Association, American Medical Association, American Medical Peer Review Association, Blue Cross and Blue Shield Association, and Health Insurance Association of America (1992).
10. *See, e.g.,* Mo. Code Regs. tit. 19, § 30-20.021(2) (D) (.3) (1993).
11. *See, e.g.,* Miss. Code Ann. § 41-9-63 (1999); Mo. Code Regs. tit. 19, § 30-20.021(2) (D) (.3) (1993); Joint Commission, Comprehensive Accreditation Manual for Hospitals, Management of Information IM 7.7 (2001).
12. *See, e.g.,* 42 C.F.R. § 405.1722(c) (1992) (Medicare Conditions of Participation); Joint Commission, Comprehensive Accreditation Manual for Hospitals, Management of Information, IM 7.1-.10 (2001).
13. 234 N.W.2d 411 (Mich. Ct. App. 1976).
14. 312 N.E.2d 614 (Ill. 1974).
15. 709 S.W.2d 872 (Mo. Ct. App. 1986).
16. American Society for Testing Materials. *1999 Annual Book of ASTM Standards, Vol 14.01* Healthcare Informatics Computerized Systems and Chemical and Material Information (1999); Health Level *Seven, Version 2.3,* www://mcis .duke.edu/standards/HL7/hl7.html.
17. 595 F. Supp 1108 (N.D. Ga. 1984).
18. 512 N.E.2d 1042, 1044 (Ill. App. 1987).
19. *Covered entity* refers to health plans, health-care clearinghouses, and healt-care providers who submit certain transactions electronically. 42 U.S.C. § 1320d (2001).
20. 45 C.F.R. § 164.526 (2001).
21. The Uniform Health Care Information Act, Wash. Rev. Code Ann. § 70.02.100.110 (West 2000).
22. Wash. Rev. Code Ann. § 70.02.170 (West 2000).

23. *See, e.g.*, ALASKA STAT. § 18.20.085 (2000) (seven years); HAW. REV. STAT. § 622-58 (2000) (seven years); MASS. GEN. LAWS ANN. ch. 111, § 70 (Supp. 1993) (thirty years); N.J. REV. STAT. ANN. § 26:8-5 (2001) (ten years for the entire record; twenty years for the discharge summary); TENN. CODE ANN. § 68-11-305 (2000) (ten years).
24. *See* MISS. CODE ANN. § 41-9-69 (1999); (retain for a period of minority plus seven years, not to exceed twenty-eight years); TENN. CODE ANN. § 68-11-305 (2000); (retain for a period of minority or mental disability, plus one year or ten years following discharge, whichever is longer).
25. 42 C.F.R. § 405.1722(d) (2000).
26. 473 So.2d 1307 (Fla. Dist. Ct. App. 1984).
27. AMERICAN HEALTH INFORMATION MANAGEMENT ASSOCIATION, Position Statement, Issue: Retention of Health Information (March 1994).
28. AMERICAN HOSPITAL ASS'N, Statement on Preservation of Medical Records.
29. *See* 40 C.F.R. § 246 (shredding or recycling) (2000); TENN. CODE ANN. § 68-11-305(c) (1) (2000) (shredding or burning).
30. *See* MISS. CODE ANN. § 41-9-75 (1999); TENN. CODE ANN. § 68-11-306 (2000).
31. *See, e.g.*, MD. HEALTH-GEN. CODE ANN. § 4-403(c) (2000) (if health-care provider dies, administrator of estate must send notice of destruction, along with statement that patient may retrieve record within thirty days of destruction, by first-class mail to the patient's last known address); OR. ADMIN. R. 333-92-095(5) (1985) (written approval of Health Division required before nursing home may destroy records of mentally retarded patients).
32. JONATHAN P. TOMES, *Healthcare Records: A Practical Legal Guide* (Kendall Hunt Publishing Co. for Healthcare Financial Management Association 1990).
33. 384 F. Supp. 821 (W.D. Ark. 1974).
34. MD. HEALTH-GEN. CODE ANN. §§ 4-401 & 4-402 (2000) (making concealment or destruction a misdemeanor offense); MICH. COMP. LAWS § 750.492(a) (2000) (making such destruction a felony offense).
35. *See, e.g.*, MISS. CODE ANN. § 41-9-79 (1999) (recommending transfer of record to other hospital; if none available, to licensing agency); TENN. CODE ANN. § 68-11-308 (2000) (requiring delivery of hospital records to Department of Health and Environment).
36. ALASKA STAT. § 18.20.085(c) (2000) (requiring hospitals to make immediate arrangements to preserve records, subject to Department of Health & Social Services' approval); HAW. REV. STAT. § 622-58(e) (2000) (same).
37. 42 C.F.R. Ch. 1, Part 2, § 2.19(b) (2000).
38. 11 U.S.C. §§ 101-1330 (2000).

Chapter 5

Access to Health Information

Learning Objectives

After reading this chapter, the learner should be able to:

1. Describe the continuum through which questions of health information ownership have passed.
2. Explain the concept of a notice of information practices.
3. Compare and contrast the terms consent and authorization with regard to a notice of information practices.
4. List the core elements of a valid release of information form.
5. Explain the principle of the minimum necessary standard.
6. Identify who is granted authority to release health information.
7. Describe the methods employed to disclose health information.
8. Explain the purpose of a redisclosure statement.
9. Compare and contrast the rights of access of patients and third parties to patient-specific health information.
10. Explain the concept of reasonable fees and the challenges made to this concept.
11. Explain the role that institutional review boards play in the access by researchers to health information involving human subjects.
12. Describe the reasons and mechanism for reporting public health threats.
13. Compare the judicial approach with the legislative approach for access to adoption records.

Key Concepts

- Adoption records
- Authorization
- Business associate
- Consent
- Institutional review board (IRB)
- Minimum necessary standard
- Notice of information practices
- Preemption
- Public health threats
- Reasonable fee
- Release of information

Introduction

Access to patient-specific health information is a complex issue governed by a variety of legal rules. Health-care providers are charged under the law with the obligation to maintain patient-specific health information in a confidential manner. At the same time, health-care providers are charged with the obligation to allow third parties and patients access to patient-specific health information, if appropriately requested. Understanding the balance between these obligations is essential to the health-care provider's practice and compliance with the laws governing access.

The law particularly targets disclosure of patient-specific health information that is deemed confidential. Confidential information (e.g., clinical data) is distinguished from nonconfidential information by the fact that the information is made available by the patient to the health-care provider during the course of their confidential relationship. By contrast, nonconfidential information (e.g., demographic data) is generally considered information that is a matter of common knowledge, with no restrictions requested by the patient. For purposes of this chapter, references to patient-specific health information are to confidential information.

Questions of access to and disclosure of patient-specific information frequently arise in the health-care context. For that reason, the health information manager must understand the legal principles governing ownership and disclosure of health information, how disclosure principles differ with respect to who seeks access to health information, and when disclosure of health information is mandated by law. With that knowledge and understanding, the health information manager can develop and implement policies and procedures addressing access and disclosure of patient-specific information.

Ownership of Health Information

Who really owns health information? Is it the patient, the health-care provider, or both? Or can health information be owned, as opposed to owning the medium in which information is stored, for example, the medical record? At this time, the law is in transition, providing no certain answer to questions of ownership of health information and the media in which it is stored. To understand why generalizations exist rather than hard and fast rules, the continuum through which ownership questions have passed must be understood.

Traditionally, the law has focused on the medium used: the paper-based medical record. Under the traditional approach, the medical record was considered the sole property of the health-care provider, and patient-specific health information was not considered separate from the medium used. Decisions on whether to allow access to the medical record fell within the sole province of the health-care provider. The health-care provider reached decisions on access through the guidance of the provider's professional association. If the association's recommendation was to prohibit access to the patient and the health-care provider did not believe otherwise, so be it.

As privacy rights were established and defined by courts and as consumer awareness blossomed, the concept developed of the patient possessing a right to his own health information contained in the medical record. Although not always clearly defined and still focusing on the medium used, the patient's right of access to the medical record and the health information contained in it could not be ignored by the health-care provider.

The trend of the future is away from focusing on the medium used and toward the protection of health information itself. This future trend places health information in a trust capacity, with the health-care provider acting as trustee for the patient's benefit to create, receive, and protect patient-specific health information. Bills promoting this view have been introduced into Congress as part of the federal government's efforts on health-care reform.[1] Currently, the law is such that answers to questions of ownership of health information fall somewhere in the middle of this continuum. See Figure 5-1. Federal regulations issued pursuant to the Health Insurance Portability and Accountability Act (HIPAA) of 1996 recognize the patient possesses a right of access to his own health information. These regulations do not, however, specify that the health-care provider acts in a trust capacity for the patient.

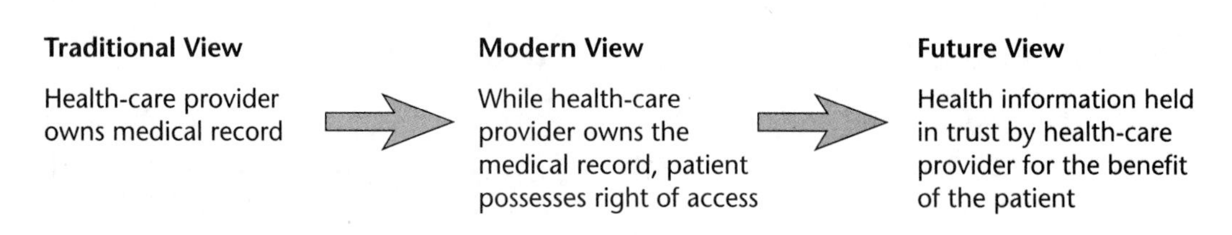

Figure 5-1. Ownership of Health Information: A Continuum

One general rule of ownership, however, is accepted in virtually all of the United States: the medical record, as a medium, is owned by the health-care provider, with the patient possessing a limited property interest in the health information contained in it. This general rule is established in some states by statutes,[2] in other states by licensing regulations,[3] and in still other states by judicial decisions.[4] When determining ownership issues in any particular situation, the health information manager must be conscious of this rule and review state law for guidance, including regulations governing specialized patient records.

Notice of Use and Disclosure

As described in Chapter 4, the medical record serves multiple uses. In addition to supporting the care provided by health-care professionals, uses traditionally unknown to the patient, such as fundraising and marketing, are involved. Federal standards for the privacy of patient-specific health information, also known as the HIPAA final privacy rule, dictate that the patient be notified of these uses and be given the opportunity to consent, reject, or request restriction of this information for any or all of the many uses the medical record serves. This notice requirement is commonly referred to as a **notice of information practices.**[5] The rule details both the content of the notice and the methods by which the patient is notified of the health-care provider's information practices. A sample notice of information practices is illustrated in Figure 5-2.

In addition to receiving a health-care provider's notice of information practices, the final privacy rule originally required that the health-care provider obtain a general **consent** (agreement) from the patient to use or disclose patient-specific health information to carry out treatment, payment, and health-care operations.[6] Many organizations in the health-care

Practice Brief—Notice of Information Practices

This notice describes how information about you may be used and disclosed and how you can get access to this information. Please review it carefully.

Understanding Your Health Record/Information

Each time you visit a hospital, physician, or other healthcare provider, a record of your visit is made. Typically, this record contains your symptoms, examination and test results, diagnoses, treatment, and a plan for future care or treatment. This information, often referred to as your health or medical record, serves as a:

- basis for planning your care and treatment
- means of communication among the many health professionals who contribute to your care
- legal document describing the care you received
- means by which you or a third-party payer can verify that services billed were actually provided
- a tool in educating heath professionals
- a source of data for medical research
- a source of information for public health officials charged with improving the health of the nation
- a source of data for facility planning and marketing
- a tool with which we can assess and continually work to improve the care we render and the outcomes we achieve

Understanding what is in your record and how your health information is used helps you to:

- ensure its accuracy
- better understand who, what, when, where, and why others may access your health information
- make more informed decisions when authorizing disclosure to others

Your Health Information Rights

Although your health record is the physical property of the healthcare practitioner or facility that compiled it, the information belongs to you. You have the right to:

- request a restriction on certain uses and disclosures of your information as provided by 45 CFR 164.522
- obtain a paper copy of the notice of information practices upon request
- inspect and copy your health record as provided for in 45 CFR 164.524
- amend your health record as provided in 45 CFR 164.528
- obtain an accounting of disclosures of your health information as provided in 45 CFR 164.528
- request communications of your health information by alternative means or at alternative locations
- revoke your authorization to use or disclose health information except to the extent that action has already been taken

Our Responsibilities

This organization is required to:

- maintain the privacy of your health information
- provide you with a notice as to our legal duties and privacy practices with respect to information we collect and maintain about you
- abide by the terms of this notice
- notify you if we are unable to agree to a requested restriction
- accommodate reasonable requests you may have to communicate health information by alternative means or at alternative locations.

We reserve the right to change our practices and to make the new provisions effective for all protected health information we maintain. Should our information practices change, we will mail a revised notice to the address you've supplied us.

We will not use or disclose your health information without your authorization, except as described in this notice.

For More Information or to Report a Problem

If have questions and would like additional information, you may contact the director of health information management at [phone number].

If you believe your privacy rights have been violated, you can file a complaint with the director of health information management or with the secretary of Health and Human Services. There will be no retaliation for filing a complaint.

Examples of Disclosures for Treatment, Payment and Health Operations

We will use your health information for treatment.

For example: Information obtained by a nurse, physician, or other member of your healthcare team will be recorded in your record and used to determine the course of treatment that should work best for you. Your physician will document in your record his or her expectations of the members of your healthcare team. Members of your healthcare team will then record the actions they took and their observations. In that way, the physician will know how you are responding to treatment.

We will also provide your physician or a subsequent healthcare provider with copies of various reports that should assist him or her in treating you once you're discharged from this hospital.

We will use your health information for payment.

For example: A bill may be sent to you or a third-party payer. The information on or accompanying the bill may include information that identifies you, as well as your diagnosis, procedures, and supplies used.

We will use your health information for regular health operations.

For example: Members of the medical staff, the risk or quality improve-

Figure 5-2. Sample Notice of Information Practices. (Reprinted with permission from the *Journal of the American Health Information Management Association*, copyright 2001.)

Practice Brief—Notice of Information Practices

ment manager, or members of the quality improvement team may use information in your health record to assess the care and outcomes in your case and others like it. This information will then be used in an effort to continually improve the quality and effectiveness of the healthcare and service we provide.

Business associates: There are some services provided in our organization through contacts with business associates. Examples include physician services in the emergency department and radiology, certain laboratory tests, and a copy service we use when making copies of your health record. When these services are contracted, we may disclose your health information to our business associate so that they can perform the job we've asked them to do and bill you or your third-party payer for services rendered. To protect your health information, however, we require the business associate to appropriately safeguard your information.

Directory: Unless you notify us that you object, we will use your name, location in the facility, general condition, and religious affiliation for directory purposes. This information may be provided to members of the clergy and, except for religious affiliation, to other people who ask for you by name.

Notification: We may use or disclose information to notify or assist in notifying a family member, personal representative, or another person responsible for your care, your location, and general condition.

Communication with family: Health professionals, using their best judgement, may disclose to a family member, other relative, close personal friend or any other person you identify, health information relevant to that person's involvement in your care or payment related to your care.

Research: We may disclose information to researchers when their research has been approved by an institutional review board that has reviewed the research proposal and established protocols to ensure the privacy of your health information.

Funeral directors: We may disclose health information to funeral directors consistent with applicable law to carry out their duties.

Organ procurement organizations: Consistent with applicable law, we may disclose health information to organ procurement organizations or other entities engaged in the procurement, banking, or transplantation of organs for the purpose of tissue donation and transplant.

Marketing: We may contact you to provide appointment reminders or information about treatment alternatives or other health-related benefits and services that may be of interest to you.

Fund raising: We may contact you as part of a fund-raising effort.

Food and Drug Administration (FDA): We may disclose to the FDA health information relative to adverse events with respect to food, supplements, product and product defects, or post marketing surveillance information to enable product recalls, repairs, or replacement.

Workers compensation: We may disclose health information to the extent authorized by and to the extent necessary to comply with laws relating to workers compensation or other similar programs established by law.

Public health: As required by law, we may disclose your health information to public health or legal authorities charged with preventing or controlling disease, injury, or disability.

Correctional institution: Should you be an inmate of a correctional institution, we may disclose to the institution or agents thereof health information necessary for your health and the health and safety of other individuals.

Law enforcement: We may disclose health information for law enforcement purposes as required by law or in response to a valid subpoena.

Federal law makes provision for your health information to be released to an appropriate health oversight agency, public health authority or attorney, provided that a work force member or business associate believes in good faith that we have engaged in unlawful conduct or have otherwise violated professional or clinical standards and are potentially endangering one or more patients, workers or the public.

Effective Date: [DATE]

Note: The above form is not meant to encompass all the various ways in which any particular facility may use health information. It is intended to get readers started insofar as developing their own notice. As with any form of this nature, the document should be reviewed and approved by legal counsel prior to implementation.

Figure 5-2 (continued). Sample Notice of Information Practices. (Reprinted with permission from the *Journal of the American Health Information Management Association*, copyright 2001.)

industry have criticized this requirement as administratively burdensome and sought to repeal or relax this requirement. At the time of this book's printing, such criticism had not been resolved. To understand this criticism, one should examine a consent form. The content requirements for a consent form in this context are illustrated in Figure 5-3. A sample consent agreement is illustrated in Figure 5-4.

1. Consent must be in plain language;
2. Inform the individual that the information may be used and disclosed to carry out treatment, payment or healthcare operations;
3. Refer the individual to the notice of information practices;
4. Inform the individual of the right to review the notice before signing the consent;
5. State that the notice may change and that the individual has a right to obtain a revised notice;
6. Inform the individual of the right to restrict use and disclosure of the information and the healthcare provider's option not to agree to the restriction;
7. State that the individual may revoke consent in writing except to the extent the healthcare provider has taken action in reliance thereon; and
8. Be signed by the individual and dated.

Figure 5-3. Content Requirements for Consent to Use and Disclose Patient-Specific Health Information to Carry Out Treatment and Payment of Health-Care Operations (45 C.F.R. § 164.506) (2001)

Furthermore, the rule requires that the health-care provider obtain written **authorization** (permission) for specific disclosures not otherwise authorized by law.[7] Many of these specific disclosures are governed by the general principles of release of information addressed later in this chapter. The difference between the consent and the authorization rests with the type of use or disclosure in question.

The HIPAA final privacy rule requires the health-care provider to obtain the patient's consent before using or disclosing the health information to carry out treatment, payment, or health-care operations. The health-care provider may even condition treatment and a health plan may condition enrollment on gaining such consent. Some exceptions do exist to obtaining prior consent before using or disclosing the health information and are illustrated in Figure 5-5. The health-care provider must document its attempts to obtain consent and the reasons that it was not obtained. Finally, the health-care provider must provide on the patient's request an accounting of the disclosures made.[8]

Practice Brief—Consent for Use or Disclosure

Consent to the Use and Disclosure of Health Information for Treatment, Payment, or Healthcare Operations

I understand that as part of my healthcare, this organization originates and maintains health records describing my health history, symptoms, examination and test results, diagnoses, treatment, and any plans for future care or treatment. I understand that this information serves as:

- a basis for planning my care and treatment
- a means of communication among the many health professionals who contribute to my care
- a source of information for applying my diagnosis and surgical information to my bill
- a means by which a third-party payer can verify that services billed were actually provided
- and a tool for routine healthcare operations such as assessing quality and reviewing the competence of healthcare professionals

I understand and have been provided with a *Notice of Information Practices* that provides a more complete description of information uses and disclosures. I understand that I have the right to review the notice prior to signing this consent. I understand that the organization reserves the right to change their notice and practices and prior to implementation will mail a copy of any revised notice to the address I've provided. I understand that I have the right to object to the use of my health information for directory purposes. I understand that I have the right to request restrictions as to how my health information may be used or disclosed to carry out treatment, payment, or healthcare operations and that the organization is not required to agree to the restrictions requested. I understand that I may revoke this consent in writing, except to the extent that the organization has already take action in reliance thereon.

☐ I request the following restrictions to the use or disclosure of my health information.

____

____

Signature of Patient or Legal Representative	Witness
Date	Notice Effective Date or Version

☐ Accepted ☐ Denied

Signature	Title	Date

Figure 5-4. Sample Consent Agreement. (Reprinted with permission from the *Journal of the American Health Information Management Association,* copyright 2001.)

1. Disclosure to public health authorities as required by law (ex. reporting of communicable disease).
2. Disclosure to governmental authority to receive reports of abuse, neglect, or domestic violence.
3. Disclosure to a health oversight agency for oversight activities as required by law, including audits and inspections.
4. Disclosure to law enforcement agencies for limited purposes, such as reporting certain types of wounds or an individual's death, which may have resulted from criminal conduct.
5. Disclosure to coroners, medical examiners, and funeral directors as required by law and as necessary to carry out their duties with respect to a decedent.
6. Disclosure for research purposes, if stringent standards are met.
7. Disclosure to avert a serious threat to health and safety.
8. Disclosure for specialized governmental functions, such as for the conduct of lawful intelligence or the protection of the President.
9. Disclosure for workers' compensation.

Figure 5-5. Exceptions to Prior Consent

In addition to the requirements of the HIPAA final rule, at least one state has passed statutes addressing the same question. Hawaii requires health-care providers to provide patients with a notice of confidentiality practices and differentiates between consents and authorizations in a manner similar to the HIPAA final privacy rule.[9] Montana and Washington have adopted the Uniform Health-Care Information Act, specifying notice to the patient of confidentiality practices.[10] In the future, other states may enact even more stringent provisions addressing the same question.

Both the federal and state governments may pass laws, rules, and regulations that address the same matter. In such instances, health information officers must determine how to reconcile federal and any state requirements. The first step in such a reconciliation process is to address the question of **preemption.** Under the preemption doctrine, certain matters are of such a national, as opposed to local, nature that federal laws preempt, or take precedence over, state laws. Accordingly, health information managers should examine carefully the content of the federal law, rule, or regulation in question to determine to what extent it addresses preemption. The terms of the HIPAA privacy rule do not *per se* preempt the laws, rules, or regulations of the various states, except where the state laws, rules, or regulations are contrary to the HIPAA privacy rule.[11] Therefore, the HIPAA privacy rule provides a floor of protections, allowing a state to enact more stringent protections. Where the state provisions are more stringent than a standard requirement or implementation specification of the HIPAA privacy rule, the health-care provider must comply with both the federal and state provisions. Compliance with both the federal and state standards is the second step of reconciliation process.

Access by or on Behalf of the Patient

Questions of access to health information by the patient or by third parties on behalf of the patient are governed by a complex web of laws and regulations. To navigate through this web, health information officers must understand the general principle of disclosure of information. From there, the health information officers must understand the differences the law makes between access by the patient and access by third parties.

General Principles of Disclosure of Information

From the general ownership rule addressed above flow two additional principles: (1) records remain within the provider's control and safekeeping and may be removed only in accordance with a court order or subpoena, and (2) the provider may not disclose or withhold health information at will. Removal of records from the provider's control is addressed in Chapter 7; the disclosure or withholding of information is addressed in this chapter.

Before any health-care provider or institution may disclose patient-specific health information, the law requires the express consent of the patient. Such expressed consent must be in writing or, where state law permits, via computer. Commonly referred to as the process for authorizing **release of information,** a valid release of information form provides health-care providers and institutions with the authority to disclose patient-specific health information to persons not otherwise authorized to receive this information.

The minimum elements that must be present to constitute a valid release of information form are governed by both federal and state law.

Health-care providers may also be guided by professional guidelines, such as that of the American Health Information Management Association.[12] Under the HIPAA final privacy rule, a valid authorization must be in plain language and contain at least the following core elements: the individual's name; a specific and meaningful description of the information to be used or disclosed; the name or other specific identification of the person or class of persons authorized to make the disclosure; the name or other specific identification of the person to whom the disclosure is to be made; an expiration date or expiration event that relates to the individual or purpose of the use or disclosure; a statement of the individual's right to revoke the authorization in writing, exceptions to the right to revoke, together with how the individual may revoke the authorization; a statement that the information used or disclosed pursuant to the authorization may be subject to redisclosure and lose its protected status; the signature and date of the individual; and if the authorization is signed by a personal representative of the individual, a description of the representative's authority to act for the individual (see Figure 5-6).[13] A valid authorization may contain additional elements or information if clinical research is involved or as

---

1. The individual's name and identifying information.
2. A specific and meaningful description of the information to be used or disclosed.
3. The name or other specific identification of the person or class of persons authorized to make the requested use or disclosure.
4. The name or other specific identification of the person or class of persons to whom the disclosure is to be made.
5. An expiration date or expiration event that relates to the individual or purpose of the use or disclosure.
6. A statement of the individual's right to revoke the authorization, the exceptions to the right to revoke, and a description of the individual may revoke the authorization.
7. A statement that the information used or disclosed is subject to redisclosure and may lose its protected status.
8. The signature and date of the individual.
9. If the authorization is signed by the individual's personal representative, a description of the representative's authority to act for the individual.

Figure 5-6. Core Elements of a Valid Release of Health Information Form

required by state law, provided that such additional elements or information are not inconsistent with the elements required under HIPAA.

Conversely, a release of information may be considered invalid if it contains any of the following defects: the expiration date has passed or the expiration event is known by the covered entity to have occurred; the authorization has not been filled out completely with respect to an element described in the core elements section; the authorization is known by the covered entity to have been revoked; the authorization lacks an element required in the core elements section; the authorization violates the compound authorization requirements; and/or any material information found in the authorization is known by the health-care provider to be false (see Figure 5-7).[14] A compound authorization is defined as an authorization for use or disclosure of patient-specific health information that has been combined with any other document. Among the limited exceptions to the use of a compound authorization are permitting an authorization for use or disclosure of information created for research to be combined with one for treatment; the combination of two or more authorizations for use or disclosure of psychotherapy notes; and where nonpsychotherapy notes are involved, a combination of authorizations as long as the health-care provider has not conditioned the provision of treatment, payment, enrollment in a health plan, or eligibility for benefits on obtaining the authorization.[15]

What information may be released is also the subject of federal law. Introduced as part of the HIPAA final privacy rule, the principle of the

---

1. The expiration date has passed, or the expiration event is known by the health-care provider to have occurred.
2. Authorization has not been filled out completely with respect to a core element.
3. Authorization is known by the health-care provider to have been revoked.
4. Authorization lacks a core element.
5. Authorization contains a compound authorization violation.
6. Any material information contained in the authorization is known by the health-care provider to be false.

Figure 5-7. Common Defects of an Invalid Release of Information Form

minimum necessary standard governs the release of patient-specific health information.[16] The principle of the minimum necessary standard requires the health-care provider to make reasonable efforts to limit the patient-specific health information to the minimum necessary to accomplish the intended purpose of the use, disclosure, or request. The health-care provider must identify those who need access to the information to carry out their duties, what category of access is needed, and what conditions, if any, are appropriate to such access. As a logical extension, those persons in the workforce for identification purposes will include all classes of employees, volunteers, student interns, and others. Further, the health-care provider is expected to develop and implement reasonable policies and procedures that limit the information released on a routine and recurring basis to the amount reasonably necessary to achieve the purpose of the disclosure. Where release is not routine or recurring, the health-care provider is expected to develop criteria designed to reasonably limit the items of patient-specific health information disclosed such that the purpose for which disclosure is sought is accomplished and review requests for disclosure on an individual basis in accordance with the criteria established.

Who may grant authority to release health information is a matter governed by state law and regulation. Generally, the authority to release information rests with (1) the patient, if the patient is a competent adult or emancipated minor; (2) a legal guardian or parent on behalf of a minor child; or (3) the executor or administrator of an estate if the patient is deceased.[17]

The question of whether one is an emancipated minor is answered by the requirements of each state's laws and/or regulations. Common conditions of emancipation include evidence that the minor is married, on active duty with the U.S. armed forces, self-supporting and living away from home, or unmarried and pregnant.[18] Where the patient has been declared incompetent by a court of law or is otherwise unable to authorize disclosure (e.g., due to coma or critical condition), state law will provide the order of individuals who may serve to authorize disclosure.

Finally, the method of disclosure must be addressed. As a general matter, state law or regulation does not specify the method of disclosure. Rather, professional guidelines and institutional practices and procedures govern. The disclosure of health information is most frequently handled by mail, but may also be accomplished through electronic transmittal, facsimile machine, or telephone where the mail method will not meet the need for urgent patient care. If handled in any of the last three ways, the health information manager should consider instituting additional safeguarding procedures. These safeguards could include encrypting data if public channels are used for electronic transmittal, creating documentation requirements for telephone disclosures, and following the guidelines of professional associations for faxing health information.[19]

One additional safeguard mandated in certain states is the inclusion of a redisclosure notice with the information sent.[20] This redisclosure notice is a statement placing the recipient on notice that the information received may be used only for the stated purpose, that the recipient is barred from redisclosing the information to third parties without the patient's authorization, and that the information should be destroyed after the stated purpose is fulfilled. The inclusion of a redisclosure notice is mandated by the federal government when information relating to alcohol or drug abuse patients is released.[21]

By the Patient

Although it may seem a somewhat elementary concept that the health information contained in the medical record belongs to the patient, and therefore the patient has a right to review and copy that information, that concept has only recently been established by the federal government pursuant to the HIPAA final privacy rule. This rule grants an individual "a right of access to inspect and obtain a copy of protected health information about the individual in a designated record set, for as long as the protected health information is maintained in the designated record set."[22] Unfortunately, the concept of patient access has not been translated into a legal right in all fifty states. The extent of the patient's access to his own health information is similar to the **continuum of ownership** issue: ranging from those states that do not address patient access at all or allow the health-care provider to determine the extent of access[23] to those that specifically grant patients access to their health records.[24] Because each state's law varies, health information managers developing policies on release of information directly to the patient must review the applicable state law, particularly if the policy is to be developed for a hospital system spanning more than one state.

Patients receiving care from health-care facilities operated by the federal government, such as Veterans Administration hospitals and Indian Health Services clinics, have greater rights of access. The Federal Privacy

Act governs patient care in those facilities and permits the patient the right of access to his own health information, to have a copy made of all or part of his record, and to correct or amend the record.[25] Unlike some federal statutes, the rights listed in the Federal Privacy Act are limited to facilities operated by the federal government and do not apply to health-care facilities that receive federal funds, such as Medicare reimbursement.

Although patients have gained greater rights of access to their health information, the rights of access are not absolute. Under certain circumstances, the health-care provider may be justified in withholding access to health information from the patient. For example, if the health-care provider determines that the release of information will have a detrimental effect on the patient, the provider may withhold the information from the patient, but may be required to provide it to a third party authorized by the patient.[26] Where withholding of health information is justified, it frequently occurs in the context of mental health treatment.

In addition to reviewing state law, the health information manager should also examine the terms of the HIPAA federal privacy rule for guidance on the time and manner of access granted to patients to review their own health information. Specific provisions govern the time frame in which the provider must act on a request, the manner in which the patient may inspect or obtain a copy of the health information and the method for review of a health-care provider's denial of a request for access.[27]

To Third Parties

As seen previously, a simple concept such as the patient being able to access his own health information does not translate into a legal right in every state. By contrast, third parties who may be perfect strangers to the patient have a right of access to the patient's health information, provided the patient has completed a valid release of information in their favor. And in certain instances, the third party may be able to access the information without patient authorization.

The extent of access and the need for patient authorization is defined by the identity of the third party seeking access. For example, if the party seeking access is the patient's attorney or insurance company, the health-care provider may disclose patient-specific health information only with the patient's authorization. Similarly, patient authorization is generally necessary before disclosure may be made to a federal, state, or local government agency.

If the patient's employer seeks access, the patient's authorization is required, unless a workers' compensation claim is involved. Where workers' compensation claims are involved, state law may provide the employer with a right of access to the information without the patient's authorization.[28]

Another example of a third party requiring patient authorization is a member of the patient's family. Although the family member may believe he possesses a right of access to the patient's health information by virtue of the family relationship, that is not the case under the law. Only with a valid release of information form may the family member legitimately gain access to the patient's health information.[29] An exception to this rule is where the family member has been appointed the patient's attorney in fact under a durable power of attorney for health care. In such an instance, the law generally allows the family member as attorney in fact to review the patient's medical record.[30]

As indicated earlier, some third parties may be provided access to patient-specific health information without first obtaining the patient's authorization. For example, health-care practitioners within the provider institution may be granted access on a need-to-know basis to perform their jobs with the patient. Similarly, surveyors with accrediting and licensing agencies may be granted access to the extent necessary to ensure compliance with standards or regulations for health information management.

Reasonable Fees

With the increasing demand for access to health information, the cost to the health-care provider to respond to such requests has increased proportionally in terms both of materials used and employee time and labor. Fortunately, the law recognizes that the health-care provider should not bear these costs free of charge to those requesting information access. State law generally permits the health-care provider to charge a reasonable fee for reproduction of the record.[31] A **reasonable fee** is defined as a fee charged by the health-care provider for the reproduction of the medical record. On the federal level, rules enacted pursuant to the Health Insurance Portability and Accountability Act clearly state that health-care providers may impose a reasonable cost-based fee for reproducing the record.[32]

The question regarding what is considered a reasonable fee has been flourishing as a matter of dispute. As health-care providers have increased reproduction charges or utilized correspondence services who set their own rates, the recipients of these charges have questioned whether the charge made is reasonable. Recipients have challenged "excessive" charges through two main approaches: filing lawsuits alleging that the charge was beyond the provider's actual costs or seeking legislative reform setting a price per page or price cap for reproduction. Both approaches have achieved mixed results, with more success achieved with legislation.[33]

The increase in challenges to reasonable fees for reproduction has emerged as a trend throughout the United States. Health information managers involved with the process of releasing information should seriously review their policies and practices to determine whether the fee charged is reasonable or falls within the limits set by rule, statute, or case law.

Access by the Researcher

Central to the rapid advancement of health care is the role of medical research. Medical research studies have measured the impact, effectiveness, quality, outcome, and costs of occupational hazards, new pharmaceuticals, and the treatment methods of chronic diseases and infectious illnesses. The results of this research have led to improved understanding and improved possibilities for the management and prevention of disease and disability.

Considerable medical research involves the study of individuals rather than the study of medical records for epidemiological purposes alone. As such, these studies are concurrent or prospective in nature, as opposed to retrospective.

Because human subjects are involved, confidentiality of patient information becomes critical. At the same time, the success of research depends in large measure on the access to health information about these subjects. The balance that must be struck between these two competing interests has been answered on the federal level through the Department of Health and Human Services and the Food and Drug Administration (FDA), which promulgate regulations governing the participation of human subjects in clinical investigations. The Department of Health and Human Services supervises investigators who receive federal funds for research; the FDA supervises clinical trials of pharmaceuticals and related medical devices.

The regulations promulgated by each agency require investigators to obtain the approval of an **institutional review board (IRB)** before involving a human subject.[34] Typically associated with a university, the IRB is a group formally designated by an institution to safeguard the rights and welfare of human subjects by reviewing, approving, and monitoring medical research. As part of the safeguards, the IRB requires the investigator to submit the research plan and informed consent form to the IRB for approval. The research plan must address, among other issues, how confidentiality will be maintained, the methods of recruiting subjects and obtaining the subject's informed consent.[35] Confidentiality protections often include maintaining research data in a locked storage area and identifying the patient in published articles by number or pseudonym only.

Any health information manager whose institution is involved with medical research involving human subjects should ensure that all requests for access to health information from investigators have the prior approval of the IRB. A request for access to patient-specific health information for research purposes that has not been previously approved, by either an IRB if human subjects are involved or a medical record committee if a retrospective review is called for, must be treated with great care. Unless patient consent has been given or patient identifying information has been removed or concealed, the health information manager should not grant the researcher access to the information sought. Furthermore, the health information manager should consider including, with *any* information released, a written statement prohibiting redisclosure without the institution's prior consent.

Access by the Business Associate

Virtually every health-care provider has at one time or another contracted with a business associate to conduct its business. In the process of doing so, certain patient-specific health information may have been disclosed to the business associate. Until recently, access to and protection of this information by the business associate was subject only to the provisions contained in contractual agreements between the parties and not to statute, rule, or regulation. With the advent of the HIPAA final privacy rule, access to and protection of that information has come under national regulation.

Under HIPAA, a **business associate** is defined as one who performs or assists in performing a function or activity involving the use or disclosure of individually identifiable health information on behalf of a covered entity.[36] A business associate is not a member of the health-care provider's workforce, such as an employee, trainee, or volunteer. Services provided by a business associate may be health related, including billing, claims processing, data analysis, utilization review, and quality assurance, or nonhealth related, including legal, actuarial, accounting, consulting, or management.

Provisions of the final privacy rule require that a health-care provider may disclose patient-specific health information to a business associate only if the provider receives satisfactory assurance that the business associate will safeguard that information. This assurance must be manifested through a written agreement, with specific provisions required.

The written agreement must establish the permitted uses and disclosures of the patient-specific health information by the business associate and indicate that the business associate may not use or disclose the information other than as expressly permitted or required by the agreement. Additionally, the agreement should require the business associate to use appropriate safeguards to prevent unauthorized use of the information and a mechanism under which unauthorized use may be reported. The agreement should indicate that the business associate must make its practices, books, and records available to the Department of Health and Human Services (HHS) to determine compliance with the privacy regulation and provide an accounting of the uses and disclosures made since receipt of the information. The agreement should bind any subcontractors or agents of the business associate to the same requirements and require the business associate to destroy or return the information at the termination of the agreement. [37]

Although the health-care provider has no duty to monitor the business associate's compliance with the terms of the agreement, the provider may be in violation of the final privacy rule if it knows of or reasonably should have known of material breaches by the business associate.[38] For that reason, health-care providers would be wise to include audit provisions in the agreement. In the event the provider learns of a material breach or repeated breaches, it should take reasonable steps to cure or end the violations, terminate the agreement, and/or report the violations to HHS.

Any health information manager whose institution is involved with business associates should ensure that the provisions of the written agreement comply with HIPAA's final privacy rule.

Access Pursuant to Reporting Laws

Access to patient-specific health information may also be necessary to safeguard the public's health. In order to prevent and lessen the occurrence of threats to public health, such as communicable diseases, virtually all states require, by either statute or regulation, the reporting of certain patient-specific health information. Because local health-care providers and institutions are in a position to observe patients posing **public health threats,** they are the most logical ones to initiate the chain of events that lead to control and prevention of these threats. For that reason, the law places a burden on health-care providers and institutions to report public health threats.

Public health threats can encompass a wide variety of health-care problems, that endanger the public health and must be reported to a public health agency. Common public health threats include communicable diseases (such as venereal diseases and AIDS),[39] child abuse,[40] injuries caused by deadly weapons,[41] fetal deaths,[42] and cancer.[43] Each state's law details its reporting requirements, including a listing of threats that must be reported, time frames within which to report the threat, and whether to disclose patient identity.

In practice, the health-care provider or institution reports these threats to the state's department of health or similar agency, which collates the data and determines what action should be taken. Where injuries by deadly weapons are concerned, the health-care provider or institution reports the incident to law enforcement personnel. Aggregate state data concerning communicable diseases are gathered by the U.S. Public Health Service, which collates and assesses the data on a national level. Working through the Centers for Disease Control, the Public Health Service publishes this information in the *Morbidity and Mortality Weekly Report.*

Every health information manager working with a health-care provider or institution that deals with public health threats must determine what mechanism is in place to report these threats. Failure of the health-care provider or institution to report public health threats may be an infraction of the law. The health information manager may wish to audit the patient's medical record for the date and time that the health-care provider reported the threat, to determine if the reporting mechanism works properly.

Access to Adoption Records

Adoption records are the medical records of the individual placed for adoption. In virtually every state, adoption records are considered confidential, and disclosure of the information contained in them may only be made pursuant to legal procedures. At the core of the access to adoption records issue are two competing interests: (1) the interests of the biological parent(s) in placing a child for adoption, often with the promise of confidentiality, and (2) the interests of the adoptee for genetic information and to satisfy curiosity about his or her natural identity. These competing interests have clashed in recent years as more and more adoptees have sought access to their adoption records, including birth records (see Figure 5-8).

The law governing access to adoption records is a mix of judicial decision and statute. For decades, courts have considered the requests of adoptees for access to their adoption records as potential impediments to the adoption process and so have discouraged granting access. Courts have erected barriers to access, such as requiring the adoptee to establish good cause for access and imposing notice and hearing requirements. Examples of good cause are specific with each court case and may include the need for genetic information to solve a medical condition or psychological trauma.[44] Notice and hearing requirements may include (1) conducting a search to determine if the biological parent(s) consents to the release of information, and (2) conducting a hearing to balance the interests of all parties.[45]

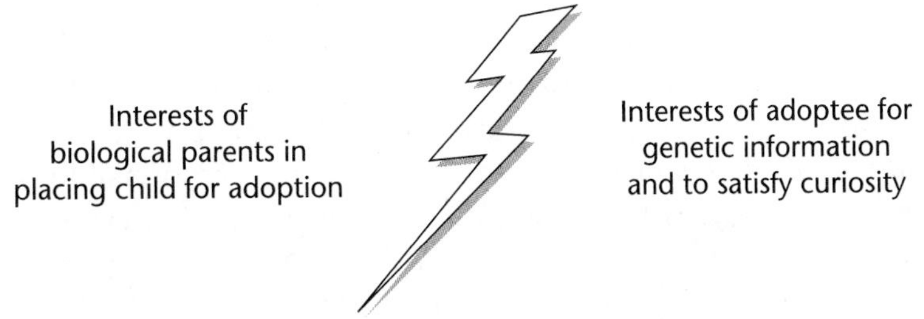

Interests of
biological parents in
placing child for adoption

Interests of adoptee for
genetic information
and to satisfy curiosity

Figure 5-8. Access to Adoption Records: Clash of Competing Interests

Because the barriers erected by courts are sometimes burdensome and difficult to overcome, adoptees have focused on state legislatures to obtain legal access to their adoption records. In some cases, legislatures have responded by easing the standards for access, by creating voluntary adoption registry services[46] or permitting independent searches for biological parents to solicit their consent for a meeting.[47] In the majority of states, the law still requires the adoptee to obtain a court order before permitting the health-care provider or institution to disclose identifying information without the consent of the biological parent.

As a matter of practice, each health information manager should determine what laws apply to adoptees in their particular state and, in consultation with counsel, develop policies and procedures to address disclosure requests. If and when the health information manager receives a request by an adoptee for information relating to his biological parents, he will be better prepared to handle the request. As a general matter, where state law bars disclosure of the information sought, the health information manager is advised to refuse the request and refer the adoptee to the agency that handled the adoption or the appropriate court having jurisdiction over adoption proceedings. Where the re-quest is accompanied by claims of an emergency nature, the health information manager should consult with counsel to determine how to assist the court in considering the request or whether to provide summary information from the record that does not include patient identification.

Conclusion

Because the proper disclosure of health information is governed by complex legal requirements, requests for access to patient-specific health information should be handled only by those with proper training and supervision. Health information managers responsible for disclosure of health information must develop, implement, and periodically revise training programs that incorporate the governing legal requirements. Such programs should address the principles raised in this chapter, particularly the differences the law makes between the categories of individuals seeking access to health information.

Case Study

You are the director of health information services at a tertiary-care hospital. You and the director of emergency room services are jointly responsible for reporting instances of communicable disease, child abuse, and cancer to the appropriate state authority. You have just completed an audit of your institution's reporting mechanism and discovered that the reporting requirements are not consistently met. The audit could not definitively establish whether the reporting never occurred or occurred but was not documented in the patient's medical record. Discuss what legal issues are present and what approaches you should take to resolve this problem.

Review Questions

1. What is the difference between confidential and nonconfidential information for purposes of access to patient-specific health information?
2. To what extent do patients possess a right to the information contained in their medical record? Explain your answer.
3. What is the difference between consent and authorization to use patient-specific health information?
4. What is the preemption doctrine, and how does it apply to patient-specific health information?
5. What are the minimum elements necessary to constitute a valid release of patient information?
6. What defects may invalidate a release of patient information form?
7. What is a compound authorization, and when is it permitted?
8. Who may grant authority to release information?
9. What is a redisclosure notice, and when is its use mandated?
10. What limitations to the Federal Privacy Act exist in terms of a patient's access to his own health information?
11. How does a family member obtain access to a patient's health information?

12. What is an institutional review board (IRB)?
13. Define a business associate, and explain how the HIPAA final privacy rule applies to a business associate.

Enrichment Activities

1. Research over the Internet notices of information practices policies, complete with forms, recommended for use by health-care organizations. Are the components of the policies consistent with the final privacy rule enacted pursuant to HIPAA? If not, what components are missing or added? Evaluate whether the policies comply with HIPAA adequately.
2. Relying on the information contained in this chapter, develop a policy for a health-care institution concerning release of patient-specific health information. What methods will you include to respond to requests for release of information? Will the methods differ based on who is making the request, what is being requested, or the urgency of the request?
3. Visit the health information management department in a local health-care facility. Review the department's procedure manual concerning release of information to determine compliance with the concepts addressed in this chapter. Observe the activities involved in processing requests for release of information. Analyze whether the department staff comply with procedures listed in the manual.

Notes

1. The Health Information Privacy Act of 1999, H.R. 1941, 106th Cong., 1st Sess. (1999) and the Fair Health Information Practices Act of 1995, H.R. 435, 104th Cong., 1st Sess. (1995), supported by the American Health Information Management Association. A similar bill was introduced in the 103rd Congress, H.R. 4077 (1994). *See also* 45 C.F.R. § 164.524 (2001).
2. LA. REV. STAT. ANN. § 40:1299.96 (West 2000); MASS. GEN. L. ch. 111, § 70 (2001); MISS. CODE ANN. § 41-9-65 (2001); TENN. CODE ANN. § 68-11-304 (2000).
3. MO. CODE REGS. tit. 19, § 30-20-011(D) (6) (1993).

4. *See, e.g., Pyramid Life Ins. Co. v. Masonic Hosp. Assoc.*, 191 F. Supp. 51 (W.D. Okla. 1961); *Rabens v. Jackson Park Hosp. Found.*, 351 N.E.2d 276 (Ill. Ct. App. 1976).
5. 45 C.F.R. § 164.520 (2001) states the general rule; 45 C.F.R. section 164.522 (2001) provides the standard for a patient to restrict use and disclosure of patient-specific health information.
6. 45 C.F.R. § 164.506 (2001).
7. 45 C.F.R. § 164.508 (2001).
8. 45 C.F.R. § 164.528 (2001).
9. 19 HAW. REV. STAT. §§ 323C-1 to -54 (2001).
10. MONT. CODE ANN. §§ 50-16-501 to -542 (2000); WASH. REV. CODE ANN. §§ 70.02.005 to 904 (2000).
11. 45 C.F.R. § 160.203 (2001).
12. The American Health Information Management Association has published minimum requirements for an acceptable authorization for disclosure of health information. MARY D. BRANDT, AMERICAN HEALTH INFORMATION MANAGEMENT ASSOCIATION, RELEASE AND DISCLOSURE, GUIDELINES REGARDING MAINTENANCE AND DISCLOSURE OF HEALTH INFORMATION (1997).
13. 45 C.F.R. § 164.508 (2001).
14. Ibid.
15. Ibid.
16. 45 C.F.R. § 165.514 (2001).
17. *See, e.g.*, LA. REV. STAT. ANN. § 13:3715.1(b) (2) (b) (West 2000).
18. *See, e.g.*, CAL. FAM. CODE § 7002 (West 2000); CONN. GEN. STAT. ANN. § 46b-150b (West 2001); MICH. COMP. LAWS ANN. § 722.4 (West 2001); NEV. REV. STAT. § 129.080 (1999); VA. CODE ANN. § 16.1-333 (Michie 2000).
19. *See, e.g.*, AMERICAN HEALTH INFORMATION MANAGEMENT ASSOCIATION, Position Statement, Issue: Facsimile Transmission of Health Information, May 1994.
20. *See, e.g.*, IOWA CODE ANN. § 228.5 (West 2001); N.Y. PUB. HEALTH LAW § 2785 (6) (b) (McKinney 2001).
21. 42 C.F.R. § 2.32 (2000).
22. 45 C.F.R. § 164.524 (2001). Exceptions to the right include information (1) found in psychotherapy notes; (2) compiled in reasonable anticipation of litigation; (3) maintained by an entity subject to the Clinical Laboratory Improvements Act; (4) maintained by a correctional institution or health-care provider acting under the direction of a correctional institution; and (5) certain categories of research.

23. Both Alabama and Kansas allow the hospital governing board to determine what access patients may have. R. Jones, *Of Professional Interest: Medical Record Access Laws,* 63 J. AMERICAN HEALTH INFORMATION MANAGEMENT ASSOC. 29 (1992).
24. Examples of states specifically permitting patients access to the health information contained in the medical record include: ALASKA STAT. § 18.23.065 (2000); CAL. HEALTH & SAFETY CODE § 123110 (West Supp. 2000); COLO. REV. STAT. ANN. §§ 25-1-801 & 802 (West 2000); CONN. GEN. STAT. ANN. § 4-104 (West 2001); FLA. STAT. ANN. § 455.241 (West Supp. 1995); HAW. REV. STAT. § 622-57 (2000); IND. CODE ANN. § 34-6-2-15 (Burns 2001); KY. REV. STAT. ANN. § 422.317 (Michie/Bobbs-Merrill Supp. 2000); LA. REV. STAT. ANN. § 40:1299.96 (West 2000); ME. REV. STAT. ANN. tit. 22 § 1711 (1999); MD. HEALTH-GEN. CODE ANN. § 4-304 (1994); MASS. GEN. LAWS ANN. ch. 112, § 12CC (West 2001); MINN. REV. STAT. ANN. § 144.335 (West 2001); MISS. CODE ANN. § 41-9-65 (2001); MONT. CODE ANN. § 50-16-541 (2000); NEV. REV. STAT. § 629.061 (1999); OHIO REV. CODE ANN. § 3701.74 (Baldwin 2001); OKLA. STAT. ANN. tit. 76, § 19 (West 2000); OR. REV. STAT. § 192.525 (1999); S.D. CODIFIED LAWS §§ 34-12-15 & 36-2-16 (2000); TENN. CODE ANN. § 68-11-304 (2000); WASH. REV. CODE ANN. § 70.02.080 (West 2000); W. VA. CODE § 16-29-1 (2000); WIS. STAT. ANN. § 146.83 (West 2001); WYO. STAT. § 35-2-611 (2001).
25. 5 U.S.C. § 552a (2000).
26. The federal government and several states sanction withholding health information in this manner, including: 45 C.F.R. § 164.520 (2001); HAW. REV. STAT. § 622-57 (2000); LA. REV. STAT. ANN. § 40:1299.96(d) (West 2000); ME. REV. STAT. ANN. tit. 22, § 1711 (West 1999); MD. HEALTH-GEN. CODE ANN. § 4-304 (2000); MASS. GEN. LAWS ANN. ch. 111, § 70 (West 2001); MINN. STAT. ANN. § 144.335.2(c) (West Supp. 2001); OHIO REV. CODE ANN. § 3701.74(c) (Anderson 2001).
27. 45 C.F.R. § 164.524 (2001).
28. *See, e.g.,* ALA. CODE § 25-5-77(b) (Supp. 2000); FLA. STAT. ANN. § 440.13(1) (C) (WEST 1991); LA. REV. STAT. ANN. § 23:1127 (West 2000); MO. REV. STAT. §§ 287.140(7) & 287.210(4) (2001); NEB. REV. STAT. § 48-120(4) (1999); S.D. CODIFIED LAWS ANN. § 62-4-45 (2000).
29. *See, e.g.,* CAL. WELF. + INST. CODE § 4514.5 (West 2000); COLO. REV. STAT. ANN. § 25-3-109(12) (West 2000); *Cannell v. Medical & Surgical Clinic, S.C.,* 315 N.E.2d 278 (Ill. App. Ct. 1974).
30. *See, e.g.,* CAL. PROB. CODE § 4678 (West Supp. 2000); GA. CODE ANN. § 31-36-10 (2000); ILL. ANN. STAT. ch. 755, para. 45/4-10 (2001); IND. CODE ANN. § 30-5-7-5 (West 2001); MO. REV. STAT. § 404.840(2) (2001); NEB. REV. STAT. § 30-3417(4) (1999); OR. REV. STAT. § 127.712 (1999).

31. *See, e.g.,* MINN. STAT. ANN. § 144.335.2(b) (West 2001) (allowing reasonable charge to patient); S.D. CODIFIED LAWS ANN. § 34-12-15 (2000) (allowing charge for actual reproduction and mailing expense); TENN. CODE ANN. § 68-11-304 (1993) (allowing charge for reasonable costs); WASH REV. CODE ANN. § 70.02.030 (2000) (allowing for reasonable charge).
32. 45 C.F. R. § 164.524 (2001).
33. *See, e.g.,* MD. HEALTH-GEN. CODE ANN. § 4-304 (2000) (allowing charge of no more than fifty centers per page); NEV. REV. STAT. § 629.061 (1999) (allowing charge of sixty cents per page for photocopies plus postage costs); WASH. REV. CODE ANN. § 70.02.010(12) (West 2000) (allowing charge not to exceed sixty-five cents per page for the first thirty pages and fifty cents per page thereafter).
34. 45 C.F.R. § 46.101 (2000) (DHHS); 21 C.F.R. § 50.1 (2000) (FDA).
35. 45 C.F.R. § 46.116 (a) (5) (2000) (DHHS); 21 C.F.R. § 50.25(a) (5) (2000) (FDA).
36. 42 C.F.R. § 164.103 ,.504 (2001).
37. 42 C.F.R. § 164.506 (2001).
38. 42 C.F.R. § 164.506 (e)(2)(iii) (2001).
39. *See, e.g.,* IDAHO CODE § 39-609 (1993); KAN. STAT. ANN. § 65-6002 (2000); MO. CODE REGS. tit. 19, § 20-20.020 (1995); S.D. ADMIN. R. 44:20 (2000).
40. *See, e.g.,* CONN. GEN. STAT. ANN. § 17a-101 (West 2001); HAW. REV. STAT. § 350-1.1 (2000); MO. REV. STAT. § 210.110 (2001); R.I. GEN. LAWS § 40-11-3.1 (2000); S.D. CODIFIED LAWS ANN. § 26-8A-6 (2000).
41. MO. REV. STAT. § 578.350 (2001).
42. *See, e.g.,* MINN. STAT. ANN. § 144.222 (2000); S.D. CODIFIED LAWS ANN. § 34-25.-32. 2 (2000); TENN. CODE ANN. § 68-3-208 (2000); VA. CODE ANN. § 32.1-264 (Michie 2000).
43. *See, e.g.,* FLA. STAT. ANN. § 385.202 (West 2000); HAW. REV. STAT. § 324-21 (2000); MD. HEALTH-GEN. CODE ANN. § 18-204 (2000); MO. REV. STAT. §§ 192.650-.657 (2001); NEB. REV. STAT. § 81-646 (2000); OHIO REV. CODE ANN. § 3701.262 (Baldwin 2001); S.D. ADMIN. R. 44:22 (2000); VT. STAT. ANN. tit. 18, § 153 (2000). The Cancer Registry Amendment Act of 1992 authorized funding to states to enhance existing cancer registries, including establishing a computerized reporting and data processing system. 42 U.S.C. § 280e (1992).
44. Examples of good cause include: *Golan v. Louise Wise Services,* 507 N.E.2d 275 (N.Y. 1987) (for treatment of a medical problem); *In re: Wilson,* 544 N.Y.S.2d 886 (App. Div. 2d 1989) (for treatment of psychological trauma substantiated by health professionals).
45. *Application of Romano,* 438 N.Y.S.2d 967, 971-72 (N.Y. Surr. Ct. 1981).

46. Many states have enacted some form of voluntary adoption registry, including: ARK. STAT. ANN. §§ 9-9-501-508 (1999); CAL. CIV. CODE §§ 224.61, 222.15 (Deering 2000); COLO. REV. STAT. § 19-5-201.5 (2000); FLA. STAT. ANN. § 63.165 (West 2000); IDAHO CODE § 39-259A (2000); IND. CODE § 31-19-18-2 (2001); LA. REV. STAT ANN. § 9:40.97 (1989); ME. REV. STAT. ANN. tit. 22, § 2706-A (1999); MASS. GEN. LAWS ANN. ch. 210, § 5D (2001); MICH. COMP. LAWS § 710.68; NEV. REV. STAT. § 127.007 (1999); N.H. REV. STAT. ANN § 170-B:19 (2001).
47. MINN. STAT. ANN. § 259.47 (West 2001); MO. REV. STAT. § 453.121 (2001); N.D. CENT. CODE § 14-15-16 (1999); TENN. CODE ANN. § 36-1-141 (2000).

Chapter 6

Confidentiality and Informed Consent

Learning Objectives

After reading this chapter, the learner should be able to:

1. Explain the interrelationship between confidentiality and privacy.
2. Identify and discuss the three sources of law on which the right of privacy is based.
3. Compare and contrast open record statutes and privacy statutes.
4. Explain the use and application of the physician–patient privilege.
5. Trace the historical development of the informed consent doctrine.
6. Discuss the concept of substituted consent and its application to minor patients.
7. Define the term *advance directive.*
8. List the obligations placed on health-care providers by the Patient Self-Determination Act.
9. Distinguish between living wills and durable powers of attorney for health care.
10. Discuss the legal protections afforded to health-care providers when treating patients in an emergency situation.
11. Compare and contrast the professional disclosure standard and the reasonable patient standard.

Key Concepts

- Advance directives
- Confidentiality
- Durable powers of attorney
- Informed consent
- Living wills
- Open record statutes
- Physician–patient privilege
- Privacy
- Privacy statutes
- Professional disclosure standard
- Reasonable patient standard
- Substituted consent

Introduction

One striking development in the delivery of health care during the twentieth century concerned **confidentiality**. From its origin in professional practice to its development into legal protections, the concept of confidentiality has served to protect patient-specific health information from disclosure. Not only have those involved with direct patient care served to protect health information, but health information managers have assumed responsibility for protecting confidential patient-specific health information. Actions by both groups to maintain confidentiality have become increasingly difficult, as demands for patient-specific information increase.

Demands for information arise not only from third-party payors and governmental entities, but also from patients themselves when deciding to consent to or forgo treatment. This demand for information has initiated a significant development in the relationship between law and medicine: the doctrine of **informed consent**.

To understand the responsibilities that confidentiality and informed consent place on health-care providers, health information officers must understand the historical development of each concept. From there, this chapter then examines the legal bases for confidentiality and the scope of the informed consent doctrine.

Confidentiality

When addressing issues of confidentiality of patient-specific health information, the focus rests on the relationship between the patient and the health-care provider. Through this relationship, the patient provides to

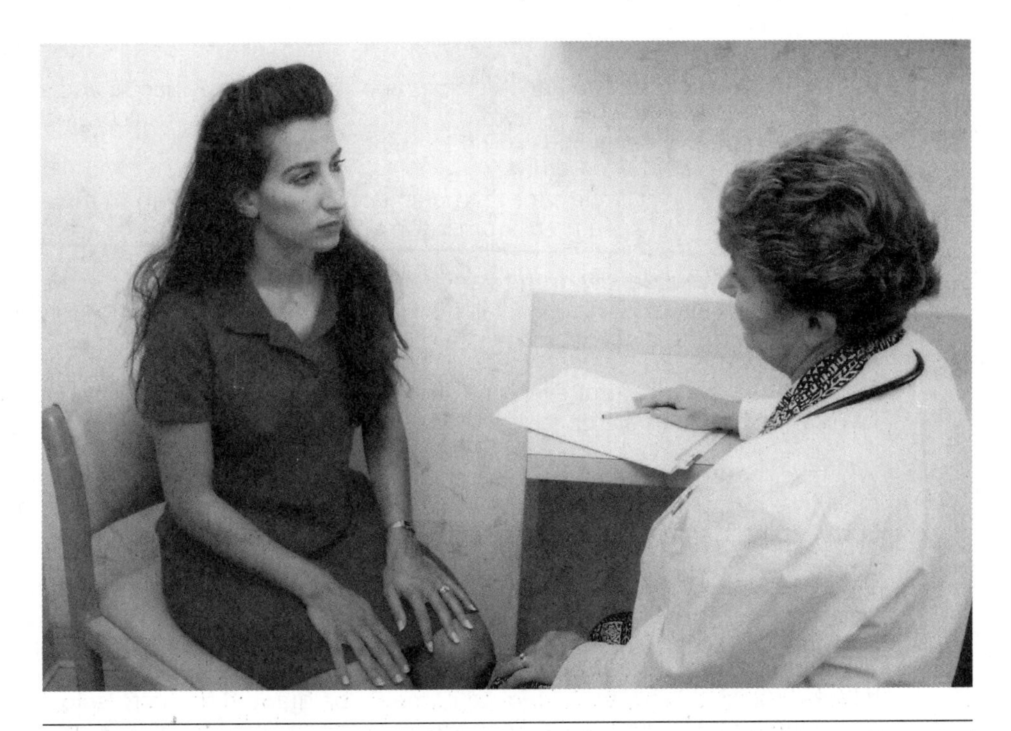

Figure 6-1. The Health-Care Provider–Patient Relationship

the health-care provider information that will assist her in diagnosing and treating the patient's symptoms. This dialogue between the patient and health-care provider is beneficial in two respects: the health-care provider gathers the data needed to make informed diagnoses and treatment decisions, and the patient provides the necessary information without fear that it will be disseminated beyond the health-care provider. (See Figure 6-1.)

The obligation of health-care providers to maintain patient information in a confidential manner is as old as medicine itself. The Oath of Hippocrates, written centuries ago, states: "What I may see or hear in the course of the treatment or even outside the treatment in regard to the life of men, which on no account one must noise abroad, I will keep to myself holding such things shameful to be spoken about."[1] The Hippocratic Oath has served as the foundation of the current medical professions' guidelines on the confidentiality of health information.[2] (See Figure 6-2.)

With the development of the health-care industry in the past century, particularly the significant changes in medical technology, the growth of

I swear by Apollo Physician and Asclepias and Hygieia and Panaceia and all the gods and goddesses, making them my witness, that I will fulfill according to my ability and judgment this oath and this covenant:

I will apply dietetic measures for the benefit of the sick according to my ability and judgment; I will keep them from harm and injustice.

I will neither give a deadly drug to anybody if asked for it, nor will I make a suggestion to this effect. Similarly, I will not give to a woman an abortive remedy. In purity and holiness I will guard my life and art.

I will not use the knife, not even on sufferers from stone, but will withdraw in favor of such men as are engaged in this work.

Whatever houses I may visit, I will come for the benefit of the sick, remaining free of all intentional injustices, of all mischief and in particular of sexual relations with both female and male persons, be they free or slaves.

What I may see or hear in the course of the treatment or even outside of the treatment in regard to the life of men, in which on no account one must noise abroad, I will keep to myself holding such things shameful to be spoken about.

If I fulfill this oath and do not violate it, may it be granted to me to enjoy life and art, being honored with fame among all men for all time to come; if I transgress it and swear falsely, may the opposite of all this be my lot.

Figure 6-2. Hippocratic Oath

government participation in health care, and the emergence of the central role of third-party payors, the amount and type of available patient-specific health information has greatly expanded. In the light of these developments, society has recognized the need for more than professionalism to protect patient-specific health information. Thus, a complex web has arisen of legal protections for patient-specific health information.

As a general matter, the underpinning to legal protections for patient-specific health information is the patient's right to **privacy**. This right to privacy is sometimes referred to as the right to be let alone and other times as the right to control personal information, depending on the source of law on which the right is based. The following sources form the foundation for rights to privacy: constitutional provisions, statutory provisions, and common law provisions, as illustrated in Figure 6-3.

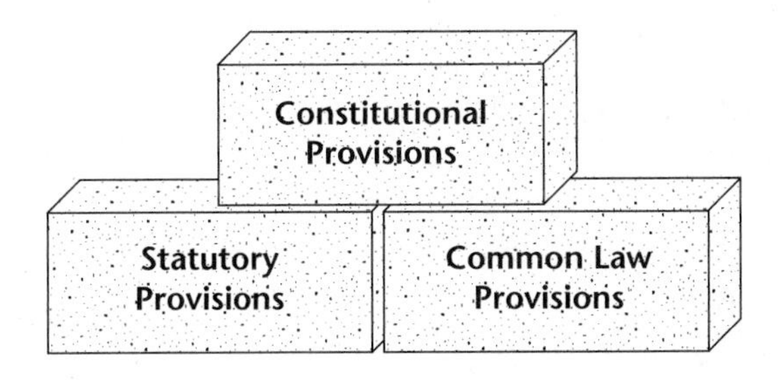

Figure 6-3. Foundation for the Rights to Privacy

Constitutional Basis

Any analysis of constitutional protections must begin with the constitution of the U.S. government. While the right to privacy is not explicitly listed in the U.S. Constitution, the U.S. Supreme Court has held that a fundamental right to privacy exists. Although the scope of the privacy right has never been clearly defined by the Supreme Court, the Court has applied it in the context of health information.

In *Whalen v. Roe,*[3] the Supreme Court examined the right to privacy in the context of New York State's effort to collect a computerized database concerning the use of certain drugs labeled as dangerous and likely to be abused. Under New York law, physicians were required to report to the state department of health the patient's name, age, and address, the names of the pharmacy and physician, and the dosage of the drug if one of the listed drugs was prescribed.

Several groups representing patients who had received the prescriptions and two physicians' associations challenged the law on grounds that it invaded the patients' privacy. In determining whether the reporting requirements amounted to a constitutional violation of the right to privacy, the Court applied a two-prong analysis relating to the patient's interests: (1) a nondisclosure prong that recognized the individual's interest in avoiding disclosure of personal matters and (2) an individual autonomy prong that recognized the individual's interest in independent decision making. The Court recognized that both patient interests existed and then balanced these interests against the state's interest in deterring drug abuse and the safeguards implemented to protect the information from subsequent disclosure. On balance, the Court concluded that the public's need for information outweighed the individual's privacy interests.

While specific to the facts of the case, the *Whalen* decision is significant for the fact that the Supreme Court recognized in it a right to informational privacy. The contours of this new right have never been fully explained, however, and are subject to further definition on the federal level. This right to privacy has also been recognized on the state level, with some states providing more explicit constitutional privacy protections than that of the federal government.[4]

Statutory Basis

On both the federal and state levels, the right to privacy has been recognized by the respective legislatures. The statutes created focus on the type of records involved, the limits placed on the use of the protected records, and whether the government or the private sector is involved.

Federal Level

Central to the federal government's efforts have been the Freedom of Information Act (FOIA)[5] and the Privacy Act of 1974.[6] Both laws apply to governmental record-keeping activities and do not focus on the activities of the private sector. The FOIA encourages access to government records and mandates disclosure upon request, absent an exception listed in the statute. By contrast, the Privacy Act presumes that certain information is confidential and may not be disclosed unless there is written consent of the individual.

In the health-care arena, these provisions come into play in the context of data held by the Social Security Administration (SSA) and the Department of Health and Human Services (HHS). Both executive branch agencies release information held by them for purposes of research and statistical studies. When releasing these data, the agencies abide by the statutory provisions listed above, including removing patient-identifying data.

Additional federal statutory confidentiality protections include the limited disclosure provisions governing drug and alcohol abuse treatment and participation in the Medicaid program.[7] These protections apply to health-care providers in the private sector who accept federal funds. For more information concerning restrictions on drug and alcohol abuse treatment programs, see Chapter 8.

State Level

Confidentiality protections on the state level fall into three categories: open record statutes, privacy statutes, and physician–patient privileges statutes. **Open record statutes** generally apply to records held by a state agency and correspond with the principles of FOIA: a presumption of disclosure absent a statutory exemption.[8] **Privacy statutes** generally correspond with the principles of the Privacy Act: a presumption of confidentiality, which may be rebutted with evidence of patient authorization to disclose information.[9]

The **physician–patient privilege** applies to the introduction of evidence at trial and is used to prevent the forced disclosure or testimony about information obtained by the health-care provider during the course of treatment. The privilege exists to encourage the patient's disclosure of relevant information to the health-care provider, no matter if that information is of an embarrassing or humiliating nature.[10] The privilege applies to both the governmental and private sectors and is generally held to rest with the patient, but may be asserted on the patient's behalf by the health-care provider to prevent forced disclosure.

Common Law Basis

Common law protections of health information essentially recognize the individual's right to bring a lawsuit for damages or injunctive relief against one who inappropriately obtains, discloses, or uses patient-specific health information. Examples of lawsuits of this type include actions for invasion of privacy, defamation, and breach of contract. Each of these lawsuits is described in detail in Chapter 3.

Informed Consent

Among the most significant developments in the relationship between law and medicine in the twentieth century is the doctrine of informed consent. From its origins in the right of privacy, this doctrine has developed into an integral part of the health-care provider–patient relationship. It has also served as the basis for federal regulations governing research involving human subjects and is reflected in consent forms used by health-care providers before treatment is rendered.

Historical Development

Where the issue of consent originally came into play, courts in the early 1900s applied the theory of battery to lawsuits brought against health-care providers.[11] As discussed in more detail in Chapter 3, battery constitutes the unauthorized touching of another. Initially, when a health-care provider did not obtain the patient's consent before treating the patient and subsequently the health-care provider touched the patient without authorization, the health-care provider was liable for battery.

As the century progressed, the focus of lawsuits addressing the consent issue changed. No longer was the question whether the patient had consented to treatment; rather, the question became whether the patient truly understood the nature and effects of the treatment for which he or she had consented. Essentially, the question centered on the quality of the consent given by the patient: Did the patient have sufficient information from which to make an informed decision?

As the focus changed, it became evident that the traditional battery theory would not suffice as a basis for these lawsuits. At the same time, courts across the country were abrogating the charitable immunity defense and refining the application of negligence principles to health-care providers. It soon became apparent that negligence principles could be applied to the consent process. Thus developed the concept of a separate legal theory: the doctrine of informed consent.

By grounding the informed consent doctrine in negligence, courts necessarily placed the focus on the health-care provider's duty of due care. As developed by the courts, the informed consent doctrine places a duty on the health-care provider to not only obtain consent to treatment but also to disclose to the patient, in an adequate manner, the nature of the treatment or procedure, the risks involved, any available alternatives, and the benefits that could reasonably be expected as a result of the treatment or procedure. The health-care provider's failure to discharge the duty to disclose sufficient information to the patient before treatment, accompanied by harm to the patient, resulted in a finding of liability for negligence.

Scope of Informed Consent Doctrine

The scope of the informed consent doctrine can be measured in several ways: who may consent to treatment, how much information the health-care provider must disclose to the patient, and what situations require

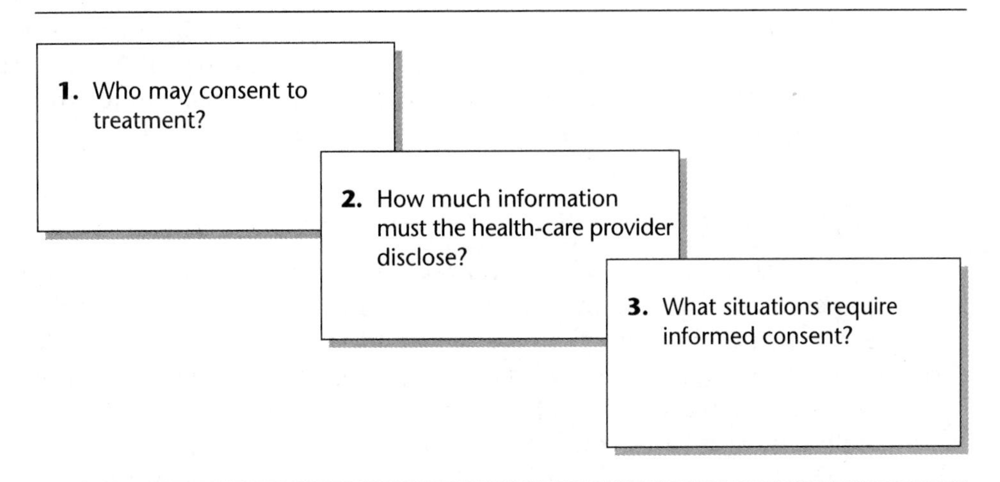

Figure 6-4. Scope of Informed Consent Doctrine

informed consent. The scope of the informed consent doctrine is illustrated in Figure 6-4.

Who May Consent to Treatment?

As a general proposition, it is the patient and the patient alone who decides whether to consent to or forgo treatment. This general proposition assumes two things: that the patient is competent under the law to consent to treatment and that an emergency situation is not present. Adult patients are presumed competent absent an adjudication of incompetency by a court of law.

For those patients in whom legal competency is clearly an issue, for example, minors and comatose patients, the law provides that an authorized person may consent to or forgo treatment on the patient's behalf. Referred to as **substituted consent**, the process allows a health-care provider to provide treatment to the patient when the patient cannot provide consent to treatment.

Minor patients

In the minor context, substituted consent given by the parent or legal guardian will apply until the minor reaches the age of majority or becomes emancipated in the eyes of the law. Examples in which emancipation would provide legal authority for the minor to give consent include marriage,[12] childbirth,[13] or entry into the armed forces.[14] Where certain medical conditions are present, state law may provide for the minor's consent even if majority or emancipation requirements are not met. Examples of these special medical conditions include pregnancy, sexually transmitted diseases, and substance abuse.[15]

Legally incompetent patients

When speaking of legally incompetent patients, the focus rests on those patients who were either never competent or were once competent but subsequently became incompetent due to illness or accident. Often, consent issues in this context involve the question of whether the patient, or someone acting on the patient's behalf, has the right to refuse treatment with the result that the patient may die. Commonly referred to as the "right to die," this issue had been present in the health-care community for many decades. It was not until the case of *Cruzan v. Director, Missouri Department of Health*[16] and responsive legislation that the country focused on the so-called right to die issue.

In *Cruzan*, the U.S. Supreme Court addressed whether life support could be withdrawn from Nancy Cruzan, a patient in a persistent vegetative state due to a car accident. The Court determined that Missouri's requirement of a showing of clear and convincing evidence of Nancy's wishes indicating that she wished life support withdrawn before the health-care provider withdrew treatment was not unconstitutional.

The national spotlight focusing on this one case eventually led to the passage of the Patient Self-Determination Act (PSDA).[17] The goal of the PSDA is "to ensure that a patient's rights to self-determination in health-care decisions be communicated and protected."[18] It requires those health-care providers who are Medicare or Medicaid certified[19] to inform their patients of the status of state law governing a patient's right to make **advance directives** for accepting or refusing health-care services and the health-care provider's written policies concerning implementation of the patients' rights. The text of the PSDA may be found in the Appendix of this book.

Advance directives are defined as written instructions recognized under state law, such as living wills or durable powers of attorney for health care, which relate to the kind of health care the patient wishes to have or not have when incapacitated. A **living will** is a document, exercised while a patient is competent, that provides direction as to medical care in the event the patient becomes incapacitated or unable to make personal decisions. A **durable power of attorney** for health care is a document that allows a competent patient to name someone else to make health-care decisions in the event the patient becomes incapacitated or unable to make personal decisions. In addition to informing the patient of the law and the provider's policy to implement it, PSDA requires the health-care provider to ensure that the patient's medical record reflects whether the patient has an advanced directive, and if so, what type. PSDA further requires the health-care provider to avoid discrimination against patients on the basis of whether the patient has executed an advance directive.

Although PSDA places new obligations on health-care providers to educate and communicate with patients, staff, and the community, it does not create or modify any substantive legal rights. It is up to each state to create or modify substantive legal rights concerning advance directives. In most states, the statutes addressing substantive legal rights grant permission to patients to use living wills, durable powers of attorney for health care, or both. A living will generally refers to a document that provides direction as to medical care in the event the patient is incapacitated or unable to make personal decisions.[20] By contrast, durable powers of attorney for health care allow a competent individual to name someone else to exercise health-care-related decisions on her behalf, when certain conditions are met.[21]

Health information managers should be aware not only of the PSDA but of fact that the U.S. Department of Health and Human Services has issued implementing regulations to PSDA and that the Joint Commission on Accreditation of Healthcare Organizations has issued standards that address advance directives.[22] Finally, health information managers should realize that the substantive legal rights governing advance directives have fifty-one possible variations, covering each state and the District of Columbia.

Emergency situations

As is self-evident, emergency situations pose difficult problems in obtaining the patient's informed consent. As a general proposition, an emergency situation is presented when the patient is unable to give consent, another person authorized to give consent on the patient's behalf is unavailable, and a delay in treatment would likely result in death or serious bodily harm to the patient.[23] Examples of emergency situations where informed consent may be difficult, if not impossible, to obtain include instances in which a person suffers sudden injury and any delay in treatment may result in increased risk to life or health and in which a patient who is undergoing treatment for a nonemergency condition experiences a worsening of the condition to the point that the patient's life is threatened.

State legislatures and courts have recognized that health-care providers confronted with these situations risk potential liability and so have created legal protections for them. These legal protections are commonly referred to as Good Samaritan laws and serve to protect health-care providers from liability for unauthorized treatment, as opposed to protection from rendering negligent treatment or intentional misconduct.[24] These laws are targeted at nontraditional settings in which health care is delivered, for example, by the side of the road after an automobile accident, as opposed to the treatment rendered by emergency room physicians. Good Samaritan statutes are addressed in more detail in Chapter 3.

Information to Be Disclosed

The extent to which information must be disclosed to the patient essentially rests with the question of whether the patient received sufficient information from which to make an informed decision. What constitutes sufficient disclosure is a matter of state law. Generally, sufficient disclosure includes information concerning the nature of the proposed procedure or treatment, the risks involved therein, any available alternatives, and the benefits that may be expected.[25] The states are split in their approach to measuring the duty of disclosure. Disclosure is measured under the law from two different perspectives: the health-care provider's and the patient's.

Frequently referred to as the **professional disclosure standard**, this standard measures what a reasonable health-care provider under the same or similar circumstances would disclose. Under this approach, expert testimony would be required to establish the parameters of the standard. Many states have adopted this standard, by statute[26] or case law.[27]

The second approach looks to the needs of the patient rather than the professional standards of the health-care provider. Here, the **reasonable patient standard** measures what material information is necessary for an average, reasonable patient to reach a decision to consent to or forgo treatment. Because it is the patient's perspective that is measured, it is unnecessary to produce expert testimony concerning the standards of practice. Several states have adopted this standard, either by statute[28] or by case law.[29]

Situations Requiring Informed Consent

Absent an emergency situation, any treatment rendered by a health-care provider involves consent of the patient, either implied or express.[30] Implied or tacit consent exists in situations in which a patient voluntarily submits to a procedure with apparent knowledge of that procedure and the procedure presents slight or no apparent risk, such as taking the patient's pulse or temperature. In these instances, the law presumes the patient has given consent.

By contrast, express consent of the patient, in the form of verbal or written informed consent, is necessary in which diagnostic or therapeutic procedures will be performed. Here, the risk of harm may or may not be readily apparent to the patient but is generally considered to be more than slight. Examples include invasive surgery, radiological therapy, or procedures that may change the body structure.

Unfortunately, no one list exists that specifies those procedures requiring informed consent. Instead, health-care providers must look to statutes, regulations, professional guidelines, and institutional requirements for guidance. And when in doubt, health-care providers are advised to take the cautious approach and obtain the patient's informed consent. In particular, health-care providers should exercise caution with regard to experimental procedures that involve human subjects. Federal statutes governing experimental procedures involving human subjects specify strict requirements for informed consent. For further information about research involving human subjects, see Chapter 5.

Conclusion

Two of the most significant developments in the relationship between law and medicine during the twentieth century are the doctrines of confidentiality and informed consent. Just as confidentiality serves to protect information conveyed by the patient to his or her health-care provider from inappropriate disclosure, informed consent serves to protect the patient from making decisions about treatment without first being provided the necessary information. Health information managers must be aware of these legal protections that have become integrated into modern health care.

Case Study

You are the director of health information services at a medium-size health-care facility providing general, emergency, and pediatric care. Because of downsizing and consolidation of managerial functions, you are also responsible for staff education in your facility. Discuss how you would structure and present an inservice program to staff members of various departments that addresses confidentiality policies and procedures of your facility, and the legal bases underlying these policies and procedures.

Review Questions

1. Compare and contrast confidentiality and privacy.
2. What are open record statutes, and which federal law do they most closely follow?
3. What are privacy statutes, and which federal law do they most closely follow?
4. When does the physician–patient privilege apply, and what is its use?
5. In what ways can the scope of the informed consent doctrine be measured?
6. Define the terms *living will* and *durable power of attorney* for health care.
7. What generally defines an emergency situation in the context of informed consent?
8. What perspectives are used to measure the professional disclosure standard and the reasonable person standard?

Enrichment Activity

Imagine you are the director of health information management at a health-care institution. Determine how your institution will address issues of patient confidentiality, including programs to educate staff on the issues of patient confidentiality. Contemplate the increased use of computerized databases and electronic means of communication and the impact these issues will have on the issue of patient confidentiality. Draft an outline of your institution's policy on patient confidentiality and plan for staff education.

Notes

1. L. EDELSTEIN, THE HIPPOCRATIC OATH: TEXT, TRANSLATION AND INTERPRETATION 3 (1943).
2. For example, the American Medical Association (AMA) has placed an ethical duty upon physicians to safeguard the communications made between physicians and patients and not disclose those communications absent patient consent. AMERICAN MEDICAL ASS'N, CURRENT OPINIONS OF THE JUDICIAL COUNCIL OF THE AMERICAN MEDICAL ASSOCIATION (1984).
3. 429 U.S. 589 (1977).
4. ALASKA CONST. art. I, § 22; ARIZ. CONST. art. II, § 8; CAL. CONST. art. I, § 1; FLA. CONST. art. I, § 23; HAW. CONST. art. I, § 6; ILL. CONST. art. I, § 6; LA. CONST. art. I, § 5; MONT. CONST. art. II, § 10; S.C. CONST. art I, § 10; WASH. CONST. art. I, § 7.
5. 5 U.S.C. § 552 (2000). In addition, bills have been introduced into Congress to provide confidentiality protection at the federal level. S.R. 1360, 104th Cong., 2d Sess. (1995); H. R. 1057, 1941, 2404, 2455, 2470, 106th Cong., 1st Sess. (1999).
6. 5 U.S.C. § 552a (2000).
7. *See* Comprehensive Alcohol Abuse & Alcoholism Prevention, Treatment & Rehabilitation Act of 1970, 42 U.S.C. § 290ee (2000); Drug Abuse, Prevention, Treatment & Rehabilitation Act, 42 U.S.C. § 290dd (2000); Medicaid Program, 42 U.S.C. § 1396 (2000).
8. *See, e.g.,* ARK. STAT. ANN. §§ 25-19-101 to -107 (Michie 2000); CAL. GOV'T CODE §§ 9070-9079 (West 2001); DEL. CODE ANN. tit. 29, §§ 10001-10005 (2000); GA. CODE ANN. §§ 50-18-70 to -74 (2000); IOWA CODE ANN. §§ 21.1 to .12 (West 2001); KY. REV. STAT. §§ 61.870 to .884 (Baldwin 2000); MICH. COMP. LAWS ANN. §§ 15.231 to .246 (West 2001); N.Y. PUB. OFF. LAW §§ 84-90 (McKinney 2000); VA. CODE §§ 2.1-340 to -346.1 (2000).
9. *See, e.g.,* CAL. CIV. CODE §§ 1798.1 to .76 (West 2001); CONN. GEN. STAT. §§ 4-190 to 4-197 (2001); IND. CODE ANN. §§ 4-1-6-1 to -9 (Burns 2001); MASS. ANN. LAWS ch. 66A, §§ 1-3 (Michie/Lawyers Co-op. 2001); MINN. STAT ANN. §§ 13.01 to .87 (West 2000); OHIO REV. CODE ANN. §§ 1347.01 to .99 (Baldwin 2000); VA. CODE §§ 2.1-377 to 2.1-386 (2000).

10. *See, e.g.,* ARK. CODE ANN. § 16-41-101, Rule 503 (Michie 2000); CAL. EVID. CODE §§ 990-995 (West 2001); DEL. R. EVID. 503; GA. CODE ANN. § 24-9-40 (2000); HAW. R. EVID. 504; KAN. STAT. ANN. § 60-427 (2000); MICH. COMP. LAWS ANN. § 600.2157 (West Supp. 2001); MISS. CODE ANN. § 13-1-21 (2000); NEB. REV. STAT. § 27-504, Rule 504 (2000); N.J. STAT. ANN. §§ 2A:84A-22.1 to :84A-22.2 (West 2001); N.M. R. EVID. 11-504; N.Y. CIV. PRAC. L. & R. 4504 (McKinney 2001); N.D. R. EVID. 503; OHIO REV. CODE ANN. § 2317.02(B) (1) (Baldwin 2001); OKLA. STAT. ANN. tit. 12, § 2503 (West 2000); S.D. CODIFIED LAWS ANN. §§ 19-13-6 to -8 (2001); VT. R. EVID. 503; WIS. STAT. ANN. § 905.04 (West 2001).
11. *See, e.g., Schloendorff v. Society of New York Hosp.,* 105 N.E. 92 (N.Y. 1914); *Rolater v. Strain,* 137 P.96 (Okla. 1913); *Pratt v. Davis,* 79 N.E. 562 (Ill. 1906).
12. *See, e.g.,* ALA. CODE § 22-8-5 (2000); ARIZ. REV. STAT. ANN. § 44-132 (2000); COLO. REV. STAT. ANN. § 13-22-103 (West 2000); KY. REV. STAT. ANN. § 214.185(3) (Michie/Bobbs-Merrill 2000); MD. HEALTH-GEN. CODE ANN. § 2-301 (2000); MINN. STAT. ANN. § 144.342 (West 2000); MISS. CODE ANN. § 93-1-5 (2000); MONT. CODE ANN. § 41-4-402 (2000); N.J. STAT. ANN. § 9:17A-1 (West 2001); N.M. STAT. ANN. § 24-10-1 (2001); N.Y. PUB. HEALTH LAW § 2504 (McKinney 2001); 35 PA. CONS. STAT. ANN. § 10101 (2000); S.C. CODE ANN. § 20-7-270 (Law. Co-op. 2000); VA. CODE ANN. § 54.1-2969 (Michie 2000).
13. *See, e.g.,* ALA CODE § 22-8-4 (2000); GA. CODE ANN. § 31-9-2 (Michie 2000); KY. REV. STAT. ANN. § 214.185(3) (Michie/Bobbs-Merrill 2000); MD. HEALTH-GEN. CODE ANN. § 2-3011 (2000); MINN. STAT. ANN. § 144.342 (West 2000); MONT. CODE ANN. § 41-1-402 (2000); N.Y. PUB. HEALTH LAW § 2504 (McKinney 2001).
14. *See, e.g.,* ALA. CODE § 22-8-4 (2000); MONT. CODE § 41-1-402 (2000).
15. *See, e.g.,* ALA. CODE § 22-8-6 (2000) (all three medical conditions); ARK. STAT. ANN. § 20-9-602 (2000) (all three medical conditions); GA. CODE ANN. § 31-9-2 (2000) (pregnancy); KAN. STAT. ANN. § 38-123 (2000) (pregnancy); MISS. CODE ANN. § 41-41-3 (2000) (pregnancy); MONT. CODE ANN. § 41-1-402 (2000) (all three medical conditions); UTAH CODE ANN. § 78-14-5 (2000) (pregnancy); VA. CODE ANN. § 54.1-2969 (2000) (all three medical conditions).
16. 497 U.S. 261 (1990).
17. 42 U.S.C. § 1396a(w) (2000).
18. 42 U.S.C. § 1396a(w) (1(A) (i) (2000).
19. The statute defines health-care providers to include Medicare- or Medicaid-certified hospitals, skilled nursing facilities, home health agencies, hospices, and HMOs. 42 U.S.C. § 1396a (a) (57) (2000).
20. States with statutes authorizing living wills include: ALA. CODE §§ 22-8A-1 to -10 (2000); ALASKA STAT. §§ 18.12.010 to .100 (2000); ARIZ. REV. STAT. §§ 36-3261 to -3262 (2000); CAL. HEALTH & SAFETY CODE §§ 4600-4673 (2001); COLO. REV. STAT. §§ 15-18-101 to -113 (2000); DEL. CODE ANN. tit. 16, §§ 2501-2509

(2000); IDAHO CODE §§ 39-4501 to -4509 (2000); IOWA CODE ANN. §§ 144A.1 to 144A.11 (2001); KY. REV. STAT. ANN. § 311.621-643 (Baldwin 2000); LA. REV. STAT. ANN. §§ 40:1299.58.1 to 40:1229.58.10 (2000); MINN. STAT. § 145B.01 to 145B.17 (West 2000); NEV. REV. STAT. §§ 449.535 to 449.690 (1993); N.M. STAT. ANN. §§ 24-7-1 to 24-7-11 (2001); OR. REV. STAT. §§ 127.505 to 127.660 (1999); S.C. CODE ANN. §§ 44-77-10 to 44-77-160 (2000) VT. STAT. ANN. tit. 18, §§ 5251-5262 and tit. 13, § 1801 (2000); W. VA. CODE §§ 16-30-1 to 16-30-13 (2000).

21. Examples of state with statutes allowing for durable powers of attorney for health care include: CAL. PROB. CODE §§ 4600 to 4806 (2001); COLO. REV. STAT. §§ 15-14-501 to 502 (2000); D.C. CODE ANN. §§ 21-2201 to 2213 (1989 & Supp. 1994); GA. CODE §§ 31-36-1 to 31-36-13 (2000); KAN. STAT. ANN. § 58-625 to 632 (2000); ME. REV. STAT. ANN. tit. 18-A, § 5-501 to -506 (1999); MISS. CODE ANN. §§ 41-41-201 TO 41-41-229 (2000); N.C. GEN. STAT. §§ 32A-8 to -27 (2000); OHIO REV. CODE ANN. §§ 1337.11 TO 1337.17 (2001); R.I. GEN. LAWS § 23-4.10-1 to -12 (2000); S.D. CODIFIED LAWS ANN. §§ 59-7-2.1 to-8 (2001); WASH. REV. CODE ANN. § 11.94.010 to .070 (2000).
22. 42 C.F.R. §§ 417.436, 431.20, 434.28 (2000); THE JOINT COMMISSION ON ACCREDITATION OF HEALTHCARE ORGANIZATIONS, Accreditation Manual, Patient Rights, RI1.2 (1995).
23. *See, e.g.,* ALA. CODE § 22-8-1 (2000); ARK. STAT. ANN. § 20-9-603 (2000); GA. CODE ANN. § 31-9-3 (2000); IDAHO CODE § 39-4303 (2000); NEV. REV. STAT. ANN. § 41A.120 (1999); PA. STAT. ANN. tit. 40, § 1301.103 (2000).
24. *See, e.g.,* CONN. GEN. STAT. § 52-557b (2001); FLA. STAT. ANN. § 768.13 (West 2000); MISS. CODE ANN. § 73-25-37 (2000); MONT. CODE ANN. § 41-1-405 (2000).
25. BARRY R. FURROW, ET AL., HEALTH LAW § 6-1 (1995).
26. *See, e.g.,* ALA. CODE § 6-5-484 (2000); ARK. STAT. ANN. § 16-114-206(b) (2000); ARIZ. REV. STAT. § 12-561, 563 (2000); DEL. CODE ANN. tit. 18, § 6852 (2000); FLA. STAT. ANN. § 766.103 (2000); IDAHO CODE § 39-4304 (2000); KY. REV. STAT. ANN. § 304.40-320 (Baldwin 2000); ME. REV. STAT. ANN. tit. 24, § 2905 (1999); NEB. REV. STAT. § 44-2816 (2000); NEV. REV. STAT. § 41A.100 (1999); N.H. REV. STAT. § 507-E:2.II (2000); N.Y. PUB. HEALTH LAW § 2805-d (2001); N.C. GEN. STAT. § 90-21.13 (1993); TENN. CODE ANN. § 29-26-118 (2000); VT. STAT. ANN. tit. 12, § 1909 (2000).
27. *See, e.g., Conrad v. Imatani,* 724 P.2d 89 (Colo. App. 1986); *Weekly v. Solomon,* 510 N.E.2d 142 (Ind. App. 1981); *Natanson v. Kline,* 350 P.2d 1093 (Kan. 1960); *Rice v. Jaskolski,* 313 N.W.2d 893 (Mich. 1981); *Baltzwell v. Baptist Med. Ctr.,* 718 S.W.2d 140 (Mo. 1986); *Collins v. Itoh,* 503 P.2d 36 (Mont. 1972); *Skripek v. Bergamo,* 491 A.2d 1336 (N.J. Super. 1985); *Hook v. Rothstein,* 316 S.E.2d 690 (S.C. App. 1984); *Bly v. Rhoads,* 222 S.E.2d 783 (Va. 1976).

28. *See, e.g.,* IOWA CODE ANN. § 147.137 (2001); N.D. CENT. CODE § 28-01-46 (1999); PA. STAT. ANN. tit. 40, § 1301.103 (2000); TEX. REV. CIV. STAT. ANN. art. 4590i, § 6.02 (1999); WASH. REV. CODE ANN. § 7.70.050(1) (2000).
29. *See, e.g., Canterbury v. Spence,* 464 F.2d 772 (D.C. Cir. 1972); *Cobbs v. Grant,* 104 Cal. Rptr. 505 (Cal. 1972); *Sard v. Hardy,* 379 A.2d 1014 (Md. 1977); *Halley v. Birbiglia,* 458 N.E.2d 710 (Mass. 1983); *Kohoutek v. Hafner,* 383 N.W.2d 295 (Minn. 1985); *Scott v. Bradford,* 606 P.2d 554 (Okla. 1980); *Wilkinson v. Vesey,* 295 A.2d 676 (R.I. 1972); *Cross v. Trapp,* 294 S.E.2d 446 (W. Va. 1982).
30. BARRY R. FURROW, ET AL., HEALTH LAW § 6-9 (1995).

Chapter 7

Judicial Process of Health Information

Learning Objectives

After reading this chapter, the learner should be able to:

1. Define the following legal terms associated with the role of a medical record in a lawsuit: evidence, admissible, and hearsay.
2. Explain why medical records are considered hearsay evidence.
3. Explain how the health information manager establishes the foundation and trustworthiness requirements for admitting the medical record into evidence.
4. List the questions typically asked of the health information manager when establishing the foundation and trustworthiness requirements.
5. Explain the use and application of the physician–patient privilege.
6. Discuss the differences among a subpoena, a subpoena ad testificandum, and a subpoena duces tecum.
7. Compare and contrast a court order authorizing disclosure of health information with a subpoena.
8. Compare and contrast the three recommended responses of a health information manager to the presentation of a subpoena.
9. Assess the steps to take when presented with an invalid subpoena duces tecum.

Key Concepts

- Admissible
- Business record exception
- Court order
- Evidence
- Foundation requirement
- Hearsay
- Physician–patient privilege
- Show cause order
- Subpoena
- Subpoena ad testificandum
- Subpoena duces tecum
- Trustworthiness requirement

Introduction

Health information contained in the medical record serves a variety of clinical and nonclinical purposes: supporting direct patient care, quality improvement activities, public health monitoring, and billing and reimbursement, to name a few. One of the most important purposes of health information contained in the medical record is as the legal document recording a particular episode of a patient's care. As such, it serves as the backbone of virtually every professional liability action and is used to establish whether the applicable standard of care was met. Other civil actions also require the admission of the medical record as evidence, including credentialing and disciplinary proceedings of physicians and other health-care professionals. Furthermore, criminal actions may require admission of the medical record to establish the cause of the victim's death, an insanity defense, or a party's physical condition, for example, blood alcohol content. These uses are illustrated in Figure 7-1.

Because of the myriad of legal protections to which health information is subject, disclosure of health information contained in the medical record may only be made pursuant to legal authority. Generally stated, health information may be disclosed only on the patient's written consent, pursuant to statutory requirements or on proper legal process. This chapter addresses those instances where disclosure is made pursuant to legal process. Health information managers must understand those instances where disclosure pursuant to legal process is appropriate or inappropriate so that they may properly respond to legal process.

- To establish the applicable standard of care
- As evidence in civil actions
- As evidence involving credentialing process
- For disciplinary proceedings of health-care professionals
- To establish the cause of death
- To determine blood alcohol content
- To support an insanity defense
- As proof of a party's physical condition

Figure 7-1. Legal Uses for the Medical Record

Medical Records as Evidence

As discussed above, the medical record serves as the legal document of a particular episode of patient care. To understand the role the medical record plays in a lawsuit, the learner must first become familiar with several legal terms that are covered in this chapter.

Lawsuits use medical records as evidence to support or discredit a party's claim. **Evidence** is defined as testimony, writings, material objects, or other things presented to prove or disprove a fact. In the context of health information, medical records may be used as evidence in civil or criminal court actions or in administrative agency proceedings.

Before a party may use the medical record as evidence to support or discredit a claim, he must determine whether the evidence is **admissible.** To be admissible, the evidence must be both pertinent and proper. What is considered pertinent and proper for use by a jury and/or a judge in reaching a decision is governed by rules of evidence. In the context of medical records, the applicable rule of evidence is the hearsay rule.

Hearsay

Hearsay is defined as out-of-court statements that are offered to prove the truth of the matter asserted. Medical records are considered hearsay evidence because the health-care providers making the statements, that is, the entries into the record, do not do so in court under oath. The complexity of bringing to court the multitude of health-care providers who made entries into a particular medical record and the cost associated with doing so make it inevitable that very few health-care providers will actually serve as witnesses in court with regard to a particular medical record. If not present in the courtroom, the witnesses cannot be subject to cross-examination. Accordingly, the majority, if not all, of the entries made in the medical record are not subject to cross-examination and are considered hearsay evidence.

Because medical records are considered hearsay evidence, they are subject to the hearsay rule, which prohibits their admission into evidence, absent an exception to the rule. The most commonly used exceptions to the rule are the **business record exception,**[1] a subset of that exception specifically governing medical records,[2] or an exception governing public or official documents.[3]

Under each of these exceptions, the party seeking to admit the medical record must meet the **foundation** and **trustworthiness requirements** of the exception. A foundation is made by establishing that the record was made (1) and kept in the ordinary course of business, (2) at or near the time the event was recorded, and (3) by a person with knowledge of the acts, events, conditions, opinions, or diagnoses appearing in it.[4] After meeting these requirements, the party seeking to introduce the record must establish the accuracy and trustworthiness of the medical record. The party accomplishes these tasks by presenting the custodian of records as a witness to explain record-keeping procedures.

The health information manager, acting as custodian of the record, must be able to testify as to both the foundation and trustworthiness requirements of the business record exception. To assist in establishing the foundation, the health information manager must possess knowledge of the requirements to create and maintain a medical record issued by governmental entities, accrediting agencies, and internal policies and procedures of the health care provider, along with knowledge of the manner in which data are recorded. To assist in establishing trustworthiness, the health information manager must possess knowledge of internal policies and procedures governing access to the medical record, and quality control techniques, such as approved methods to make corrections to and use abbreviations in the record. If computerized patient records are involved, additional steps are necessary to establish the foundation and trustworthiness requirements. For more information concerning computerized patient records, see Chapter 11.

In a typical situation, the health information manager testifies at either a deposition or at trial. In both situations, the health information manager is placed under oath and answers a series of questions designed to establish the foundation and trustworthiness requirements. If the health information manager is presented with a subpoena duces tecum, the health information manager will present and deliver the original or a copy of the medical record to the requesting party, in the case of a deposition, or to the court, in the case of trial. A sample listing of questions typically presented to the health information manager acting as custodian of records is found in Figure 7-2.

Privilege

In addition to overcoming the hearsay rule, a party wishing to admit the medical record as evidence must overcome application of the privilege doctrine. A privilege is the legal right to keep certain information confidential and protect it from subpoena, discovery, or introduction into evidence at trial. A privilege will be considered waived if the confidentiality

---

1. State your full name and business address.
2. Are you the custodian of records for [name of health-care provider]?
3. In answering these questions, have you made a full and complete search of [name of health-care provider]'s patient record for patient [name of patient]?
4. Have you presented today a true, complete, and accurate copy of all [name of health-care provider]'s records for patient [name of patient]?
5. If not, please state as accurately as possible all such documents that are not presented today and the reason(s) therefor.
6. Are all entries contained in the records presented today made by [name of health-care provider] or his employees in the ordinary course of business?
7. If not, please identify which document or entry presented today is not made in the ordinary course of [name of health-care provider]'s business.
8. What procedures are taken to ensure the accuracy of the records you have presented today?

Figure 7-2. Sample Questions Presented to the Custodian of Records

is breached, through either carelessness or deliberate disclosure by the party holding the privilege.[5]

In the context of health information contained in the medical record, the most frequently used privilege is the **physician–patient privilege.** Other privileges, such as the attorney–client and attorney work product privileges, are used in the context of health information contained in incident reports. For more information concerning the application of these other privileges, see Chapter 9.

The physician–patient privilege is created by statute and is used to prevent the forced disclosure of, or testimony about, information obtained by the health-care provider during the course of treatment.[6] The privilege exists to encourage the patient's disclosure of relevant information to the health-care provider, no matter if that information is of an embarrassing or humiliating nature. The privilege is generally held to rest with the patient, but may be asserted on the patient's behalf by the health-care provider to prevent forced disclosure.

The privilege frequently applies in situations in which the health-care provider is a party to the lawsuit. It generally does not apply in criminal actions, will contests, and physician licensure proceedings. Whether the health-care provider should assert the physician–patient privilege is a question to be answered with the assistance of legal counsel.

Responses to Legal Process

The general rule of ownership of health information states that the health-care provider owns the medium in which health information is stored, the medical record, with limited property interests possessed by the patient. From this rule flows the principle that the record must remain within the provider's control and safekeeping and may be removed only in accordance with proper legal process. Both subpoenas and court orders constitute proper legal process.

When faced with a subpoena or a court order, the health information manager is placed in the difficult position of how to respond. Should he release the requested records, refuse to release the requested records, or excise those portions of the records that the health information manager determines are protected and release the remainder? If the health information manager fails to respond to the subpoena, he exposes the health-care provider to potential contempt of court charges. If the health information manager improperly releases the records, he may subject the health-care provider to liability for breach of confidentiality. Only upon a determination that a valid subpoena or court order has been presented and that a valid legal defense against disclosure does not exist should the health information manager release the requested records. This section addresses subpoenas and court orders and the methods used to respond to them.

Subpoenas

The most common legal process a health-care provider will encounter is being served with a subpoena. A **subpoena** is a command issued by a court or other authorized official to appear and/or present certain documents and other things. A subpoena commanding the appearance of a witness to give testimony is called a **subpoena ad testificandum.**[7] A subpoena commanding the production of books, documents, and other things is called a **subpoena duces tecum.**[8] A subpoena duces tecum is often used in the context of health information management, commanding the custodian of the records to produce a particular record at trial or deposition and provide testimony as to the authenticity of the record produced. An example of a subpoena duces tecum in a civil case brought in federal court is illustrated in Figure 7-3.

Certain elements are common to all valid subpoenas and are listed in Figure 7-4. Subpoenas may vary in certain respects, depending on whether the subpoena was issued by a federal or state court. For example, a subpoena issued by a federal court may be issued only by the clerk of the federal court under seal of the court.[9] By contrast, subpoenas issued in state court are issued pursuant to state rules, which may allow noncourt officials to issue subpoenas, such as a notary public or someone appointed by the state court to take testimony.[10] Subpoenas also differ concerning provisions of advance notice. In the federal court, no provision exists requiring advance notice for a subpoena in connection with discovery;[11] in state court, advance notice for a discovery subpoena may be required.[12] Finally, subpoenas may differ as to witness fees, with fees given in federal court often greater than those given in state court actions.[13] Health information managers dealing with subpoenas should become familiar with the requirements of a valid subpoena for their particular jurisdiction.

AO 88 (Rev. 1/94) Subpoena in a Civil Case

Issued by the
UNITED STATES DISTRICT COURT
DISTRICT OF

V.

SUBPOENA IN A CIVIL CASE

CASE NUMBER:[1]

TO:

☐ YOU ARE COMMANDED to appear in the United States District Court at the place, date, and time specified below to testify in the above case.

PLACE OF TESTIMONY	COURTROOM
	DATE AND TIME

☐ YOU ARE COMMANDED to appear at the place, date, and time specified below to testify at the taking of a deposition in the above case.

PLACE OF DEPOSITION	DATE AND TIME

☐ YOU ARE COMMANDED to produce and permit inspection and copying of the following documents or objects at the place, date, and time specified below (list documents or objects):

PLACE	DATE AND TIME

☐ YOU ARE COMMANDED to permit inspection of the following premises at the date and time specified below.

PREMISES	DATE AND TIME

Any organization not a party to this suit that is subpoenaed for the taking of a deposition shall designate one or more officers, directors, or managing agents, or other persons who consent to testify on its behalf, and may set forth, for each person designated, the matters on which the person will testify. Federal Rules of Civil Procedure, 30(b)(6).

ISSUING OFFICER SIGNATURE AND TITLE (INDICATE IF ATTORNEY FOR PLAINTIFF OR DEFENDANT)	DATE

ISSUING OFFICER'S NAME, ADDRESS AND PHONE NUMBER

(See Rule 45, Federal Rules of Civil Procedure, Parts C & D on Reverse)

[1] If action is pending in district other than district of issuance, state district under case number.

(continues)

Figure 7-3. Subpoena in a Civil Case: A U.S. Government Document

AO 88 (Rev. 1/94) Subpoena in a Civil Case

PROOF OF SERVICE

	DATE	PLACE
SERVED		

SERVED ON (PRINT NAME) MANNER OF SERVICE

SERVED BY (PRINT NAME) TITLE

DECLARATION OF SERVER

I declare under penalty of perjury under the laws of the United States of America that the foregoing information contained in the Proof of Service is true and correct.

Executed on ____________________
DATE

SIGNATURE OF SERVER

ADDRESS OF SERVER

Rule 45, Federal Rules of Civil Procedure, Parts C & D:

(c) PROTECTION OF PERSONS SUBJECT TO SUBPOENAS.

(1) A party or an attorney responsible for the issuance and service of a subpoena shall take reasonable steps to avoid imposing undue burden or expense on a person subject to that subpoena. The court on behalf of which the subpoena was issued shall enforce this duty and impose upon the party or attorney in breach of this duty an appropriate sanction which may include, but is not limited to, lost earnings and reasonable attorney's fee.

(2) (A) A person commanded to produce and permit inspection and copying of designated books, papers, documents or tangible things, or inspection of premises need not appear in person at the place of production or inspection unless commanded to appear for deposition, hearing or trial.

(B) Subject to paragraph (d)(2) of this rule, a person commanded to produce and permit inspection and copying may, within 14 days after service of subpoena or before the time specified for compliance if such time is less than 14 days after service, serve upon the party or attorney designated in the subpoena written objection to inspection or copying of any or all of the designated materials or of the premises. If objection is made, the party serving the subpoena shall not be entitled to inspect and copy materials or inspect the premises except pursuant to an order of the court by which the subpoena was issued. If objection has been made, the party serving the subpoena may, upon notice to the person commanded to produce, move at any time for an order to compel the production. Such an order to compel production shall protect any person who is not a party or an officer of a party from significant expense resulting from the inspection and copying commanded.

(3) (A) On timely motion, the court by which a subpoena was issued shall quash or modify the subpoena if it

(i) fails to allow reasonable time for compliance;

(ii) requires a person who is not a party or an officer of a party to travel to a place more than 100 miles from the place where that person resides, is employed or regularly transacts business in person, except that, subject to the provisions of clause (c)(3)(B)(iii) of this rule, such a person may in order to attend trial be commanded to travel from any such place within the state in which the trial is held, or

(iii) requires disclosure of privileged or other protected matter and no exception or waiver applies, or

(iv) subjects a person to undue burden.

(B) If a subpoena

(i) requires disclosure of a trade secret or other confidential research development, or commercial information, or

(ii) requires disclosure of an unretained expert's opinion or information not describing specific events or occurrences in dispute and resulting from the expert's study made not at the request of any party, or

(iii) requires a person who is not a party or an officer of a party to incur substantial expense to travel more than 100 miles to attend trial, the court may, to protect a person subject to or affected by the subpoena, quash or modify the subpoena, or, if the party in whose behalf the subpoena is issued shows a substantial need for the testimony or material that cannot be otherwise met without undue hardship and assures that the person to whom the subpoena is addressed will be reasonably compensated, the court may order appearance or production only upon specified conditions.

(d) DUTIES IN RESPONDING TO SUBPOENA.

(1) A person responding to a subpoena to produce documents shall produce them as they are kept in the usual course of business or shall organize and label them to correspond with the categories in the demand.

(2) When information subject to a subpoena is withheld on a claim that it is privileged or subject to protection as trial preparation materials, the claim shall be made expressly and shall be supported by a description of the nature of the documents, communications, or things not produced that is sufficient to enable the demanding party to contest the claim.

Figure 7-3. *(continued)*

1. Name of court where lawsuit is brought
2. Names of the parties to the lawsuit
3. Docket number of the case
4. Date, time, and place of the requested appearance
5. Specific documents to be produced if a subpoena duces tecum is involved
6. Name and telephone number of attorney who requested the subpoena
7. Signature, stamp, or seal of the official empowered to issue the subpoena
8. Witness fees, where provided by law

Figure 7-4. Common Elements of a Valid Subpoena

Court Orders

In addition to subpoenas, health information managers may be presented with court orders authorizing disclosure of patient-specific health information. A **court order** differs from a subpoena in that the court order authorizes disclosure that would otherwise be prohibited by statute and regulation. A subpoena cannot authorize disclosure that would otherwise be prohibited by statute and regulation; a subpoena is subject to any and all legal defenses created by statute, regulation, and common law. The method used to apply for a court order authorizing disclosure is subject to regulation and rules of court and may vary by jurisdiction.

In certain situations, such as where the treatment of substance abuse is present, disclosure of portions of the medical record or the record in whole is mandated only upon presentation of both a subpoena duces tecum and a court order.[14] The components of a court order authorizing disclosure in such a situation are illustrated in Figure 7-5.

A variation of a court order is a show cause order. A **show cause order** is a court decree directing a person or organization to appear in court and explain why the court should not take a proposed action. If the person or organization fails to appear or sufficiently persuade the court to take no action, the court will take the action originally proposed. In the health information context, show cause orders may be issued in the event of no response to the subpoena or court order originally issued.

---

1. Name of court issuing order authorizing disclosure
2. Names of the parties to the lawsuit
3. Docket number of the case
4. Limitations for disclosure of only those components of the patient's records that are essential to fulfill the objective of the order
5. Limitations for disclosure to those persons whose need for information is the basis for the order
6. Any other limitations on disclosure that serve to protect the patient, the physician–patient relationship, and/or the treatment given, such as sealing the court proceeding from public scrutiny
7. Signature of judge authorizing disclosure

Figure 7-5. Components of a Valid Court Order Authorizing Disclosure

Response Methods

Before ever being presented with a subpoena or court order, the health information manager should have in place a policy and procedure addressing how to respond. This policy should be developed with the advice of the health-care provider's legal counsel and should address the division of labor between the health information manager and counsel. Where the instances of subpoenas are minimal, it may be appropriate for the health information manager to consult with or forward to counsel all subpoenas received. Where instances of subpoenas are not minimal, involvement of counsel each time may be cost-prohibitive and impractical, and the health information manager could handle all subpoenas, referring to counsel only those that present problems.

As an initial matter, the health information manager should not automatically assume that every subpoena presented requires the release of the information requested. If such an assumption is made and the information released is subject to a valid legal defense such as the physician–patient privilege, the health information manager subjects the health-care provider to potential liability for improper release of records. The health information manager should first determine whether subpoenas issued in his particular jurisdiction also require valid written consent given by the patient before release is made.[15] The health information manager should also determine whether the information requested involves treatment for substance abuse, mental health, or AIDS—all areas subject to strict confidentiality protections.

One case illustrating the difficulties of responding to a subpoena for health information subject to strict confidentiality protections is *John Roe v. Jane Doe.*[16] In *Roe*, a physician received both a subpoena and a signed release of information authorizing release of information regarding the patient's workers' compensation claim. The physician complied with the subpoena by forwarding the patient's entire medical record to the requesting attorney.

In the patient's subsequent lawsuit for breach of confidentiality, the court held that the physician improperly disclosed her patient's HIV status and was liable for punitive damages. Specifically, the court noted that the signed release of information that accompanied the subpoena was not sufficient under New York law to permit disclosure of HIV information. Only a signed release of information that specifically authorized release of HIV information and use of a form developed or approved by the State of New York would have permitted such disclosure. For more details concerning disclosure of HIV information, see Chapter 10.

If after determining that the information requested cannot be released because of the confidentiality restrictions listed previously or because of the potential for another valid legal defense, the health information manager has several choices of how to respond. First, he may refer these problematic subpoenas to the health-care provider's legal counsel for assistance. If the health-care provider has been named a party in the lawsuit, prompt referral of the subpoena to counsel is always in order. The counsel in turn has several choices, including (1) responding by letter to the requesting attorney informing him of the health-care provider's refusal to release the requested information; (2) filing with the court a motion to quash the subpoena; or (3) where appropriate, advising the health information manager to release the requested information in whole or in part. If the court denies counsel's motion to quash the subpoena, it will issue a court order authorizing release of the requested information.

A second option is for the health information manager to contact the requesting attorney and make a noncommittal response acknowledging the confidentiality restrictions under which the health-care provider operates. The health information manager should then forward to the requesting attorney a predrafted release form to be signed by the patient that complies with all applicable confidentiality restrictions. Upon receipt of this completed release form, the health information manager may then release the requested information.

A third available option is to excise those portions of the medical record that the health information manager determines are protected and release the remainder. When exercising this option, the health information manager is advised to inform requesting counsel that he complied with the subpoena in part and that the nonreleased information is subject to confidentiality protections barring release without a court order or a valid consent given by the patient.

At no time should the health information manager ignore the subpoena. Substantial penalties exist for failing to obey a subpoena, including fines and contempt of court proceedings.[17] If the health information manager questions the validity of the subpoena or whether it should be honored, consultation with the health-care provider's counsel to determine how to proceed is in order.

Conclusion

In the course of any given day, a health information manager may be presented with either a court order authorizing disclosure of health information, a subpoena requesting health information, or both. In order to respond to these situations, the health information manager must possess knowledge of the similarities and differences between these types of legal process and the role a medical record plays in a lawsuit. Armed with this knowledge, the health information manager can develop policies and procedures that both protect the health-care provider and comply with applicable legal requirements.

Case Study

You supervise the correspondence unit of the health information services department of a medical center. Today, you received a subpoena duces tecum from an attorney, demanding either the originals or copies of all medical records concerning Mary Smith, who allegedly is or was a patient of the medical center. The subpoena lacks sufficient information for you to determine whether Mary Smith is or was a patient in your facility. The subpoena is not accompanied by a valid authorization to release information for Mary Smith, as required in your state. How should you respond to the subpoena?

Review Questions

1. What are the legal uses of the medical record?
2. Are the entries made in the medical record ordinarily subject to cross-examination? Why or why not?
3. What questions are typically presented to the custodian of records in order to introduce a medical record into evidence?
4. What legal processes may be used to remove the medical record from the health-care provider's safekeeping?
5. Compare and contrast a subpoena, a subpoena ad testificandum, and a subpoena duces tecum.
6. Should the health information manager assume that each subpoena presented requires the release of the information requested? Why or why not?
7. How should the health information manager handle an invalid subpoena duces tecum?

Enrichment Activity

Engage in a role-playing activity with another student. One student should act as the health information manager and another as an attorney. The attorney should present the health information manager with a series of questions designed to establish the foundation and trustworthiness requirements in order to admit a medical record into evidence.

Notes

1. *See, e.g.*, Federal Business Records Act, 28 U.S.C. § 1732(a) (2000) (general business record exception); FED. R. EVID. 803(6) (general business record exception); ARK. R. EVID. 803(6); CAL. EVID. CODE § 1271 (West 2001); DEL. R. EVID. 803(6); FLA. STAT. ANN. § 90.803(6) (West 2000); IOWA CODE ANN. § 622.28 (West 2000); KAN. STAT. ANN. § 60-460(m) (2000); MASS. GEN. LAWS ANN. ch. 233, § 78 (West 2000); N.J. R. EVID. 803(c) (6); R.I. R. EVID. 803(6).

2. *See, e.g.*, GA. CODE ANN. § 24-7-8 (Michie 2000); 725 ILCS 5/115-5.1 (Smith-Hurd 2001); IND. CODE ANN. § 34-43-1-4 (West 2001); NEV. REV. STAT. § 51.135(2) (1994).
3. *See, e.g.*, ARK. R. EVID. 803(8); DEL. R. EVID. 803(8); FLA. STAT. ANN. § 90.803(8) (West 2001); HAW. R. EVID. 803(b) (8); KAN. STAT. ANN. § 60-460(o) (2000); N.J. R. EVID. 803(c) (8); R.I. R. EVID. 803(8).
4. FED. R. EVID. 803(6).
5. 23 CHARLES A. WRIGHT & KENNETH W. GRAHAM, JR., FEDERAL PRACTICE AND PROCEDURE: EVIDENCE § 93 (1980).
6. *See, e.g.*, ARK. CODE ANN. § 16-41-101 (Michie 1999); CAL. EVID. CODE §§ 990-995 (West 2000); GA. CODE ANN. § 24-9-40 (Michie 2000); KAN. STAT. ANN. § 60-427 (1983); MICH. COMP. LAWS ANN. § 600.2157 (West 2001); MISS. CODE ANN. § 13-1-21 (Supp. 2001); NEB. REV. STAT. § 27-504 (1989); N.J. STAT. ANN. §§ 2A:84A-22.1 to :84A-22.2 (West 2001); OHIO REV. CODE ANN. § 2317.02(B) (1) (Baldwin 2001); OKLA. STAT. ANN. tit. 12, § 2503 (West 2000); S.D. CODIFIED LAWS ANN. §§ 19-13-6 to -8 (2000); WIS. STAT. ANN. § 905.04 (West 2001).
7. BLACK'S LAW DICTIONARY 1440 (7th Ed. 1999).
8. *Id.*
9. FED. R. CIV. P. 45(a).
10. *See, e.g.*, ALA. R. CIV. P. 45(a); KY. R. CIV. P. 45.01; MO. SUP. CT. R. 57.09(b) TENN. R. CIV. P. 45.01; VT. R. CIV. P. 45(a).
11. FED. R. CIV. P. 45(a).
12. *See, e.g.*, MO. SUP. CT. R. 30 (providing three days' notice).
13. *Compare*, 28 U.S.C. § 1821 (2000); FED. R. CIV. P. 45(c) (offering $40 per day including travel time) with ARK. R. CIV. P. 45(d) (offering $30 per day) and MO. REV. STAT. § 491.280.1 (2001); MO. SUP. CT. R. 57.09(c) (offering $3 per day for county residents; $4 for out-of-county residents).
14. 42 C.F.R. § 2.61(a-b) (2000).
15. Such is the case in Ohio where information subject to the physician–patient privilege may not be released pursuant to a subpoena without presentation of a valid consent given by the patient. *Pacheco v. Ortiz*, 463 N.E. 2d 670, 671 (Cuyahoga Cty. 1983); *see also, Henry v. Lewis*, 102 A.D. 2d 430 (N.Y. App. Div. 1984); *People v. Bickham*, 431 N.E.2d 365 (Ill. 1982).
16. 599 N.Y.S.2d 350 (N.Y. App. Div. 1993).
17. *See, e.g.*, ARK. R. CIV. P. 45(g); CAL. CIV. PROC. CODE § 202(h) (West 2001); DEL. R. CIV. PROC. 45(f); HAW. R. CIV. PROC. 45(f); MO. REV. STAT. § 491.140-.200 (2001); MO. S. CT. R. 57.09(e).

Chapter 8

Specialized Patient Records

Learning Objectives

After reading this chapter, the learner should be able to:

1. Summarize the difference between specialized patient records and general medical records.
2. Discuss the regulations governing patient identification and their practical application.
3. Compare and contrast release of information forms used in an ordinary health-care setting with those used in a substance abuse setting.
4. Identify those instances where disclosure of health information of substance abuse treatment may be made without written patient consent.
5. Compare and contrast a court order authorizing disclosure of patient-specific information with a subpoena duces tecum.
6. Discuss procedures for handling a court order authorizing disclosure and a subpoena duces tecum.
7. Explain the difference between the official record and the personal record in the mental health/developmental disability context.
8. Identify the sources of legal requirements in the home health-care context.
9. Summarize the benefits and risks associated with genetic information.

Key Concepts

- Disclosure with patient authorization
- Disclosure without patient authorization
- Genetic information
- Official record
- Patient identification
- Patient notice
- Personal record
- Release of information
- Specialized patient records
- Treatment program

Introduction

Although all health information must be treated with care, certain categories of health information demand special treatment. In particular, the health information of those patients undergoing treatment for certain illnesses, such as substance abuse or mental illness, or in nonacute-care settings, such as the patient's home, are subject to legal requirements that differ from those of an acute-care setting. For purposes of this chapter, health information records for these illnesses or in these settings are referred to as **specialized patient records.**

One distinguishing aspect between specialized patient records and general medical records is the nature of the information present in the record. Specialized patient records contain not only truly medical information, but also therapeutic mental and emotional information. The volume of this therapeutic mental and emotional information is often greater than that contained in a general medical record, as in substance abuse cases in which information may be recorded about the patient's coming to grips with her problem. Such a variety of information, combined with the lengths of stay of many of these patients, creates a voluminous medical record, thereby raising storage concerns, which in turn implicate record retention policies.

Specialized patient records also differ concerning who makes entries in the record. In a general medical record, entries are made by professionals who are licensed and certified, such as the physician who admitted the patient and gave orders directing her care, the nurse who administered medications, and the physical therapist who noted the patient's progress. These health-care providers are governed by statutes, rules and regulations, and professional guidelines that address the manner in which they treat a patient and how to document that care properly.

By contrast, a specialized patient record involving substance abuse or mental health will not only include entries by those professionals listed above but also by paraprofessionals, such as teachers, if the patient is a juvenile, or counselors with no license or certification but experience with the illness in question. These paraprofessionals play a role in the treatment of the patient and therefore must document their role in patient care. In many instances, the licensing authority regulating the facility providing the treatment only regulates entries in the record in the context of professionals rendering treatment. In such instances, the question becomes whether the licensing authority permits entries in the record by paraprofessionals and, if so, what rules and regulations govern those entries.

Finally, the health information of those patients who receive treatment for substance abuse or a mental illness are subject to stricter confidentiality requirements than the health information of those patients receiving medical care in an acute-care setting. For example, confidentiality requirements in the context of substance abuse often provide that the health-care facility cannot confirm that the patient is, has been, or ever was a patient at the facility, absent the patient's permission to do so.

Because of these differences, the health information manager must be aware of the legal requirements to which specialized patient records are subject. By understanding these requirements, the health information manager can create effective policies that manage specialized patient records while addressing legal concerns and issues.

Drug and Alcohol Abuse

As a general rule, most legal questions associated with health information management cannot be answered by looking to federal law. One exception to this rule exists in the context of drug and alcohol abuse treatment. In such a context, federal law speaks directly to the handling of health information.

Two federal laws place restrictions on the disclosure and use of substance abuse patient records: the Drug Abuse Prevention, Treatment and Rehabilitation Act addressing drug abuse patient records[1] and the Comprehensive Alcohol Abuse and Alcoholism Prevention, Treatment and Rehabilitation Act of 1970 addressing alcohol abuse patient records.[2] Both laws delegate to the secretary of health and human services the power to promulgate rules and regulations imposing restrictions on these records.

The rules and regulations[3] that the secretary has promulgated apply to all treatment programs that receive federal assistance.[4] A **treatment program** is defined to include entities whose sole purpose is to provide alcohol or drug abuse diagnosis or treatment. The definition also includes general medical-care facilities *if* (a) there is an identified unit for diagnosis, treatment, or referral or (b) medical personnel or other staff whose primary function is to provide such services and who are identified as such providers. Because the federal assistance can be either direct or indirect, virtually every substance abuse program operated in the United States is subject to these laws.[5]

The federal regulations at issue are broad in scope and detail and address many issues central to management of health information. All health information managers working in the substance abuse area must become familiar with these regulations. The theme underlying these regulations is that health information contained in patient records is confidential; therefore, only **disclosure with patient authorization,** should be permitted. Thus, this discussion focuses on two main areas: confidentiality and release of information, and only briefly addresses other issues.

Confidentiality

Patient Identification

Under the applicable regulations, confidentiality of health information is much stricter than that in an acute-care setting. The regulations restrict identification of a patient who is in a facility or component of a facility publicly identified as providing substance abuse treatment. Acknowledgment of the presence or past presence of a patient can be made only with the patient's written consent or subject to a court order entered in compliance with the regulations.[6]

In practice, the issue of **patient identification** comes into play because of the number of inquiries treatment programs receive concerning their patients. The applicable regulations place an unconditional obligation on the programs not to identify in any way the patients they treat or have treated. These regulations do not, however, prevent a program from disclosing that a patient is not and never was a patient with their program. And the regulations do permit acknowledgment of a patient's presence if the facility is not publicly identified as only a substance abuse facility and if acknowledgment would not reveal that the patient is a substance abuser.[7]

The contradiction presented by the regulations raises a practical dilemma: if some inquiries are answered with the response that the law prevents disclosure that a person currently is or previously was a patient, and other inquiries are answered that the person currently is not and previously was not a patient, it will not take much detective work to determine whether a person is or was a patient in the treatment program. The regulations address this dilemma in a backhanded way. The regulations suggest that an inquiring party may be informed of the regulations and advised that disclosure of patient-specific information is restricted by these regulations, without giving away that the restriction applies to any particular patient. As a practical matter, health information managers may wish to adopt a uniform method of answering these inquiries, subject to the advice of legal counsel.

Patient Notice

Patients must be given notice of federal confidentiality requirements upon admission to the program or soon after. This **patient notice** must include a written summary of the federal law and regulations.[8] The regulations allow programs to develop their own notices or use a sample notice. This sample notice is illustrated in Figure 8-1. Because the regulations require unconditional compliance, it is important that every treatment program document in each patient's medical record that such notice was given and the time frame in which it was given.

Release of Information

Federal regulations governing the disclosure of patient information fall into three categories: (1) disclosures made with written patient authorization, (2) those made without written patient authorization but pursuant to federal regulation, and (3) those made subject to a valid court order.

Disclosure with Written Patient Authorization

Release of information form

Disclosure of patient information in the substance abuse context involves the use of a **release of information** form, a document that permits the dissemination of confidential health information to third parties. To be valid, the completed written authorization form must meet the requirements of

The confidentiality of alcohol and drug abuse patient records maintained by this program is protected by Federal law and regulations. Generally, the program may not say to a person outside the program that a patient attends the program, or disclose any information identifying a patient as an alcohol or drug abuser unless:

(1) The patient consents in writing;
(2) The disclosure is allowed by a court order; or
(3) The disclosure is made to medical personnel in a medical emergency or to qualified personnel for research, audit, or program evaluation.

Violation of the Federal law and regulations by a program is a crime. Suspected violations may be reported to appropriate authorities in accordance with Federal regulations.

Federal law and regulations do not protect any information about a crime committed by a patient either at the program or against any person who works for the program or about any threat to commit such a crime.

Federal laws and regulations do not protect any information about suspected child abuse or neglect from being reported under State law to appropriate State or local authorities.

Figure 8-1. Sample Notice: Confidentiality of Alcohol and Drug Abuse Patient Records
(42 C.F.R., Ch. 1, Part 2 § 2.22(d) (2001))

the regulations. Similar to the components of a valid general release of information form, a release of information form in the substance abuse context must identify the patient, the program that should release the information, the program or person who should receive the information, what information is to be disclosed, and include the patient's signature and date. In addition, the consent must identify the purpose of the disclosure, include a statement indicating that the consent is subject to revocation at any time, and include a date, event, or condition upon which the authorization will expire if not revoked before. The components of a valid authorization are illustrated in Figure 8-2.

The regulations allow programs to develop their own forms that comply with the regulations or use a sample form. This sample form, illus-

A written authorization to a disclosure under these regulations must include:

(1) The specific name or general designation of the program or person permitted to make the disclosure.

(2) The name or title of the individual or the name of the organization to which disclosure is to be made.

(3) The name of the patient.

(4) The purpose of the disclosure.

(5) How much and what kind of information is to be disclosed.

(6) The signature of the patient and, when required for a patient who is a minor, the signature of a person authorized to give consent under § 2.14; or, when required for a patient who is incompetent or deceased, the signature of a person authorized to sign under § 2.15 in lieu of the patient.

(7) The date on which the consent is signed.

(8) A statement that the consent is subject to revocation at any time except to the extent that the program or person which is to make the disclosure has already acted in reliance on it. Acting in reliance includes the provision of treatment services in reliance on a valid consent to disclose information to a third party payor.

(9) The date, event, or condition upon which the consent will expire if not revoked before. This date, event, or condition must ensure that the consent will last no longer than reasonably necessary to serve the purpose for which it is given.

Figure 8-2. Components of a Valid Authorization
(42 C.F.R., Ch. 1, Part 2 § 2.31(a) (2001))

trated in Figure 8-3, contains reference to the signature of the parent or guardian where required. The question of whether a minor can authorize disclosure of health information in the substance abuse context is dependent on whether the applicable state law permits the minor to consent for treatment. Where the minor can apply for and obtain substance abuse treatment on her own behalf, she may also authorize disclosure of health information. Conversely, where state law requires parental consent to

The following form complies with paragraph (a) of this section, but other elements may be added.

1. I (name of patient) Request Authorize:
2. (name or general designation of program which is to make the disclosure)
3. To disclose: (kind and amount of information to be disclosed)
4. To: (name or title of the person or organization to which disclosure is to be made)
5. For (purpose of the disclosure)
6. Date (on which this consent is signed)
7. Signature of patient
8. Signature of parent or guardian (where required)
9. Signature of person authorized to sign in lieu of the patient (where required)
10. This consent is subject to revocation at any time except to the extent that the program which is to make the disclosure has already taken action in reliance on it. If not previously revoked, this consent will terminate upon: (specific date, event, or condition).

Figure 8-3. Sample Authorization Form
(42 C.F.R., Ch. 1, Part 2, § 2.31(b) (2001))

treatment, the authorization to disclose health information must contain signatures of both the minor patient and the parent or guardian.

A release of information form that does not comply with the regulations is not valid. Examples of invalid release forms include those in which any of the elements are missing, the consent period has expired or is known to have been revoked, or the form contains information that the health information manager knows is false or reasonably should know is false. Health information managers should develop policies on how to respond to invalid authorization forms after first reviewing the regulations and speaking with legal counsel as necessary.

Notice accompanying disclosure

Another difference between a general release of information and that used for substance abuse programs is the regulation prohibiting redisclosure. Federal regulations prohibit the person or facility receiving the patient information from further disclosing the information unless the patient has given written consent addressing this redisclosure. A notice prohibiting redisclosure must accompany any disclosure of patient-specific information.

In this situation, the regulations do not give any freedom to the program to develop the notice prohibiting redisclosure. Rather, each program must use the statement listed in the regulation. This statement is illustrated in Figure 8-4.

In the light of the unconditional compliance required by the regulations, it is important that each treatment program releasing patient information make special efforts to ensure that the receiving party understands that the patient information it receives is confidential and not available for redisclosure. At minimum, the statement prohibiting redisclosure must accompany any disclosure of patient information. Whether additional efforts should be made, such as placing a stamp on each page indicating that no further dissemination is allowed, is a policy question subject to time and cost constraints and the advice of counsel.

This information has been disclosed to you from records protected by Federal confidentiality rules (42 CFR part 2). The Federal rules prohibit you from making any further disclosure of this information unless further disclosure is expressly permitted by the written consent of the person to whom it pertains or as otherwise permitted by 42 CFR part 2. A general authorization for the release of medical or other information is NOT sufficient for this purpose. The Federal rules restrict any use of the information to criminally investigate or prosecute any alcohol or drug abuse patient.

Figure 8-4. Notice Prohibiting Redisclosure
(42 C.F.R., Ch. 1, Part 2 § 2.32 (2001))

Disclosure without Written Patient Authorization

As the regulations illustrate, the sensitive nature of patient information in the substance abuse context requires release of patient information by written authorization. The regulations recognize only limited exceptions to the written authorization requirement.

Medical emergencies

The first exception applies to medical emergencies. Patient-identifying information may be released without written consent to medical personnel providing emergency treatment. The emergency treatment is defined as "treating a condition which poses an immediate threat to the health of any individual and which requires immediate medical intervention."[9]

One potential medical emergency may involve an error in manufacturing or packaging of drugs. Such disclosure would be made to Food and Drug Administration (FDA) personnel where there is reason to believe that an individual's health would be threatened because of an error in manufacturing, labeling, or selling a drug under the FDA's jurisdiction. The FDA uses this patient information to notify patients and their physicians of potential dangers.

In every instance where a release is made pursuant to a medical emergency, the treatment program must document the disclosure in the patient record. This documentation must include the name of the medical personnel to whom disclosure was made and their affiliation to any health-care facility, the name of the person making the disclosure, the date and time of disclosure, and the nature of emergency or error.[10]

Research activities

The second exception applies to scientific research activities that meet specific requirements. Patient-specific information may be disclosed for research purposes only after the treatment program director determines that the researcher is qualified to conduct the research and has a research protocol that both ensures security of the information disclosed and prohibits redisclosure. The researcher may not identify individual patients in reports and may disclose patient-identifying information only back to the treatment program.[11]

Audit activities

Audits of patient-specific information by qualified organizations and individuals may be conducted without written patient consent if regulatory requirements are met. Access to the information may be provided to persons (1) acting on behalf of a federal, state, or local governmental agency that provides financial assistance to the treatment program, or by law regulates the treatment program, (2) acting on behalf of third-party payors, peer review organizations, or private organizations providing financial assistance, or (3) qualified to conduct the audit, as determined by the program director.

After meeting these qualifications, the auditor must agree in writing that the information gathered in the audit will be used only for audit or evaluation purposes or to investigate or prosecute crimes or other activities, as authorized by court order. The auditor must also agree in writing that she will disclose patient-specific information back to the treatment program only. Finally, if copies of records are made or if records are removed from the program's premises, the auditor must agree in writing to maintain the information in accordance with certain security requirements and destroy patient-specific information upon completion of the audit. A peer review organization acting on behalf of Medicare or Medicaid may redisclose patient-identifying information to the Medicare/Medicaid program.[12]

Disclosures Pursuant to Court Orders

In the course of any given day, a health information manager at a substance abuse treatment program may be presented with either a court order authorizing disclosure of patient-specific information, a subpoena requesting patient-specific information, or both. Court orders and subpoenas are issued for a variety of reasons: to investigate or prosecute a crime, to protect against an existing threat or serious bodily injury, or to present evidence of a patient's substance abuse treatment in a legal proceeding where the patient has placed her treatment at issue.

It is important to understand the differences between these two legal documents. A court order authorizes disclosure of patient-specific information that would otherwise be prohibited by statute and regulation. It does not, however, *require* the disclosure of this information. A subpoena or subpoena duces tecum is a command to appear and/or present certain documents and other things. A subpoena or subpoena duces tecum *alone* does not authorize disclosure of information that would otherwise be prohibited by statute and regulation. In combination, however, these documents *mandate* disclosure of patient-specific information unless a valid legal defense exists against disclosure.[13]

The method used to apply for a court order authorizing disclosure is subject to regulation and is illustrated in Figure 8-5. The components of a valid court order authorizing disclosure are presented in Figure 8-6. Court orders authorizing disclosure will only be issued upon a finding of good cause: there exists no other way to obtain the information and the public interest and need for disclosure outweighs the potential impact on the patient.

How a health information manager handles these court orders and subpoenas in practice is a matter governed by both federal regulation and common sense. For example, a request by a law enforcement official or related agency for patient information that is not accompanied by a court order authorizing disclosure must be treated under the regulations like requests seeking patient identification addressed previously in this chap-

---

(a) Application: The application must use a fictitious name such as John Doe to refer to the patient and may not contain or otherwise disclose any patient identifying information unless the patient is the applicant or has given written consent or the court has ordered the record sealed from public scrutiny.

(b) Notice: The patient and the person holding the records from whom disclosure is sought must be given adequate notice in a manner which will not disclose patient identifying information to other persons and an opportunity to file a written response to the application or appear in person for the limited purpose of providing evidence.

(c) Review of Evidence: Any oral argument, review of evidence, or hearing on the application must be held in the judge's chambers or in some manner which ensures that patient identifying information is not disclosed to anyone other than a party to the proceeding, the patient, or the person holding the record, unless the patient requests an open hearing in a manner which meets the written consent requirements of these regulations. The proceeding may include an examination by the judge of the patient records referred to in the application.

Figure 8-5. Procedures for Applying for Court Orders Authorizing Disclosure (42 C.F.R., Ch. 1, Part 2 § 2.64 (2001))

An order authorizing disclosure must:

(1) Limit disclosure to those parts of the patient's record which are essential to fulfill the objective of the order;
(2) Limit disclosure to those persons whose need for information is the basis for the order; and
(3) Include such other measures as are necessary to limit disclosure for the protection of the patient, the physician–patient relationship and the treatment services; for example, sealing from public scrutiny the record of any proceeding for which disclosure of a patient's record has been ordered.

Figure 8-6. Components of a Valid Court Order Authorizing Disclosure (42 C.F.R., Ch. 1, Part 2 § 2.64(e) (2001))

ter: with a noncommittal response acknowledging the confidentiality restrictions under which the treatment program operates. The mere fact that the request is made by a law enforcement official is not sufficient to overcome the restrictions imposed by the regulations.

Similarly, a subpoena served upon the treatment program by an attorney without a court order does not require under the regulations automatic disclosure of the information sought. That is not to say that the subpoena should be ignored. Rather, health information managers should develop a procedure for handling these situations, such as contacting the attorney upon receipt of the subpoena, informing him of the regulations prohibiting disclosure, and notifying him that a court order is necessary before the health information manager will disclose the information. Other policy considerations may include determining how to handle a court appearance, if one is necessary, and notifying the attending therapist of the subpoena and requesting her review of the record to determine whether disclosure is in the patient's best interest.

Miscellaneous Issues

Effect of State Laws

Although federal law directly regulates substance abuse patient records, these regulations expressly recognize that the states will play a role in regulating these types of records. This recognition allows the laws and regulations of the different jurisdictions (state and federal) to coexist, as opposed to excluding the states from any role.

State law and regulation may be equal to, less restrictive than, or more restrictive than federal law. Where a conflict between federal and state law appears, whichever law is stricter will apply.[14] Where a matter is not addressed by federal law, the state law will apply. For example, the federal regulations do not prohibit a patient's access to her own health information.[15] The health information manager must look to the provisions of state law to determine whether the treatment program must provide the patient access to her own health information. For more information regarding access to health information, see Chapter 5.

Disposition of Records

For a variety of reasons, a treatment program may be discontinued or acquired by another program. In those situations, the regulations expressly address the disposition of substance abuse records. Under the regulations, the records must be purged of patient-identifying information or destroyed *unless* the patient's written consent is obtained to transfer the record or the applicable statute of limitations requires that the records be maintained for a period beyond the closure or transfer.

If the transfer has not been authorized and the records must be retained for the statute of limitations period, the records must be placed in a sealed envelope or other container and labeled as follows:

> Record of [insert name of program] required to be maintained under [insert citation to statute, regulation, court order, or other legal authority requiring that records be kept] until a date not later than [insert appropriate date][16]

The regulations require that a responsible person hold these sealed and marked records in confidence until the end of the retention period specified on the label. Upon expiration of the retention period, the responsible person must destroy the records.

Enforcement and Penalties

Because one of the purposes of the regulations is to ensure that patients who seek treatment for substance abuse are not more vulnerable due to availability of their patient record than those who do not seek treatment, the regulations provide for an enforcement mechanism and criminal penalty for violations. The regulations assume that all federally assisted substance abuse programs will comply with the restrictions that the regulations impose. Any violation of the regulations may be reported to the United States attorney for the district in which the violation occurred or to the FDA if a methadone program is involved. Upon conviction, any person who violates the regulations may be fined no more than $500 if a first offense and no more than $5,000 for each subsequent offense.

Mental Health and Developmental Disability Care

The treatment of patients with mental illness and/or developmental disabilities[17] takes place in a variety of settings: inpatient psychiatric hospitals, residential treatment facilities, and therapists' offices, to name a few. Although the settings may vary, many of the legal questions concerning mental health and developmental disability information are the same as those involved in health information in general: requirements for accurate and timely documentation, retention of medical records, and confidentiality of health information. Although many similarities exist, two main differences separate health information in these contexts from that of a general medical context: (1) additional requirements for record content and (2) more stringent privacy requirements.

Content Requirements

Documentation in the mental health and developmental disability fields often involves situations not present in a general medical record. For example, these settings may involve changes in the patient's supervision (from seclusion to use of restraints, privileges, passes, and discharge), significant legal events (commitment orders, interaction with police), and the presence of suicide attempts. Furthermore, restrictions on patient rights may become necessary under certain circumstances. As a matter of both law and good medical practice, each of these situations necessitates proper documentation in the medical record.

For any psychiatric facility receiving Medicare funds, the Medicare Conditions of Participation govern. These regulations establish standards for documenting the development of assessment and diagnostic data, psychiatric evaluation, treatment plan, recording patient progress, discharge plan, and summary.[18]

Frequently, state mental health codes specify documentation requirements in these situations. Special attention must be accorded these codes in order for the health-care provider to be in compliance with state law. For example, the applicable state law may specify that a treatment facility devise a written program plan for each patient describing the patient's problems, precise goals of treatment, and the measures to be employed to reach those goals.[19] Where restraints are applied to a patient, the clinical record must reflect each use of restraint and its reason.[20] Similarly, any limitation on the patient's right to correspondence, visitors, phone calls, or access to a spiritual adviser must be documented in the clinical record, along with the reason for the limitation.[21] Any use of special treatment procedures such as electroshock therapy and neuroleptic medication also requires documentation.[22]

In addition to statutory and regulatory requirements, accrediting standards may mandate certain documentation requirements. For example, the Joint Commission on Accreditation of Healthcare Organizations (JCAHO) promulgates standards for facilities offering mental health, mental retardation, and developmental disability services. In addition to the standard documentation requirements, JCAHO requires documentation of the patient's legal status and the involvement of family members in the patient's treatment program.[23]

Another significant departure from a general medical record involves the existence of two separate records: (1) the official or public record maintained by the treatment facility and (2) the personal record maintained by the clinician. The **official record** contains that information necessary to document the patient's care and treatment: history and mental status exam, consent forms, treatment plans, physician orders, laboratory results, and so forth. This is the record required to be maintained by law.

By contrast, the **personal record** maintained by the clinician consists of notes in the clinician's sole possession that give the clinician's viewpoint of the patient and their communications. The clinician's personal record does not substitute for progress notes in the official record and is kept separate from the official record. There is no legal requirement that a personal record be maintained in addition to the official record. In some jurisdictions, a personal record maintained by a clinician is considered to be the clinician's private property and work product, and may not be subject to discovery in a legal or administrative proceeding.[24]

Privacy Restrictions

As important as confidentiality and release of information are to health information professionals, they are particularly critical to the performance of health information professionals practicing in the mental health and developmental disability fields. This is so because of the additional legal restrictions under which these fields operate.

Patient Identification

As with facilities offering substance abuse treatment, facilities offering mental health and developmental disability treatment are subject to strict confidentiality requirements. The fact that an individual is, was, or will be a patient at the facility may not be disclosed absent patient consent.[25] This type of restriction poses the same practical dilemma as in the substance abuse treatment contest: how to answer inquiries into patient status. As in that context, the health information manager should develop policies that do not tolerate any disclosure of patient-specific information absent patient consent.

Release of Information

Patient-specific information recorded and communications made in the course of providing mental health or developmental disability services are considered confidential and may not be disclosed except as provided by law. Disclosure may be made pursuant to a patient's written authorization, without a patient's written authorization under limited circumstances, or pursuant to a court order. Because no one federal law addresses the disclosure issue, state law must be reviewed. Due to the comprehensive nature of the Illinois Mental Health and Developmental Disabilities Confidentiality Act, it will serve as illustration throughout this section. In practice, the health information manager must review the law of the state in which treatment is given to determine the governing requirements.

Disclosure with written patient authorization

To be valid, a release of information form must be in writing and meet the specifications of state law. For example, the Illinois act specifically addresses the content of the authorization form. These directives include the person to whom disclosure is to be made, the purpose for disclosure, the nature of the information to be disclosed, the right to inspect and copy the information to be disclosed, the consequences of refusal to authorize, an expiration of authorization date, the right to revoke authorization at any time, and the signatures and date of the patient and of a witness who can attest to the identity of the patient. Any revocation of authorization must be in writing and witnessed. Whatever action taken pursuant to the authorization form and the authorization form itself must then become part of the record.[26]

As in the substance abuse context, any information disclosed pursuant to the patient's written authorization may not be redisclosed to another party, absent patient authorization. The health information manager in practice must determine what steps should be made to notify the recipient of this prohibition on redisclosure. These steps should be made part of written policy and procedure.

Disclosure without written patient authorization

Patient-specific information may be disclosed without patient authorization only where statutory or regulatory authority allows disclosure. Similar to the substance abuse context, state law may allow **disclosure without patient authorization** to health-care personnel within the treatment facility or under the treating clinician's supervision.[27] So that disclosure without patient authorization is made only to those health-care personnel with a need to know, the health information professional should formulate a release of information policy that specifically lists departments or individuals affiliated with the treatment facility who meet the need to know test.

Disclosure without written patient authorization may also be permitted by state law to persons conducting peer review, an attorney defending the treatment facility, and any agency that has custody of the recipient.[28] Further, such disclosure may be made to the parents or legal guardian of the resident, to law enforcement officers, or to the court in a judicial proceeding.[29] Because the authority to disclose without patient authorization is based on state law, the health information professional should become familiar with the applicable state law.

Disclosure pursuant to court order

Just as in the substance abuse context, the health information professional may be presented with a subpoena or court order authorizing disclosure of mental health or developmental disability information.[30] How the health information manager responds is a matter governed by state law and policy of the treatment facility. Under no circumstances, however, should either of these documents be ignored.

Home Health Care

As in any other portion of the health-care delivery system, health information in the home health-care setting is subject to legal considerations. Unfortunately, no one comprehensive law exists that addresses the legal requirements for home health care. Rather, the legal requirements arise from a myriad of sources: the Medicare Conditions of Participation, state law and regulation, and accrediting standards. Although each source is separate, they must be reviewed together to obtain an understanding of the legal requirements governing home health care.

For any home health-care agency receiving Medicare funds, the Medicare Conditions of Participation govern. These regulations outline the qualifications for home health agency staff and detail the rights of patients treated by that staff. The regulations require that the patient be informed of her rights in advance of or during the initial treatment, and that the agency maintain documentation of that notification. The regulations also specify that all clinical records maintained by the home health agency are confidential and that the agency must advise the patient of its policies and procedures regarding the disclosure of clinical records.[31]

In addition to these regulations, home health agencies must meet the requirements of state law. State law may consist of statute, regulation, or both. The applicable state law frequently contains many of the same provisions found in the Medicare regulations. For example, Florida's Home Health Services Act tracks many of the same provisions as the Medicare Conditions of Participation but adds more specificity in certain areas. Under the Florida statute, the contents of the clinical records include:

> [P]ertinent past and current medical, nursing, social and other therapeutic information, the plan of treatment, and other such information as is necessary for the safe and adequate care of the patient.[32]

The statute also addresses confidentiality and disclosure of information, specifying that the patient's written consent or that of the patient's guardian must be obtained before health information may be disclosed.[33]

Regulations are often found in the context of the state-administered Medicaid program or the licensing requirements for home health-care agencies. For example, Tennessee's licensing regulations for home health agencies include details on record content, retention, and security safeguards.[34]

Where state laws or regulations do not specifically address home health care, the health information manager should determine whether county requirements govern. These requirements would typically be issued by the county's department of health or social services.

Although accrediting standards and professional guidelines do not have the force of law, they may be used in establishing the proper standard of care in a negligence action against the home health agency. For that reason, the health information manager should pay close attention to these accrediting standards and professional guidelines. Both the Joint Commission on Accreditation of Healthcare Organizations and the Community Health Accreditation Program (CHAP) promulgate standards for community-based and hospital-based organizations offering home health services.[35] And professionals working for home health agencies are guided by the requirements of their respective professional organizations regarding confidentiality of information.

Health information managers dealing with home health-care agencies and their patient records should become familiar with federal regulations, state licensing laws and regulations, accrediting standards, and professional guidelines. It is particularly important to be aware of the differing legal requirements among states if the home health-care agency provides care to patients in more than one state so that the home health-care agency is acting in compliance with state law.

Genetic Information

Another form of specialized patient record is **genetic information**. Unlike mental health or substance abuse patient records, genetic information may not exist as a separate and distinct patient record. Rather, this information may be contained in any form or part of a medical record. Because it can be found in many different places, the potential exists for many persons to have access to this information. While genetic information may revolutionize health care by predicting diseases and revealing cures, its sensitive nature poses special challenges for protecting the confidentiality of this information and its potential for wrongful use.

Genetic information in the simplest sense means information about an individual or family obtained from a genetic test or an individual's DNA sample.[36] It differs from other health information in that it is not a current or past picture of a person's health; rather, it is a look into the person's health future.

Science has obtained this information in large measure through the work of the Human Genome Project. With funding from the U.S. Congress, the Human Genome Project is a joint effort of the U.S. Department of Energy and the National Institutes of Health. Its mission is to map and characterize each human gene.[37] As discoveries are made, research material is made available to the public on the project's GenBank web site.[38]

Health-care providers can use these research materials to assist a patient's well-being. Should a genetic test reveal that a patient has a gene for a disease that has not yet manifested itself, the health-care provider may increase diagnostic surveillance of the patient, thereby improving the patient's quality of life or chances for survival. A genetic test may also indicate that a patient is merely a carrier of a gene for a specific disease. In this case, the disease will likely not manifest itself in the patient but may manifest itself in the patient's offspring.

Benefits such as these are counterbalanced with concerns about potential misuse. Employers who gain access to their employees' genetic information may reach incorrect and damaging conclusions about the employees and take action accordingly. Health insurers may consider coverage decisions based on the potential for future manifestation of a given disease. Child custody battles could involve consideration of a parent's genetic disposition for future disease. As these concerns illustrate, it is important that genetic information be protected and used wisely.

At the federal level, concern over the misuse of genetic information in an insurance coverage decision was so widespread that Congress addressed it by passing the Health Insurance Portability and Accountability Act of 1996 (HIPAA).[39] HIPAA specifically prohibits genetic information, absent a diagnosis of a condition, from being considered a preexisting condition for health insurance purposes. HIPAA also prohibits health insurers from charging an individual a higher premium than others in a group because of the existence of genetic information. In addition to legislation, an executive order at the federal level prohibits departments and agencies of the executive branch from using genetic information in any hiring or promotion action.[40] The order also prohibits the departments and agencies from requesting or requiring genetic test results from applicants or current employees.

Various states have addressed these concerns through legislation prohibiting genetic discrimination and access to genetic information. Missouri law prohibits health insurers from requesting genetic information, inquiring into whether a person has taken or refused a genetic test, and inquiring into the results of any genetic test.[41] California law prohibits health insurers from seeking, using, or maintaining genetic information for any nontherapeutic purposes and from discriminating in the renewal of policies based on genetic characteristics.[42] Arizona law considers the results of genetic testing confidential and protects a person from being compelled to disclose the identity of an person who has taken a genetic test or the results of that test.[43] Maryland law prohibits health insurers from requesting or requiring the results of a genetic test for use in underwriting. It further requires that testing results may be released only on the written authorization of the subject of the genetic test.[44] Wisconsin law prohibits health insurers from conditioning the provision of insurance coverage or benefits or the setting of rates on genetic testing information.[45] As these examples illustrate, state legislatures have engaged in a high level of activity dealing with issues surrounding genetic information.

The health information manager's responsibility to safeguard patient-specific health information is heightened when genetic information is involved. Health information managers dealing with genetic information must remain aware of legislation at both the federal and state levels if they are to protect this information from a breach of confidentiality or improper use.

Conclusion

In order to manage specialized patient records properly, it is critical that the health information professional understand the different legal requirements that govern these specialized patient records. These legal requirements arise from a myriad of sources: statutes, regulations, accrediting standards, and professional guidelines. All must be reviewed together so that the health information professional can create effective policies that manage specialized patient records while addressing legal concerns and issues.

Case Study

You are the director of health information services in a major medical center that maintains both a psychiatric unit and a substance abuse unit in addition to general medical and surgical units. Your facility plans to join a computer network with fifteen hospitals throughout the state, which will allow online access to laboratory data, regardless of which facility performed the lab work. None of the other fifteen facilities offer psychiatric or substance abuse treatment. Identify and discuss the confidentiality issues present with such a network in the light of the statutory, regulatory, and accrediting requirements governing patients treated in these units.

Review Questions

1. What are the types of specialized patient records covered in this chapter and their distinguishing characteristics?
2. Why should substance abuse treatment programs comply with the regulations governing release of patient information?
3. What would influence a substance abuse program's decision whether to make additional efforts beyond the governing regulations to safeguard the release of patient information?
4. Documentation of what types of situations may be present in a mental health or developmental disability context that may not be present in a general medical record?
5. Why should genetic information be protected from access by the general public?
6. What is the definition of genetic information?
7. How does the Health Insurance Portability and Accountability Act apply to genetic information?

Enrichment Activities

1. Tour a substance abuse facility in your local area. Observe the method by which patients receive notice of federal confidentiality requirements,

how requests for identification of patients are handled by the facility's staff, and the manner in which the prohibition against redisclosure of patient-specific health information is handled. Compare your observations against the information you learned in this chapter concerning these areas. If a tour of such a facility is unavailable, engage in a group discussion where the group develops the facility's method of patient notification of confidentiality requirements, the method for handling patient identification requests, and the manner in which it handles the redisclosure prohibition.

2. Prepare an outline for an inservice education presentation to healthcare staff describing the special protections accorded to substance abuse patient records.

Notes

1. 21 U.S.C. § 1175, later amended and transferred to 42 U.S.C. § 290ee-3 (2000).
2. 42 U.S.C. § 4582, later amended and transferred to 42 U.S.C. § 290dd-3 (2000).
3. These regulations are titled Confidentiality of Alcohol and Drug Abuse Patient Records and can be found at 42 C.F.R. Ch. 1, Part 2, §§ 2.1-2.67 (2001).
4. Federal assistance means not only direct financial assistance but also includes: tax-exempt status, receipt of tax-deductible contributions, authority to dispense controlled substances under the Controlled Substances Act, and licensure or certification by a part of the federal government. 42 C.F.R., Ch. 1, § 2.12(b) (2001).
5. These regulations do not apply to programs maintained by the Veterans Administration because those programs are governed by separate law and regulation. *See* 38 U.S.C. § 4132 (2001).
6. 42 C.F.R. Ch. 1, § 2.13 (2001).
7. 42 C.F.R. Ch. 1, § 2.13(c) (2) (2001).
8. 42 C.F.R. Ch. 1, § 2.22 (2001).
9. 42 C.F.R. § 2.51(a) (2001).
10. 42 C.F.R. § 2.51(a-c) (2001).
11. 42 C.F.R. § 2.52(a-b) (2001).
12. 42 C.F.R. § 2.53(a-d) (2001).
13. 42 C.F.R. § 2.61(a-b) (2001).

14. 42 C.F.R. § 2.20 (2001).
15. 42 C.F.R. § 2.23(a) (2001).
16. 42 C.F.R. § 2.19(b) (2001).
17. Developmental disability commonly refers to a disability attributed to mental retardation, cerebral palsy, epilepsy, autism, or other similar condition.
18. 42 C.F.R. § 482.61(a-e) (2001).
19. Minn. Stat. Ann. § 253B.03.7 (West 2000); Nev. Rev. Stat. § 433.494 (1999).
20. Minn. Stat. Ann. § 253B.03.1 (West 2000).
21. Minn. Stat. Ann. §§ 253B.03.2-.4 (West 2000).
22. Minn. Stat. Ann. §§ 253B.03.6-.6b (West 2000).
23. Joint Commission on Accreditation of Healthcare Organizations, Accreditation Manual for Mental Health, Chemical Dependency and Mental Retardation/Developmental Disabilities Services, Standard IM.7.2.2 & IM.7.2.4 (1995).
24. *See, e.g.*, Ill. Comp. Stat., ch. 740, para. 110/3 (2001).
25. *See, e.g.*, N.J. Stat.Ann. § 30:4-24.3 (2001); N.M. Stat. Ann. § 43-1-19 (2000).
26. Ill. Comp. Stat. ch. 740, para. 110/5 (2001).
27. *See, e.g.*, Ill. Comp. Stat. ch. 740, para. 110/9 (2001); N.M. Stat. Ann. § 43-1-19 (2000).
28. Ill. Comp. Stat. ch. 740, para. 110/6-/9.1 (2001).
29. N.D. Cent. Code § 25-16-07 (1999).
30. Ill. Comp. Stat. ch. 740, para. 110/10 (2001).
31. 42 C.F.R., Ch. IV, §§ 484.1-.52 (2001).
32. Fla. Stat. Ann. § 400.491 (2001).
33. Fla. Stat. Ann. § 400.494 (2000).
34. Tennessee Comp. r. & Regs. 1200-8-26-.06 (2001).
35. Joint Commission on Accreditation of Healthcare Organizations, Accreditation Manual for Home Care, Management of Information (1995); Community Health Accreditation Program, Inc., Standards of Excellence for Home Care Organizations (1993).
36. Or. Rev. Stat. §§ 659.036 & 659.227 (1999).
37. NHGRI, Understanding Our Genetic Inheritance: The US Human Genome Project; The First Five Years: Fiscal Years 1991–1995. Available at www.nhgri.nih.gov/hgp/hgp_goals/5yrplan.html.
38. Available at www.ncbi.nlm.nih.gov/Genbank/index.html.
39. 42 U.S.C. § 1320d (2001).

40 . Exec. Order No. 13145, 65 Fed. Reg. 6877 (2000).

41 . MO. REV. STAT.. § 375.1303 (2001).

42 . CA. CIVIL CODE § 56.17 (West2001)(nontherapeutic purposes ban) & § CAL. HEALTH & SAFETY CODE § 1374.7 (West 2001) (genetic discrimination ban).

43 . ARIZ. STAT.. § 12-2802 (2000).

44 . MD. CODE ANN.., (INS.) § 27.909 (2001).

45 . WIS. STAT. ANN. § 631.89 (West 2001).

Chapter 9

Risk Management and Quality Management

Learning Objectives

After reading this chapter, the learner should be able to:

1. Compare and contrast risk management with quality management.
2. Trace the growth and development of risk management.
3. Explain how the three components of patient record requirements relate to risk management.
4. Define an incident report.
5. List the purposes an incident report serves.
6. Differentiate between discovery and admissibility of incident reports.
7. Compose a scenario that illustrates how an incident report may be protected by the attorney–client privilege.
8. Differentiate between the two aims of peer review statutes: privilege and immunity.
9. Analyze the variations of peer review statutes.
10. Identify the reporting requirements of the Health Care Quality Improvement Act.

Key Concepts

- Admissible
- Confidentiality
- Discovery
- Incident report
- Peer review privileges
- Proper documentation
- Quality management
- Risk management

Introduction

Most legal issues concerning health information management focus on patient-specific health information given and obtained during the course of patient care. Accordingly, the focus of this book has centered on health information contained in patient medical records. While the majority of a health information manager's practice focuses on such information, such a practice focus is not exclusive. Health information management practice also addresses nonpatient records.[1]

Two nonpatient record areas in which the health information manager plays a vital role are risk management and quality management. Both are methods of quality control that exist in virtually every hospital and health-care facility. Both are distinct improvement techniques; the extent to which they are integrated varies by health-care facility. This chapter will not provide an all-encompassing look at risk management and quality management; rather, it will concentrate on the legal bases and requirements for those programs. Further details regarding forms to use and exact methods to employ are left to the broader teaching of quality improvement and management.

Risk Management

General Principles

To understand the health information manager's role in risk management, the learner must understand the definition and evolution of risk management. As a general matter, **risk management** is defined as a management function designed to achieve two purposes: (1) to identify areas of operational and financial risk or loss to a health-care facility, and its patients, visitors, and employees; and (2) to implement measures to lessen the effects of unavoidable risks and losses, prevent recurrences of those risks or losses, and cover inevitable losses at the lowest cost.[2] A risk management program is outcome oriented, focusing on the potential risks to the health-care facility and the methods used to avoid those risks. In other words, risk management looks at specific incidences to assist in determining what activities should be avoided and how to do so.

The growth and development of risk management in the health-care field can be traced to a number of different influences, foremost among them the loss of the doctrine of charitable immunity. For most of this century, health-care institutions were shielded from liability for the negligent acts of their employees by the doctrine of charitable immunity. Beginning in the mid-1960s, the doctrine was slowly dismantled through court decisions such as the landmark case of *Darling v. Charleston Community Memorial Hospital.*[3] State legislatures followed the lead set by the court system and abolished the doctrine by statute. Without the protection afforded by the charitable immunity doctrine, health-care institutions became exposed to an increasing number of lawsuits brought against them. Details regarding the doctrine of charitable immunity and its relationship with liability principles are addressed in Chapter 3.

The growth of risk management was also aided by several other forces. First, the so-called medical malpractice crisis of the 1970s brought to the attention of many health-care executives the reality that an increase in the number of medical malpractice lawsuits against their facility could result in not only damage awards but also higher insurance premiums. Second, the Joint Commission on Accreditation of Healthcare Organizations (JCAHO) began to require hospitals to implement risk management programs in their institutions.[4] Third, state legislatures became involved, establishing by statute minimum requirements for risk management programs in hospitals or delegating that task to administrative agencies.[5] As all of these forces converged on health-care institutions, executives realized that the risk management principles already in use in the business community could be applied to the health-care community.

Because of its evolution, risk management as a management function necessarily varies by institution. In terms of lines of organizational authority, risk managers may be considered part of the facility's safety department, its finance department, or its operations team. Where a facility operates with in-house counsel, the risk manager may report to that entity. In terms of who serves as a risk manager, the individual may have background in the legal, nursing, health information management, and/or insurance fields. One constant in risk management, however, is the role of health information managers.

Health information managers play a role in a risk management program in at least two ways: through the traditional method of enforcing patient record requirements and through the use of incident reports.

Patient Record Requirements

Health information managers have traditionally influenced the risk management process by implementing, enforcing, and educating health-care providers about patient record requirements. This education role centers on three areas: documentation, security, and confidentiality.

Documentation

The health information manager cannot stress too heavily the importance of **proper documentation** to reduce risk. Because a medical record serves as the legal record of a particular episode of a patient's care, it is the backbone of every professional liability action. As such, it is used to prove what did or did not happen in a particular case and to establish whether the applicable standard of care was met. A properly documented medical record benefits a health-care provider's defense in a lawsuit; a poorly documented medical record hinders the health-care provider's defense.

A properly documented medical record is both timely and complete, meaning that all entries in the record are authored and authenticated and reflect the total care actually rendered to the patient. In addition, the record meets the appropriate requirements for record content, including the use of approved abbreviations and methods to correct the record where necessary. Further details concerning the requirements of a timely and complete medical record are addressed in Chapter 4.

With proper documentation, the risks to a health-care facility may be reduced in a number of ways. For example, complete documentation of a patient's condition, including accurate information about adverse incidents that happened to the patient during treatment (e.g., a medication error), assists the caregiver in rendering appropriate treatment, thereby reducing risk to both the patient and the health-care facility. In addition, corrections to the record made according to proper methods reduce risk to the health-care facility because it may be concluded that the facility's purpose was to correct a mistake in the documentation of the patient's treatment and not to conceal information. Finally, a complete, timely, and accurate record reduces risk at trial because the health-care provider's defense ability is tremendously enhanced.

Security

Security of health information falls within the traditional role of the health information manager. Security issues regarding a risk management program center on the availability of medical records for purposes of patient care, access to patient-specific health information by or on behalf of the patient, and the retention of medical records.

The ready availability of a medical record to health-care personnel cannot be understated: various medical disciplines use the medical record as a method to communicate about the patient's illness and course of treatment during a particular episode of patient care. And should the patient subsequently require care, health-care providers rely on information from prior medical records to assist in the diagnosis and treatment of the patient. Failure to make medical records available during a current or subsequent episode of patient care may result in harm to the patient and exposure of the health-care provider to liability.[6] Such risk can be reduced by actively managing the availability of medical records for purposes of patient care.

Availability of medical records concomitantly involves the question of access to health information by or on behalf of the patient. Questions of access are governed by a complex web of laws and regulations, addressed in detail in Chapter 5. Because of this complexity, requests for access to patient-specific health information should be handled only by those with proper training and supervision. Careful management of these requests reduces risk to the health-care facility by ensuring that only those with a right to know have access to patient-specific health information. Careful management also lessens the potential for liability due to improper disclosure of health information.

Availability of medical records also involves the question of how long medical records should be retained. At minimum, health care facilities reduce the risk of a lawsuit for negligent loss of records by retaining records for the minimum period specified under statute and regulation. Additionally, if records are retained offsite by a commercial contractor due to storage constraints, risk may be reduced by including restrictions in the written contract that address confidentiality safeguards and indemnification in the event of unauthorized disclosure. Finally, when the health-care facility can no longer maintain medical records beyond the controlling statute and regulation period, it can reduce the risk of civil and criminal liability by ensuring that all record destruction is conducted in the ordinary course of business according to institutional policy. For further information, see Chapter 4.

Confidentiality

Long a matter closely associated with health information managers, confidentiality is central to reducing risk. **Confidentiality** is the obligation of the health-care provider to maintain patient information in a manner that will not permit dissemination beyond the health-care provider. The health-care community has for decades considered the confidentiality of health information a matter of utmost importance. The failure of health-care providers to respect confidentiality, combined with greater public awareness of the adverse effects of unauthorized disclosure of health information, may have an impact on risk management programs through an increased number of lawsuits. Such lawsuits generally allege violations of the right to privacy, breach of confidentiality, and/or breach of contract.

One lawsuit illustrating the risks associated with not maintaining confidentiality is *Estate of Behringer v. Medical Center at Princeton.*[7] In *Behringer,* a physician on staff at the hospital was treated at the hospital and diagnosed with acquired immunodeficiency syndrome (AIDS). After news of the doctor's diagnosis was circulated among the hospital staff and his patients, the physician sued the hospital for breach of the duty to maintain the confidentiality of his diagnosis. The court found in his favor, noting that the hospital failed to take reasonable precautions to ensure that his diagnosis and medical records were held confidential.

Risks of such lawsuits may be lessened through education of health-care professionals concerning the professional and legal obligations to maintain confidentiality. Beyond education, a health-care institution may reduce risk by adhering to and enforcing its policies regarding the confidentiality of patient information.

Incident Reports

As discussed previously, proper documentation in the medical record includes recording adverse incidents that occur during an episode of patient care. Such documentation in the medical record is separate and distinct from an incident report, which is a risk management technique used to describe and manage an adverse incident. Understanding this difference is essential to the proper functioning of a risk management program.

Definition and Purposes

To describe an incident report accurately, the learner must first understand what an incident is. A hospital incident is defined as

> any event or circumstance not consistent with the normal routine operations of the hospital and its staff or the routine care of a patient. It may be an error, an accident, or a situation which could have, or has, resulted in injury to a person or damage to hospital equipment or property.[8]

Incidents may encompass a variety of events, such as a medication error, a slip and fall, the loss of a patient's belongings, or an equipment malfunction affecting the patient. The incident is not limited to patients alone, but may also affect the health-care provider, its employees, or a visitor. Because the incident is not routine and could or did result in injury to a person or damage to equipment or property, it is considered adverse.

The **incident report** is the documentation of the adverse incident, whether done on a paper form or through a computerized database with access highly controlled. The report describes the incident itself, including the time, date, and place of occurrence, along with the condition of the subject of the incident (patient, employee, or visitor), statements or observations of witnesses, and any responsive action taken. The report differs from the medical record in that if poorly developed, it may also include subjective statements or opinions concerning fault or the circumstances surrounding the incident. By contrast, the medical record consists of a basic recounting of facts, devoid of personal opinion or subjective statements. Because the presence of this additional information in the incident report is inconsistent with the purposes of a medical record, the medical record should not incorporate the incident report. Rather, the incident report should be filed separately from the medical record.

An incident report serves multiple purposes: to document fully the circumstances surrounding the incident, to identify situations that may lead to litigation, to educate health-care personnel in order to prevent future incidents, and to create a database for monitoring the number and types of incidents. The first two purposes relate to the traditional notion of risk management because they serve to alert the health-care provider's attorney and insurance carrier to specific incidences that may lead to a claim against the health-care provider. The second two purposes relate not only to risk management but also to quality assurance: in addition to identifying specific incidences of risk, incident reports also permit the health-care provider to study patterns of activity to determine which practices should be altered and how to fashion training programs to achieve the optimum result.

These multiple purposes are best served if the incident report is completed as soon as practicable after the incident, when memories are fresh. By completing the report in a timely fashion, the health-care provider hastens the availability of the report to its attorney, insurance carrier, and quality assurance department for review and evaluation. And it is the availability of the report to the provider's attorney that will determine whether the report is discoverable and admissible in the event of litigation.

Discoverability and Admissibility

Because an incident report details the event that caused injury to the patient, employee, or visitor, it is one of the most important sources of information to the parties involved in a lawsuit against the health-care provider. Whether the report becomes available to the plaintiff will be determined by the rules of evidence governing discovery and admissibility and the privileges that attach these rules.

Discovery is the process used by parties to obtain information that relates to the subject matter of a lawsuit or an administrative agency proceeding. Discovery occurs before trial and involves identifying and locating books, documents, or other tangible things and persons relating to the subject matter at issue. The information to be discovered may relate to claims or defenses for either side of the lawsuit and is made by a formal request, such as through written interrogatories.[9] Information is considered discoverable if the applicable rules require disclosure of the information upon the formal request of a party.

The fact that certain information may be discovered does not automatically mean that the information may be admitted into evidence at trial.[10]

Information is considered **admissible** into evidence at trial if the applicable rules establish that the information is both pertinent and proper for the judge and/or jury to consider when deciding the issues involved in the lawsuit. As a general matter, incident reports are governed by the hearsay rule of evidence and its exception covering business records. Detailed material addressing the hearsay rule and business record exception is contained in Chapter 7.

The existence of an incident report does not automatically mean that a party to the lawsuit may either discover or admit the report. In order to discover or admit the report, the party must overcome the application of privileges. A privilege is the legal right to keep certain information confidential and protect it from subpoena, discovery, or introduction into evidence at trial. A privilege will be considered waived if the confidentiality is breached, through either carelessness or deliberate disclosure by the party holding the privilege.[11]

In the context of incident reports, the most frequently used privilege is the attorney–client privilege. Other privileges, such as the attorney work product privilege, have met with very limited success when applied to incident reports.[12] Because courts have increasingly rejected use of the attorney work product privilege in this context, the work product privilege will not be addressed here.

The attorney–client privilege protects communications made between attorneys and their clients from disclosure to third parties. It is designed to facilitate full and open communication between attorneys and their clients by assuring clients that the communication will remain confidential. To fall within the privilege, certain criteria must be met: an attorney–client relationship must be established and the client must make the communication in confidence for the purpose of obtaining legal advice from the attorney.[13]

Whether an incident report will be protected by the attorney–client privilege generally centers on the question of whether the report was made for the benefit of the attorney alone or whether dissemination of the report to others, such as the insurance carrier or internal quality assurance department, will defeat the privilege. In some jurisdictions, the report is not protected if disseminated to anyone other than the attorney;[14] in other jurisdictions, as long as the report is not placed in the medical record and dissemination is limited to the attorney and the health provider's insurance carrier, the report is protected.[15]

To guarantee protection of the privilege, the health information manager must work to ensure that the incident report is not placed in the medical record. This can be accomplished not only through standard medical record reviews, but also through involvement in developing the provider's written policies and procedures governing incident reports. Such policies and procedures should address (1) the content of the report, including labeling it as confidential and addressing it to the health-care provider's attorney; (2) the limited dissemination of the report inside and outside the health-care institution; and (3) the training of staff to properly complete the report.

In summary, every health information manager must understand the applicable rules of discovery, admission of evidence, and the attorney–client privilege within the health-care provider's jurisdiction, whether or not the health information manager is formally involved in the health-care provider's risk management program. Without such an understanding, the health information manager may act inadvertently to allow placement of the incident report in the medical record, with the result that the attorney–client privilege is lost and the report may be both discovered and admitted into evidence in a particular case. In addition, the health information manager loses the opportunity to educate fellow health-care personnel on the proper methods to complete the incident report.

Quality Management

The second area in which the health information manager plays a vital role concerning nonpatient records is **quality management**. Quality management has long been a part of the health information manager's role in the health-care delivery system. Over the past decade, various terms and methods have been applied to describe quality management, including *performance improvement, continuous quality improvement, total quality management, quality control, quality review, and problem detection*. While each of these terms or methods differs from the one preceding it, all fall within the umbrella of quality management.

As with risk management, quality management is an improvement technique that health-care providers use. Although similar databases may be involved, quality management significantly differs from risk management. Quality management is a clinical function, focusing on how to improve patient care. It looks at patterns of activity to define optimum performance and determine how to achieve them. As such, quality management is primarily process oriented rather than outcome oriented. By contrast, risk management looks at specific incidences of risk or loss to determine which activities to avoid. Risk management focuses primarily on the outcome, not the process.

Quality management activities in health-care institutions are conducted under the control and direction of peer review committees. These committees are composed of health-care professionals who are charged with the responsibility for evaluating, maintaining, and/or monitoring the quality and utilization of health-care services.[16] Peer review committees typically discharge this responsibility through audit and review of patient information against established guidelines. Where a pattern emerges indicating that the established guidelines were not met, the peer review committee determines what further action should be taken, including education and training of staff.

Peer Review Privileges

An effective quality management program benefits a health-care institution by allowing neutral evaluators the opportunity to provide useful feedback and recommendations designed to improve patient care. To achieve this benefit, the committee members must fully participate and offer candid criticism of the information they review. Yet, health-care institutions cannot force health-care professionals such as physicians to participate in peer review activities where the institution's medical staff acts as a semi-autonomous body. Furthermore, health-care professionals may hesitate to honestly analyze or criticize a colleague if the analysis or criticism they make will be published or otherwise disclosed. Finally, participation and candor may be inhibited by the fear of lawsuits charging defamation, or violations of antitrust laws, or the loss of patient referrals.

To address these concerns, state legislatures have passed peer review statutes. The aims of these statutes are twofold: (1) to protect the deliberations and records of peer review committees from access by nonparticipants and (2) to protect participants in peer review activities from civil liability. Not all statutes address both aims; however, most statutes address the first aim.[17] Under the first aim, peer review deliberations and records are considered "privileged," that is, protected from subpoena, discovery, or introduction into evidence. Under the second aim, participants are considered "immune" from monetary liability in the event of a lawsuit or other legal proceeding.

Because **peer review privileges** are a matter of state statute, the protections they afford necessarily vary from state to state.[18] For example, many of the statutes passed in the 1970s protected only peer review activity that took place in hospitals. As new entities such as health maintenance organizations became involved in health care, peer review statutes were revised to afford these entities the same protections afforded hospitals.[19] Nonetheless, some states have failed to revise their statutes to include these new entities, making it likely that peer review activities conducted by these entities fall outside the scope of the statute's protections.

State statutes also vary regarding the definition of peer review activity. Some statutes do not define the term beyond general language such as records and proceedings; other statutes explicitly state which documents and materials fall within their protections.[20] As a general rule, a statute's failure to include an explicit definition of what peer review activity is protected will result in excluding some activities from that protection. Certain activities commonly associated with peer review activity, such as the credentialing process, could therefore fall outside the scope of the statute's protection.

The statutes further vary by the nature of civil immunity afforded to participants. Some statutes provide absolute immunity from all suits,[21] while others provide only qualified immunity if a defamation action is brought.[22] Where immunity is granted, the law assumes that the participant acted in good faith. If a plaintiff can demonstrate that the participant acted with malice, the participant is no longer shielded from liability.

In addition to statutory variations, the peer review privilege may vary by the way in which courts have interpreted it. Many statutes give courts the authority to require disclosure under certain exceptional circumstances, such as a criminal action brought against a health-care provider accused of a felony. Each situation varies, but courts generally order disclosure in those cases where the information sought is essential to protect the public interest and the information cannot be obtained from another source.[23]

Every health information manager involved in quality management activities should understand the statutory peer review privilege as it applies in his or her jurisdiction. Such an understanding will assist the health information manager in ensuring that the health-care provider's quality management policies and procedures conform to the law and preserve the confidentiality of peer review materials.

National Practitioner Data Bank

Closely interwoven with any quality management program is the physician disciplinary process. Conclusions reached during peer review activities may directly bear on a health-care institution's decision to limit or discontinue a physician's practice in the institution or otherwise discipline a physician. And in some health-care institutions, the peer review committee is charged with direct responsibility over the professional disciplinary process. For those persons involved with decisions concerning staff privileges and disciplinary actions, it is necessary to understand the requirements of the Health Care Quality Improvement Act.

Passed in 1986, the Health Care Quality Improvement Act is designed to improve the exchange of information about decisions relating to the professional competence and conduct of physicians, dentists, and other health-care practitioners.[24] The desired result of such an exchange of information is an improvement in the quality of medical care through restrictions on the ability of certain physicians and dentists to change locations without disclosing previous incompetent performance or misconduct. The act accomplishes this result through the use of the National Practitioner Data Bank and complex reporting and query requirements. The U.S. Department of Health and Human Services has published regulations further defining the reporting and query requirements.[25]

Information concerning professional competence and conduct is reported to the National Practitioner Data Bank by hospitals, medical societies, licensing boards, prepaid medical practices, and other health-care entities involved in peer review activities. Specific information contained in the Data Bank includes data concerning malpractice payments, licensure actions, and adverse actions such as the loss of staff privileges of physicians and dentists in all fifty states. Figures 9-1 through 9-5 illustrate the types of information that must be reported to the Data Bank.

With these data available in the Data Bank, health-care entities such as hospitals are required to query the data bank whenever receiving an application for a position on the medical staff. Once admitted to the medical staff, the health-care entity must continue to query the Data Bank every two years concerning each staff member. The act presumes that receipt of information concerning incompetence or misconduct will result in the denial, restriction, or termination of staff privileges.

Health-care institutions that have taken steps to restrict a physician's privileges or otherwise discipline a physician through peer review

1. The physician's or licensed health-care practitioner's name, date of birth, work address and, if known, home address and social security number
2. The name of each professional school attended and the year of graduation
3. For each professional license, the license number, the field of licensure, and the name of the state or territory in which the license is held
4. The physician's or licensed health-care provider's Drug Enforcement Administration registration number, if known
5. The payment amount, date of payment, and whether the payment is for a judgment or a settlement
6. The name, if known, of any hospital with which the physician or licensed health-care practitioner is associated
7. A description of the acts or omissions and injuries or illnesses upon which the action or claim was based
8. Other information as required by the secretary of health and human services from time to time after publication in the *Federal Register* and an opportunity for public comment

Figure 9-1. Requirements for the Reporting of Medical Malpractice Payments

activities have been subject to lawsuits. Health-care institutions faced with these lawsuits have found protection through the act's grant of qualified immunity.

Actions taken by health-care institutions to restrict staff privileges, when those actions are the result of peer review activities, may be protected by the act from liability. Under the act, those who participate in peer review activities are immune from civil damage actions if the statute's fairness and reporting requirements are met.

Health information managers involved in questions of physician staff privileges and disciplinary actions face the challenge of understanding the complex reporting and query requirements of the act and its implementing regulations. The health information manager's successful integration of the reporting and query requirements into the credentialing and disciplinary process will result not only in compliance with the law but also in improvement in the quality of patient care.

1. The physician's or dentist's name, date of birth, work address and, if known, home address and social security number

2. Name of each professional school attended and the year of graduation

3. For each professional license, the physician's or dentist's license number, the field of licensure, and the name of the state or territory in which the license is held

4. The physician's or dentist's Drug Enforcement Administration registration number, if known

5. A description of the acts or omissions or other reasons for the action taken

6. A description of the board action, the date the action was taken, and its effective date

7. Classification of the action in accordance with a reporting code adopted by the secretary of health and human services

8. Other information as required by the Secretary from time to time after publication in the *Federal Register* and an opportunity for public comment

Figure 9-2. Requirements for the Reporting of Sanctions Taken by Boards of Medical Examiners

Actions based on professional competence or professional conduct:

(a) which revoke or suspend or otherwise restrict a physician's or dentist's license;

(b) which censures, reprimands, or places on probation a physician or dentist; or

(c) under which a physician's or dentist's license is surrendered

Figure 9-3. Reportable Actions Taken by the Boards of Medical Examiners

Actions taken by health-care entities:

(a) which adversely affect the clinical privileges of a physician or dentist for a period longer than 30 days; or

(b) which involve the acceptance of the surrender of clinical privileges or other restriction by a physician or dentist

Figure 9-4. Reportable Actions Taken by Health-Care Entities: Clinical Privileges

1. The physician's or dentist's name, date of birth, work address and, if known, home address and social security number
2. Name of each professional school attended and the year of graduation
3. For each professional license, the license number, the field of licensure, and the name of the state or territory in which the license is held
4. The physician's or dentist's Drug Enforcement Administration registration number, if known
5. A description of the acts or omissions or other reasons for privilege loss or surrender
6. A description of the entity's action, the date the action was taken, and its effective date
7. Other information as required by the secretary of health and human services from time to time after publication in the *Federal Register* and an opportunity for public comment

Figure 9-5. Requirements for the Reporting of Adverse Actions Taken by Health-Care Entities

Conclusion

As this chapter demonstrates, complex legal requirements govern a health-care provider's risk management and quality management programs. The health information manager's knowledge of these requirements will influence the success of the health-care provider's programs. Key to that influence is the ability to apply that knowledge to a particular situation. Health information managers face that challenge by educating the health-care provider's staff concerning patient record requirements, protecting incident reports from discovery, and reporting adverse actions regarding clinical privileges. In each example, the health information manager applies legal principles to real-life situations. For these reasons, health information managers must understand the legal bases and requirements of risk management and quality management.

Case Study

You are a health information manager closely involved with risk management at General Hospital, a teaching institution. Beginning this July, the hospital will incorporate presentations by hospital employees into its Grand Rounds series of lectures. You have been asked to present the lecture covering risk management. Compose a presentation addressing the legal aspects of risk management, particularly concentrating on patient record requirements and incident reports.

Review Questions

1. What are the general principles of risk management?
2. How does a properly documented medical record reduce the risk of a health-care facility?
3. Compare and contrast the ready availability of a medical record in the risk management context.
4. How does the concept of patient confidentiality relate to the concept of reducing risk?
5. What are the advantages of completing an incident report as soon as practicable after an incident?
6. What is a privilege, and how can it be waived?
7. Explain the concept of a peer review committee and its duties.
8. What is the National Practitioner Data Bank, and how does a health-care institution use the data it contains?

Enrichment Activities

1. Interview the official responsible for processing applications to join the medical staff at a local health-care facility. Discuss what consideration is given to the information held by the National Practitioner Data Bank in processing those applications. Examine whether the steps followed

by the facility are consistent with the requirements of the Health Care Quality Improvement Act and its implementing regulations.

2. Review articles in health-care journals concerning risk management. How do the discussions address incident reports, and discoverability and admissibility issues? Compare the information in these articles with the concepts covered in this chapter, and discuss these with your instructor.

Notes

1. By nonpatient records, I refer to those records addressing the issues of quality control in a health-care setting such as incident reports and peer review documents.
2. BARRY R. FURROW ET AL., HEALTH LAW, Ch. § III at 49 (1987).
3. 211 N.E.2d 253 (Ill. 1965), *cert. denied,* 383 U.S. 946 (1966).
4. JOINT COMMISSION, COMPREHENSIVE ACCREDITATION MANUAL FOR HOSPITALS, Performance Improvement, PI.3.1 (2001).
5. *See e.g.,* ALASKA STAT. § 18.20.075 (2000); FLA. STAT. ANN. § 395.0197 (West 2000); MD. HEALTH-GEN. CODE ANN. § 19-319(g) (2000); N.C. GEN. STAT. § 131E-96 (1999); R.I. GEN. LAWS § 23-17-24 (2000).
6. *See, e.g., Butterfield v. Okubo,* 831 P.2d 97 (Utah 1992) (unavailability to emergency room physician of infant's past medical records concerning breathing difficulties resulted in liability for failing to prescribe appropriate treatment).
7. 592 A.2d 1251 (N.J. Super. Ct. 1991).
8. JOHN F. MONAGLE, RISK MANAGEMENT: A GUIDE FOR HEALTH CARE PROFESSIONALS 29 (1985).
9. FED. R. EVID. 26(b) (1).
10. *See, e.g.,* FLA. STAT. ANN. § 395.0197(4) (West 2000) (incident reports "shall be subject to discovery, but shall not be admissible as evidence in court").
11. 23 CHARLES A. WRIGHT & KENNETH W. GRAHAM, JR., FEDERAL PRACTICE AND PROCEDURE: EVIDENCE § 93 (1980).
12. *See, e.g., Kay Laboratories, Inc. v. District Court,* 653 P.2d 721 (Colo. 1982) (rejecting attorney work product privilege); *Weiner v. Memorial Hosp.,* 453 N.Y.S.2d 142 (1982) (rejecting attorney work product privilege).
13. MCCORMICK ON EVIDENCE (John W. Strong ed., 4th ed. 1992).

14. *See Kay Laboratories, Inc. v. District Court,* 653 P.2d 721 (Colo. 1982); *Bernardi v. Community Hosp. Ass'n.,* 443 P.2d 708 (Colo. 1968).
15. *See, e.g., Sierra Vista Hosp. v. Shaffer,* 56 Cal. Rptr. 387 (1967); *Sligar v. Tucker,* 267 So.2d 54 (Fla. Dist. Ct. App. 1972); *Community Hosps. of Indianapolis, Inc. v. Medtronic,* 594 N.E.2d 448 (Ind. Ct. App. 1992); *Enke v. Anderson,* 733 S.W.2d 462 (Mo. Ct. App. 1987); *Clark v. Norris,* 734 P.2d 182 (Mont. 1986).
16. The composition and responsibilities of peer review committees are defined by both statute and accrediting agencies, such as the Joint Commission on Accreditation of Healthcare Organizations. *See, e.g.,* CONN. GEN. STAT. ANN. § 19a-17b (West 1997); HAW. REV. STAT. ANN. § 624-25.5 (2000); KAN. STAT. ANN. § 65-4915 (2000); MO. REV. STAT. § 537.035(2) (2000); JOINT COMMISSION, COMPREHENSIVE ACCREDITATION MANUAL FOR HOSPITALS, Medical Staff, MS.8 (2001).
17. In fact, some statutes expressly deny immunity to peer review participants while simultaneously affording protection to peer review materials. *See, e.g.,* CAL. HEALTH & SAFETY CODE § 1370 (West 2000).
18. This portion of the text draws heavily on Robert W. McCann, Protecting the Confidentiality of Peer Review Information, JOURNAL OF THE AM. HEALTH INFO. MGMT. ASS'N., Dec. 1993, at 52–56, and is cited with permission of the American Health Information Management Association.
19. *See, e.g.,* ARIZ. REV. STAT. ANN. § 36-445-01 (2001) (hospitals and outpatient surgical centers); DEL. CODE ANN. § 1768 (2000) (hospitals, medical societies, health maintenance organizations); OHIO REV. CODE ANN. § 4731.224 (Baldwin 2000) (hospitals and ambulatory surgical centers); TENN. CODE ANN. § 63-6-219 (1999) (medical societies, health-care institutions, health maintenance organizations, preferred provider organizations).
20. *Compare* ARIZ. REV. STAT. ANN. § 36-445.01 (West 2001) ("all proceedings, records and materials prepared in connection with the reviews"); CONN. GEN. STAT. ANN. § 38-19a(d) (West 1997) ("the proceedings of a medical review committee conducting a peer review"); R.I. GEN. LAWS § 5-37.3-7 (2000) ("the proceedings and records of medical peer review committees"); *with* D.C. CODE ANN. § 32-505 (1999) ("the files, records, findings, opinions, recommendations, evaluations, and reports of a peer review body"); IOWA CODE ANN. § 147.135 (West 1993) ("all complaint files, investigation files, reports, and other investigative information relating to licensee discipline or professional competence in the possession of a peer review committee"); KAN. STAT. ANN. § 65-4915 (2000) ("the reports, statements, memoranda, proceedings, findings and other records of peer review committees").
21. *See, e.g.,* CONN. GEN. STAT. ANN. § 19a-17b (West 1997); DEL. CODE ANN. § 1768 (2000); IOWA CODE ANN. § 147.135 (West 2000); MO. REV. STAT. § 537.035 (2000); OR. REV. STAT. § 41.675 (1999).

22. *See, e.g.*, ALA. CODE § 6-5-333 (2001); ARIZ. REV. STAT. ANN. §§ 36-2401(3) & -2402(b) (2001); FLA. STAT. ANN. § 766.101(4) (West 2000); TENN. CODE ANN. § 63-6-219(c) (1999); W. VA. CODE § 30-3C-2 (2000).
23. *See, e.g.*, D.C. CODE § 32-505(a) (3) (2000).
24. 42 U.S.C. §§ 11101-11152 (2000).
25. 45 C.F.R. §§ 60.1-.14 (2001).

Chapter **10**

HIV Information

Learning Objectives

After reading this chapter, the learner should be able to:

1. List the tests used to identify and/or confirm positive HIV results.
2. Identify and explain the three component steps of the voluntary testing process.
3. Compare and contrast court-ordered HIV/AIDS testing with HIV/AIDS testing pursuant to statutory authority.
4. Describe the situations in which employers may require HIV/AIDS testing of employees.
5. Describe the types of restrictions that confidentiality statutes and ethical guidelines place on HIV/AIDS information.
6. Explain the rationale for mandatory testing of health-care employees.
7. Analyze the limits on disclosure of HIV/AIDS information concerning the patient and the health-care provider.

Key Concepts

Anonymous testing
Confidentiality statutes
Employment challenges
Ethical guidelines
Improper disclosure
Mandatory testing
Voluntary testing

Introduction

Acquired immunodeficiency syndrome (AIDS) has emerged as one of the most pressing public health threats. An estimated 1 million persons in the United States are infected with the human immunodeficiency virus (HIV), the virus that develops into AIDS.[1] At the present time, no vaccine exists to prevent infection with HIV nor does a cure exist for AIDS.

As the public health threat posed by AIDS has increased, certain misunderstandings have emerged. Individuals unknowledgeable about the methods of transmission of the disease have created a climate of fear. From this fear has emerged a stigmatization of, and discrimination against, those suffering from AIDS and HIV.

Legislatures across the United States have responded to the stigma and discrimination experiences of AIDS and HIV sufferers, as well as the public health threat, with a complex mix of legislation. This legislation has addressed testing and reporting requirements and confidentiality concerns. The court system has also responded to the AIDS experience, particularly within the context of mandatory testing of health-care workers and improper disclosure of HIV status.

Health information managers handling patient-specific health information relating to HIV and AIDS must understand the complex legal rules to which this information is subject. By understanding the law applicable to this information, the health information manager is better able to respond to the demands for information made by patients, hospital administrators, researchers, and government agencies.

Testing

Background Information about HIV/AIDS

HIV is a retrovirus that attacks and suppresses a person's immune system. It is transmitted in a limited number of ways: through intimate sexual contact, exposure to infected blood or blood components, or passed from mother to child in utero or through breast milk. In the earlier stages of the disease, HIV-infected individuals may experience fever, swollen lymph nodes, weight loss, night sweats, decreased appetite, and diarrhea. As the disease process progresses, the individual is more likely than the average person to experience great difficulty in fighting other infectious diseases, such as Kaposi's sarcoma, *Pneumocystis carinii* pneumonia, and herpes zoster.

It is impossible to know when or if an infected individual will experience the onset of symptoms. Symptoms generally surface on a gradual basis and progress through various stages. Eventually, the individual may fully develop AIDS and die from the disease.

While no one test has been developed that isolates the virus, a variety of tests have been developed to detect the presence of HIV antibody and antigen in blood and body fluids. The most commonly used, the enzyme-linked immunosorbent assay (ELISA), detects the presence of HIV in serum or plasma. If a positive result arises from the ELISA test, medical protocols generally call for the health-care provider to confirm the result by performing a second test on the same specimen. Tests used to confirm positive results include the Western blot assay, the radioimmunoprecipitation assay (RIPA), and the indirect immunofluorescence assay (IFA). If positive results are confirmed by a second test, the individual is considered seropositive for HIV.

Voluntary Testing

The vast majority of HIV testing conducted in the United States involves **voluntary testing.** In the context of managing health information, voluntary testing encompasses three areas: consent for testing, delivery of pretest information, and disclosure of test results.

Voluntary testing necessarily implies that the individual to be tested has consented to the testing. This implication has been incorporated into state statutes requiring the individual's written informed consent before testing.[2] In addition, states receiving federal funds under the HIV Health Care Services Program must require persons requesting others to be tested for HIV to obtain a written, signed consent from the individuals to be tested.[3]

In addition to written informed consent, most states place a burden on the health-care provider ordering the HIV test to deliver certain pretest information to the individual to be tested. Often referred to as pretest counseling or consultation, common requirements include distributing information about the type of tests involved, the testing methodology employed, the meaning of the test results, the methods of transmitting the disease, and the methods of reducing risk of transmission.[4]

Once the test results become available, the health-care provider must contact the tested individual with the results. The disclosure of test results is also the subject of state regulation. Commonly referred to as posttest counseling or consultation, the disclosure process generally involves four parts: (1) the test results and the possible need for additional testing; (2) the meaning and importance of the test results; (3) the methods to reduce further transmission, including partner notification programs; and (4) referral to available health-care services and support groups.[5] Where the test results are positive for HIV, the health-care provider is required to report the identity of the patient to the appropriate public health authorities unless an exception to the reporting requirement applies.

Mandatory Testing

The concept of **mandatory testing** involves a decision by the legislature or a court to force an individual to receive testing for some health reason without granting the individual the right to refuse. In the context of individuals with positive HIV status or AIDS, mandatory testing generally falls into either of two categories: court-ordered testing or testing pursuant to statutory authority.

State law empowers courts to issue orders to protect the public good. AIDS and HIV status are no exception. A court may order testing of an individual if the court has determined by clear and convincing evidence that the individual is reasonably believed to be infected with HIV and is a serious and present health threat to others. Such court-ordered testing does not allow the individual the right to refuse testing.[6]

Statutory authority mandating testing generally targets groups perceived as presenting a public health threat. In some states, prisoners entering or being discharged from correctional facilities must undergo testing without the right to refuse.[7] In addition, some states require sexual offenders who are convicted or have pleaded guilty or nolo contendere and whose crime included sexual intercourse to undergo testing without the right to refuse.[8]

One group that has been targeted for mandatory testing is employees, with mixed results. Some states permit employee testing only on a voluntary basis, with consent and confidentiality issues addressed in the statute.[9] Other states prohibit HIV testing of employees altogether.[10] Some states prohibit HIV testing of employees as a general matter but allow mandatory testing in certain defined situations.

These situations generally involve the employee's ability to perform a particular job in a safe manner. The first situation follows from employment discrimination law and involves a bona-fide occupational qualification to the job in question. To meet the bona-fide occupational qualification, the law places the burden on the employer to demonstrate that the HIV test is job related and necessary to determine an individual's qualifications for a particular job.[11] And in some cases, the law places the burden on the employer to show that no reasonable accommodation short of HIV testing exists.[12]

The second situation follows from handicap discrimination law and involves classifying HIV status and AIDS as a handicap. For states classifying HIV and AIDS in that manner, testing may be mandated where public health authorities determine that the infected individual would pose a direct threat to the safety or health of others.[13]

After determining that the employer may mandate HIV testing in the employment setting in some states, the next question involves the employer's right to use the HIV test results in making employment decisions. Here, the law is less clear. Only one state, North Carolina, appears to sanction the employer's ability to reject job applicants on the basis of a confirmed HIV-positive test result.[14] Whether other states will grant employers such authority remains to be seen.

Anonymous Testing

Many persons in society have elected not to undergo AIDS/HIV testing for fear of learning of a positive result and the possibility of discrimination. In an effort to encourage individuals to avail themselves of HIV testing, some states have passed laws allowing individuals to undergo anonymous testing.[15]

Anonymous testing entails a system that assigns a unique identifier, such as a number or coding system, to the individual. That identifier replaces the individual's signature on the consent form and name on the vial containing the blood sample. It is that identifier, not the individual's name, that is reported to the public health authorities with the test result. Anonymous testing is unavailable in some circumstances, such as testing to determine eligibility to donate blood, plasma, semen, or other human tissue.[16]

Patient Confidentiality

The health-care community has long considered the confidentiality of patient information a matter of utmost importance. This concern, combined with greater public awareness of the adverse effects of unauthorized disclosure of health information, has resulted in the creation of specific legal protections to govern the confidentiality of health information. Although all states consider health information confidential to some extent, the need to provide greater protection to health information concerning HIV status and AIDS has been legally recognized in the majority of states.[17]

As a general rule, **confidentiality statutes** place restrictions on identifying both the patient tested and the test result. Disclosure of the patient's identity or the test result may be made only to the subject of the test or her legally authorized representative, a person designated in a legally effective release of information, the health-care provider's staff directly involved in the patient's care, or the appropriate public health authority. In the case of mandatory testing by statute or court order, the relevant statute or court order will specify additional individuals who may receive the test results and/or the subject's identity.[18] Legal prohibitions exist against passing along or redisclosing information concerning an individual's HIV status to other parties, unless authorized by law.[19] Where unauthorized disclosure of test results or the subject's identity occurs, the injured person may bring a civil suit for damages.[20]

One case illustrating these principles is *John Roe v. Jane Doe*.[21] In *Roe*, the patient informed his physician of his positive HIV status during an office visit for treatment of unrelated symptoms. He specifically asked and received assurances from his physician that his HIV status would be treated confidentially. Subsequently, his physician received a subpoena from the patient's employer along with a signed release of information authorizing release of information regarding the patient's workers' compensation claim. The physician complied with the subpoena by forwarding the patient's entire medical record to the requesting attorney.

Roe then sued his physician for breach of confidentiality, negligence, and breach of contract. The court held that the physician improperly disclosed her patient's HIV status and was liable for punitive damages. Specifically, the court noted that the open-ended release of information form accompanying the subpoena was insufficient to permit disclosure of HIV information for two reasons: (1) New York law required that the release form specify authorization of the release of HIV information, which the form at issue did not address; and (2) New York law mandated use of a release of information form developed or approved by the commissioner of health, and the form at issue did not meet this requirement. The court also faulted the physician for releasing the patient's medical records without including a statement prohibiting redisclosure of the patient's HIV information. As the *Roe* case demonstrates, a standard release of information may be insufficient to authorize release of HIV information.

In addition to legal restrictions, confidentiality protections may also be provided by **ethical guidelines**, which are standards of conduct issued by professional organizations to guide their memebers' future course of action. They are sometimes used to establish the standard of care in a negligence action. For example, the American Medical Association (AMA) has determined that the medical profession's obligation to maintain confidentiality of an individual's HIV status does not cease upon the death of the individual. In response to physicians' concerns that identification of a patient's cause of death as involving HIV or AIDS may result in adverse effects upon the character of the deceased patient or upon family members and friends, the AMA has promulgated ethical guidelines for use in determining when it is appropriate for a physician to include AIDS/HIV-related information in the autopsy report.[22] As discussed in earlier chapters, a professional association's guidelines may be used to establish the appropriate standard of care in a negligence action.

Legal Challenges

Most lawsuits addressing the AIDS/HIV issue fall into one of two categories: challenges of health-care employees to mandatory testing and challenges to the improper disclosure of AIDS/HIV status.

Employment Challenges

The rationale for requiring testing of health-care employees for AIDS/HIV arises from the context of infection control policies. Hospitals have long been charged under state regulations and accrediting standards with establishing a system for reporting infections among their patients and employees.[23] The infection control procedures that have resulted are aimed at protecting the health of both the patient and the employee.

These policies are also aimed at shielding the health-care institution from liability from actions alleging negligent transmission of a communicable disease by an employee. Courts have held health-care institutions liable for the transmission of other infectious diseases by employees, such as when a nurse passed the tuberculosis virus to a newborn infant.[24] Health-care institutions in turn have determined that this potential for liability justifies their efforts to screen their employees for communicable diseases, including AIDS/HIV.

The infection control policies of health-care institutions, which include screening of employees for infectious diseases, generally concentrate on employees with direct patient-care responsibilities. Where testing for AIDS/HIV is concerned, testing should be based on a reasonable belief that the individual employee has been exposed to HIV.

Legal challenges to this testing generally arise where the employee was terminated for refusing to undergo HIV testing. Claims brought under these lawsuits, referred to as **employment challenges,** include arguments that refusal to undergo testing is protected by the federal Rehabilitation Act and the constitutional prohibitions against unreasonable searches and seizures. Constitutional challenges may be brought in this context only if the employer is a public, not private, institution subject to the constitutional restraints on state action.

One of the first cases addressing both of these arguments in the health-care employment setting was *Leckelt v. Board of Commissioners.*[25] In *Leckelt,* the court upheld the employer's actions in requiring HIV testing and discharging the employee for refusing to undergo such testing. The court determined that the law prohibited discrimination, not testing, and that the testing used by the hospital was not a discriminatory action but a constitutionally reasonable one.

One case illustrating the success of a constitutional challenge to mandatory HIV testing is *Glover v. Eastern Nebraska Community Center.*[26] In *Glover,* employees of a multicounty health services agency treating retarded persons objected to the agency's mandatory HIV and hepatitis B testing policy on grounds that the testing constituted an unreasonable search and seizure. The court agreed that such mandatory testing was not justified because the risk of transmission posed to the agency's patient was virtually nonexistent.

As these cases illustrate, any employer seeking to impose mandatory HIV testing should consider utilizing a nondiscriminatory testing program based on a reasonable belief that the employee has been exposed to HIV. At the same time, the employer must demonstrate that the employee poses a serious risk of transmitting the disease to patients.

Improper Disclosure Challenges

One of the greatest fears facing an HIV-infected individual is the possibility of **improper disclosure,** meaning that HIV status may be disclosed to third persons without consent. Improper disclosure of HIV status may result in adverse effects to the individual, including negative judgments about the individual's character, friends, and family. When the confidentiality protections created by statute and professional standards fail, the aggrieved individual may consider filing a lawsuit asserting a violation of the right to privacy, breach of confidentiality, and/or breach of contract. Lawsuits filed under these circumstances have included HIV-infected individuals who are patients and health-care providers.

As discussed in the *Roe* case earlier in this chapter, physicians have been held liable for breaches of confidentiality and contract where they failed to comply with the applicable legal requirements restricting access to their patient's HIV information. Where the health-care provider is the HIV-infected individual, the protections afforded by the legal restrictions on access to HIV information are not as clear. From one perspective, the health-care provider is a patient who should be able to avail herself of all the confidentiality protections the law provides. From the opposite perspective, an HIV-infected health-care provider may pose serious risks to any patient upon whom she performs invasive procedures. For that reason, the patient is entitled to know the health-care provider's HIV status. Such patient notification has been recommended by the Centers for Disease Control.[27]

One case illustrating the first perspective is *Estate of Behringer v. Medical Center at Princeton.*[28] In *Behringer,* a physician sought medical treatment for pneumonia at the Princeton Medical Center. Between the time of admittance and discharge, his positive HIV status and subsequent diagnosis of AIDS was widely circulated among the medical center's staff. When he returned to his medical practice, he found that many of his patients had elected to see other physicians after learning through the medical community that he was HIV positive.

Behringer sued the medical center, raising a claim of breach of the duty to maintain the confidentiality of his diagnosis. The court found in his favor, noting that the medical center owed a duty to Behringer as a patient to take reasonable precautions to maintain the confidentiality of his diagnosis and that the duty was breached when the diagnosis became public knowledge.

In the *Behringer* case, the legal questions focused on the health-care provider in his capacity as a patient seeking treatment. Where the HIV-infected health-care provider is providing patient care as opposed to solely seeking treatment, the confidentiality protections afforded under the law are not as stringent. One case illustrating this concept is *In re: Milton Hershey Medical Center.*[29] In that case, a physician in a joint residency program between two medical centers was accidentally cut when operating on a patient. The resident voluntarily tested for HIV, with a positive result later confirmed by subsequent tests. The medical centers then petitioned a Pennsylvania court for permission to disclose information of the resident's positive HIV status to the patients who were potentially affected and to certain physicians on the medical staffs.

The court granted the medical centers' request, finding that the resident's interest in maintaining his privacy was outweighed by the interests of the medical centers in protecting the public's health and that of their patients in particular. The court ordered a very selective and limited disclosure of the resident's identity, using a pseudonym for disclosure to the patients and using the resident's real name for disclosure to only those physicians associated with his residency program. The court also narrowly tailored the information disclosed to the patients to include only the fact that the resident who participated in certain types of procedures was HIV positive and that the medical centers offered counseling and HIV testing.

As these cases demonstrate, the strict limits on disclosure of an individual's HIV status imposed by law may be enforced through lawsuits. Where the affected individual is the patient, the courts generally enforce the laws to benefit the patient's privacy interests. Where the affected individual is a health-care provider, however, exceptions to these strict limits exist that may warrant disclosure despite the health-care provider's opposition. In such a situation, courts generally perform a balancing test, weighing the privacy interests of the health-care provider against the interests of the provider's patients and the public in general to know the risks to which they are subject. Where the health-care provider's privacy interests are outweighed by the competing interests of patients and the public, courts will find that a compelling need exists that warrants disclosure of HIV information, however limited in scope.

Conclusion

As this chapter demonstrates, HIV/AIDS information is subject to stricter confidentiality protections than that afforded health information in general. These protections include statutory requirements covering the manner in which testing is conducted, whether on a voluntary, mandatory, or anonymous basis. Legal restrictions also apply to the way in which HIV/AIDS information is managed, including limits on identifying the individual tested and the test result, specifications for legally effective authorizations to release information, and prohibitions on redisclosure of HIV information. Health information managers must understand the legal restrictions relating to HIV and AIDS in their state in order to handle this sensitive information properly.

Case Study

You are the director of health information services at General Hospital, supervising several employees who release health information. As a community service, your facility recently launched a new HIV/AIDS outreach program. Because of the anticipated increase in patients with HIV/AIDS, you have decided to reexamine your policies and procedures governing release of information. Discuss what points should be included in the policies and procedures, particularly how employees should handle inadequate requests for release of information and subpoenas concerning HIV/AIDS information.

Review Questions

1. What are the similarities and differences of voluntary testing, mandatory testing, and anonymous testing?
2. What restrictions apply to the disclosure of a patient's identity or test result?
3. How does the infection control system relate to employee testing for HIV/AIDS?

4. Describe the difficulties faced by an HIV/AIDS patient whose infected status is disclosed without the patient's consent.
5. What interests would a court balance when faced with a request to require disclosure of HIV/AIDS status?

Enrichment Activity

Research over the Internet policies offered by professional associations concerning how to handle HIV/AIDS information. Look for recommendations on how health-care facilities should handle requests for release of information and maintain patient confidentiality despite the efforts of the media or the public to obtain this protected information. Compare and contrast those policies, and discuss them with your instructor and fellow students.

Notes

1. Centers for Disease Control, U.S. Department of Health & Human Services, HIV/AIDS Surveillance: Mid-Year Edition (June 2001).
2. For example, Illinois' AIDS Confidentiality Act imposes a requirement for written patient consent. S.H.A. 410 ILCS 305/4 (2001). Missouri law requires insurers who mandate HIV testing as a condition of obtaining insurance to obtain the written consent of the applicant to be tested. MO. CODE REGS. tit. 4, § 190-14.140(2) (A) (2000). Other states requiring written consent include: ARIZ. REV. STAT. ANN. § 20-448.01(B) (2000); CAL. HEALTH & SAFETY CODE § 120990 (West 2000); CONN. GEN. STAT. ANN. § 19a-582(a) (West 2001); LA. REV. STAT. ANN. § 40:1300.13(A) (West 2000); MONT. CODE ANN. § 50-16-1007(1) (2000); N.Y. INS. LAW § 2611 (a) (McKinney 2001); OHIO REV. CODE ANN. § 3901.46(B) (1) (Baldwin 2001); 35 PA. CONS. STAT. ANN. § 7605(a) (2001).
3. 42 U.S.C. § 300(ff) (61) (b) (2001).
4. *See, e.g.,* CAL. CODE REGS. tit. 22, § 41149; CONN. GEN. STAT. ANN. § 19a-582(c) (West 2001); FLA. ADMIN. CODE ANN. r. 10D-93-070(4); ILL. ADMIN. CODE tit. 77, §§ 697.110 & .300(d); MO. CODE REGS. tit. 19, § 20.26.030(2) (1990); N.C. ADMIN. CODE tit. 15A, r. 19A.0202 (9-10).
5. *See, e.g.,* CAL. CODE REGS. tit. 22, § 41150; CONN. GEN. STAT. ANN. § 19a-582(d) (West 2001); FLA. ADMIN. CODE ANN. r. 10D-93.070(7); ILL. ADMIN. CODE tit. 77,

§ 697.300(f); Mo. Code Regs. tit. 19, § 20.26.030(2) (D) (1990); N.C. Admin. Code tit. 15A, r. 19A.0202(9-10).

6. *See* Conn. Gen. Stat. Ann. § 19a-582(e) (8) (West 2001); Ga. Code Ann. § 31-17A-3 (2001); Mo. Rev. Stat. § 191.674(1) (2001).
7. *See, e.g.,* Idaho Code § 39-604 (2000); Mich. Comp. Laws Ann. § 791.267(2) (West 2001); Mo. Rev. Stat. § 191.659 (2001).
8. *See* Conn. Gen. Stat. Ann. § 54-102b (West 2001); Fla. Stat. Ann. § 775.0877(1) (West 2000); Me. Rev. Stat. Ann. tit. 5, § 19203-A(5) (West 1999); Mo. Rev. Stat. § 191.663 (2001); Or. Rev. Stat. § 135.139(2) (1999); S.C. Code Ann. § 16-3-740 (Law. Co-op 2000).
9. These states have passed statutes imposing general restrictions on HIV testing of employees: Colo. Rev. Stat. § 25-4-1401 (2000); Del. Code Ann. tit. 16 § 1202 (2000); S.H.A. 410 ILCS 305/3 (2001); Iowa Code § 216.6 (2000); Me. Rev. Stat. Ann. tit. 5 § 19204-B.1 (1999); Mo. Rev. Stat. 191.653 (2000); W. Va. Code § 16-3C-1 (2000).
10. *See* Cal. Health & Safety Code § 120975 (West 2000); Haw. Rev. Stat. § 325-101(c) (2000); Mass. Gen. Laws Ann. ch. 111 § 70F (West 2001).
11. *See* N.M. Stat. Ann. § 28-10A-1.A (Michie 2001); Tex. Health & Safety Code Ann. § 81.102 (West 1999); Wash. Rev. Code § 49.60.172 (West 2000).
12. Fla. Stat. Ann. § 760.50(3) (c) (West 2000); Ky. Rev. Stat. Ann. § 207.135(2) (b) (Michie/Bobbs-Merrill Supp. 2000).
13. *See* Ga. Code Ann. § 31-17A-2 (2001); N.C. Gen. Stat. § 130a-148(h) (2000); R.I. Gen. Laws § 23-6-22 (2000); Wis. Stat. Ann. § 103.15(2) (West 2001).
14. N.C. Gen. Stat. § 130A-148(i) (1&2) (1992).
15. *See, e.g.,* Haw. Rev. Stat. § 325-16(b) (3) (2000); Iowa Code Ann. § 141A.7 (West 2001); Kan. Stat. Ann. § 65-6007 (2000); La. Rev. Stat. Ann. § 1300.13.E (West 2000); Me. Rev. Stat. Ann. tit. 5, § 19203-B (West 1999); Mich. Comp. Laws Ann. § 333.5133(9) (West 2001); Mo. Rev. Stat. § 191.686 (2000).
16. *See, e.g.,* S.H.A. 410 ILCS 305/6 (2001); Iowa Code Ann. § 141.7 (West 2001); La. Rev. Stat. Ann. § 40:1300.13.F(1) (West 2000).
17. Alaska Stat. § 09.25.120 (1994); D.C. Code Ann. § 7-131 (2000); N.C. Gen. Stat. § 130A-143 (2000); Utah Code Ann. § 26-6-27 (2001).
18. *See, e.g.,* Cal. Penal Code § 1524.1(g) (West 2000); Conn. Gen. Stat. Ann. § 19a-583(a) (10) (West 2001); Ga. Code Ann. § 24-9-47 (r & t) (2001); 410 ILCS 305/9(g) (2001); Me. Rev. Stat. Ann. tit. 5, § 19203(10) (West 1999).
19. *See* Ala. Code § 22-11A-54 (2001); Conn. Gen. Stat. Ann. § 19a-583(b) (West 2001); Ga. Code Ann. § 24-9-47(b) (2001); 410 ILCS 305/9 (2001); La. Rev. Stat. Ann. § 1300.14(A & D) (West 2000); Mo. Rev. Stat. § 191.656 (2000).

20. *See* CAL. HEALTH & SAFETY CODE § 120980 (West 2000); MO. REV. STAT. § 191.656(6) (2000).
21. 599 N.Y.S.2d 350 (N.Y.App. Div. 1993).
22. AMERICAN MEDICAL ASSOCIATION COUNCIL ON ETHICAL & JUDICIAL AFFAIRS, CONFIDENTIALITY OF HUMAN IMMUNODEFICIENCY VIRUS STATUS ON AUTOPSY REPORTS (1992).
23. *See, e.g.,* ILL. ADMIN. CODE tit. 77, § 690.100B(b) Infection Control, IC, 1-.62 (2001) (1) (1985); JOINT COMMISSION, COMPREHENSIVE ACCREDITATION MANUAL FOR HOSPITALS, Infection Control, IC, 1-.62 (2001); AMERICAN HOSPITAL ASSOCIATION, INFECTION CONTROL IN THE HOSPITAL 22 (4th ed. 1979).
24. *Taaje v. St. Olaf Hosp.,* 271 N.W. 109 (Minn. 1937); *see also, Kapuschinsky v. United States,* 248 F. Supp. 732 (D.S.C. 1966) (nurse passed infection to newborn infant); *Helman v. Sacred Heart Hosp.,* 381 P.2d 605 (Wash. 1963) (nurse passed staphylococcus infection to patient).
25. 714 F. Supp. 1377 (E.D.La. 1989), *aff'd,* 909 F.2d 820 (5th Cir. 1990).
26. 867 F.2d 461 (8th Cir. 1988), *cert. denied,* 493 U.S. 932 (1989).
27. Centers for Disease Control, U.S. Department of Health & Human Services, Recommendations for Preventing Transmission of Human Immunodeficiency Virus & Hepatitis B Virus to Patients During Exposure-Prone Invasive Procedures, July 12, 1991, at 5.
28. 592 A.2d 1251 (N.J. Super. Ct. Law Div. 1991).
29. 595 A.2d 1290 (Pa. Sup. Ct. 1991), *aff'd,* 634 A.2d 159 (Pa. 1993).

Chapter 11

Computerized Patient Records

Learning Objectives

After reading this chapter, the learner should be able to:

1. Identify the reasons supporting the transformation to a computerized patient record.
2. Compare and contrast the three broad categories of law and regulation governing the creation and storage of a computerized patient record.
3. Discuss the business record exception to the hearsay rule and its application to a computerized patient record.
4. Evaluate the role of the health information manager in meeting the requirements of the business record exception.
5. List the types of lawsuits that may arise from a breach of confidentiality of a computerized patient record.
6. Compare and contrast physical security, personnel security, and risk prevention techniques.
7. Evaluate risk prevention techniques associated with computerized patient record systems.
8. Identify the electronic tools that have transformed the health-care field's business processes.
9. Compare and contrast the security issues associated with the use of the Internet and e-mail.
10. Explain why the field of telemedicine has not advanced more rapidly.

Key Concepts

- Admissibility
- Authentication
- Authorship
- Business record exception
- Clinical information system
- Computerized patient record (CPR)
- Digital imaging
- Electronic mail
- Internet
- Patient record system
- Personnel security
- Physical security
- Risk prevention techniques
- Telemedicine

Introduction

Since the mid-1980s, health information managers have been working to transform the traditional paper-based patient record into a **computerized patient record (CPR).** This transformation has succeeded in a limited number of health-care facilities. Many other health-care facilities have incorporated some health data into a computerized database, allowing easier access to these data. In the future, the vision of a completely computerized patient record will become real and commonplace and not the exception to the rule.

The reasons for transformation to a computerized patient record are many and are illustrated in Figure 11-1. First and foremost among those reasons is the availability and accessibility of clinical data stored in an electronic format. Ever-increasing demands for more detailed and sophisticated patient data have highlighted the need for quick access to a wide variety of clinical data. These demands emerge not only from within the health-care facility but also from outside the facility: external forces such as regulatory agencies, accrediting organizations, and insurance companies request increasingly detailed patient data. The traditional paper medical record simply cannot keep pace with these demands.

Forces external to health-care providers have also placed the issue of computerized patient records at center stage. For example, the federal government's efforts in health-care reform have centered on improving health-care delivery through the use of computerized patient records.[1] And the Institute of Medicine has recommended that all health-care providers adopt a computerized patient record as their standard medical record.[2]

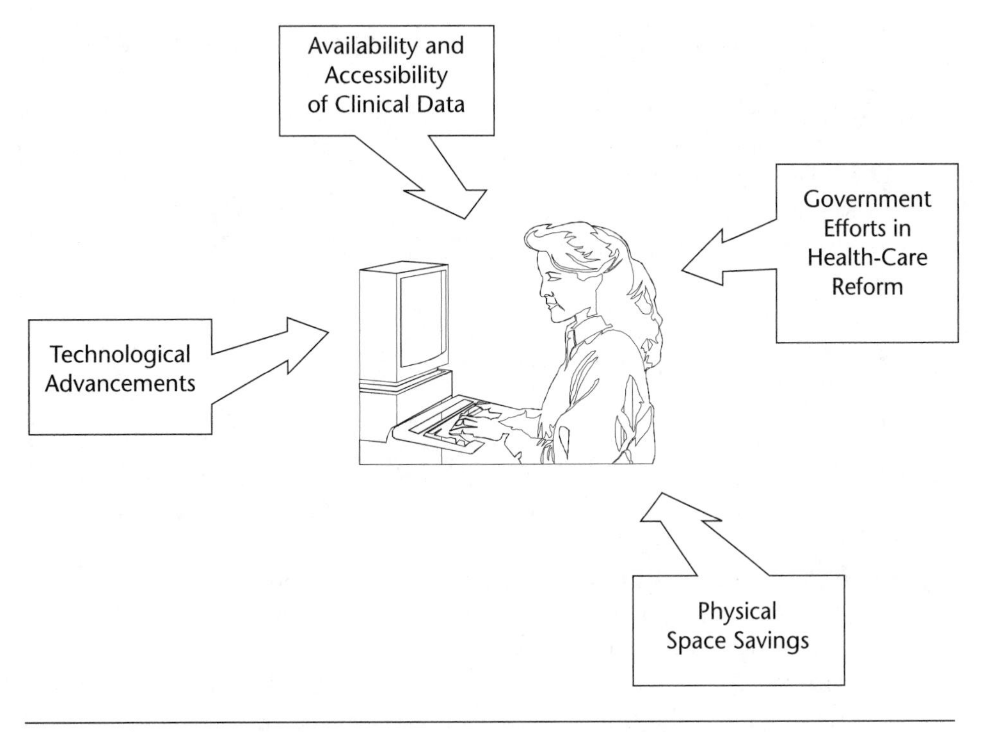

Figure 11-1. Reasons for the Transformation to a CPR

Additionally, computerized patient records offer physical space savings. The health information manager's role will shift from paper management to information management. Budgeting operating costs for storage conceivably will be reduced. This format difference translates into potential cost savings because of the possible reduction in administrative costs.

Fortunately, advancements in technology have made computerization of health information possible. These advances include, but are not limited to, integrated patient-care information systems, optical disk technology, and electronic data interchanges. Additionally, electronic tools have influenced the manner in which the health-care industry has conducted itself from a business perspective. An extensive body of literature currently exists addressing the technological aspects of a computerized patient record and its impact on the health information management department. Therefore, this chapter concentrates on the legal issues involved in computerization of patient-specific data.

After completing this chapter, the health information manager should be able to recognize the legal issues present in computerized patient records that may affect accreditation, licensure, and liability. By understanding the legal issues, the health information manager is one step closer to properly evaluating, selecting, and implementing an information system that not only satisfies the needs of the health-care organization but also sufficiently addresses legal issues and concerns.

Accreditation and Licensure Issues

Licensing authorities and accrediting organizations play a major role in the life of a health-care provider: the state licensing authority authorizes the provider to practice in a particular state, and the accrediting organization sets standards for each provider's compliance. For this reason, it is important to understand the impact these bodies have on health-care providers considering the transformation to a computerized patient record. Although the federal government has begun to address issues concerning electronic transmission of health information, much work remains to be done. Until such time as the federal government completes its efforts on health-care reform, the standards and restrictions of licensing authorities and accrediting organizations will also govern how the transformation to a computerized patient record will occur.

The basis of any discussion of a computerized patient record involves accurate definitions of the terms. Computerized patient records are generally considered to be records created, authenticated, stored, and retrieved by computers. To be more specific, a computerized patient record is defined as:

> [A]n electronic record that resides in a system specifically designed to support users by providing accessibility to complete and accurate data, alerts, reminders, clinical decision support systems, links to medical knowledge, and other aids.[3]

Other terms commonly used in discussions of a computerized patient record are defined by the Institute of Medicine as follows:

> A **patient record system** is the set of components that form the mechanism by which patient records are created, used, stored, and retrieved. It includes people, data, rules and procedures, processing and storage devices, . . . and communication and support facilities.

> A **clinical information system** has a central focus of clinical data, not financial or billing information. Such systems may be limited in their scope to a single area of clinical information (e.g., lab data) or they may be comprehensive and cover virtually every facet of clinical information pertinent to patient care (e.g., computer-based patient record systems).[4]

For learning purposes, this chapter addresses the patient record in an electronic form as a computerized patient record or CPR.

Any health information manager evaluating and selecting a CPR must closely examine the requirements and limits that licensing authorities and accrediting bodies place on a computerized patient record. This section examines those requirements and limits in the context of the creation, storage, and authentication of health information electronically.

Creation and Storage

The first question the health information manager must consider is whether the creation and storage of patient-specific information in an electronic medium is even authorized by the state law or the appropriate licensing authority. A review of the applicable law reveals that any of three answers may apply: (1) the computerized patient record may be expressly authorized, (2) the statutes or regulations may be silent on the question, or (3) the statutes or regulations seemingly prohibit the use of a computerized patient record. These answers are illustrated in Figure 11-2.

Unfortunately, very few states expressly authorize the creation and storage of a patient record electronically. Five states that specifically address this issue by statute are Hawaii, Indiana, Lousiana, Nevada, and Tennessee. Statutes in Hawaii and Louisiana authorize computerization of medical records.[5] In Indiana, state law specifically authorizes the recording

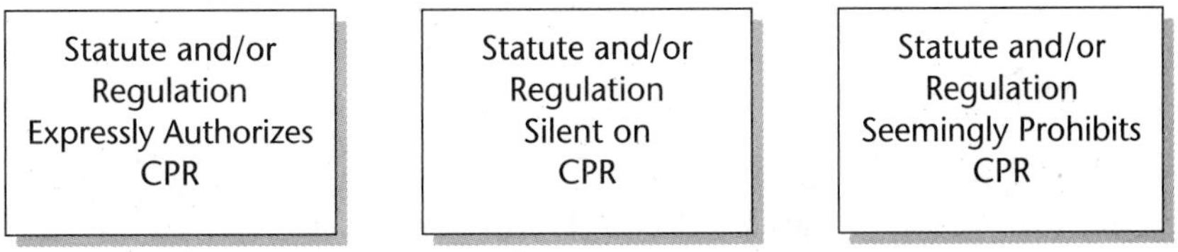

Statute and/or Regulation Expressly Authorizes CPR

Statute and/or Regulation Silent on CPR

Statute and/or Regulation Seemingly Prohibits CPR

Figure 11-2. State Law Grants Authority to Create and Store Patient-Specific Data in Electronic Form

of hospital medical records using an electronic imaging system.[6] Nevada law permits the creation and storage of health-care records in a computer system that limits access to those records.[7] Under Tennessee law, the term *hospital record* is defined to include electronic data.[8] Where the statute does not address the question, the authorization may be found in administrative regulation. For example, the administrative regulations of Montana, Oregon, and Washington allow permanent records to be kept in computerized form.[9]

What is more frequently the case is state law or regulation that leaves the question open. In such an instance, the applicable statute or regulation may authorize specific media, such as hard copy, abstracts, or microfilm, *and* also include a catchall phrase such as "other usable forms" or "acceptable form."[10] The use of catchall phrases like these implies that an electronic patient record may be authorized for use by a health-care provider. Such an implication may not give much comfort, however, to a health information manager investing scarce financial resources in a computerized patient record system. To determine whether the phrase in the statute or regulation actually authorizes the use of a computerized patient record, the health information manager must learn the licensing authority's interpretation of the phrase.

Finally, some states expressly require the storage of patient records in certain media, such as an original file or microfilm.[11] Express requirements of specific media for creation and storage of patient records, standing by themselves, seemingly prohibit the use of a CPR. Again, the health information manager should check with the appropriate licensing authority to determine its interpretation of the requirement. If the licensing authority's interpretation follows the language of the requirement strictly, automating patient-specific data may be prohibited in that particular state. The health information manager who chooses to implement a computerized patient record system despite this prohibition may place the health-care provider's license in jeopardy.

Authentication

As discussed in Chapter 4, all entries recorded in the patient record must be authored and authenticated. **Authorship** identifies the health-care provider who has made an entry in the record, in writing, by dictation, by keyboard, or by keyless data entry. **Authentication** confirms the entry, either by written signature, initials, or computer-generated signature code. This confirmation implies that the entry as recorded is accurate. Such entries in the record must have been made contemporaneously with the occurrence of the event. Because of the nature of a CPR, the timeliness of the entry can be established automatically, as can the timeliness of any corrections or updates. Moreover, the CPR can establish the identity of the person making or correcting an entry, assuming that computer passwords are not shared or biometric identification techniques are used. Corrections to entries made in the CPR are addressed in detail in Chapter 4.

For a computerized patient record, such authentication is represented by an electronic signature. Any statute or regulation that expressly authorizes the use of a computerized patient record, such as those discussed earlier in this chapter, would permit authentication by electronic signature. Conversely, a state's statute or regulation requiring a physician's signature to authenticate a medical record, without expressly authorizing use of a computer key or code as an electronic signature, poses a potential barrier to computerization. Where the statute or regulation is not clear, the licensing authority's interpretation of the statute or regulation will serve as the guide to proper authentication.[12]

Electronic signatures are also addressed by the Electronic Signatures in Global and National Commerce Act of 2001.[13] This act applies to the use of electronic signatures in international and national commerce. It states that electronic signatures may not serve as a legal bar to contracts or other records involved in interstate and foreign commerce. Courts have not yet interpreted this act to determine whether the transfer of health information to support reimbursement constitutes interstate commerce. Assuming that such a determination is reached, this act would support authentification of entries made in the record by computer key.

Accrediting bodies, by contrast, expressly recognize authentication by computer methods. Both the Medicare Conditions of Participation and the Joint Commission on Accreditation of Healthcare Organizations permit authentication of entries made in the record by computer key.[14] It then rests with the health-care organization to utilize a software program that establishes the electronic signature as unique to the author and to represent the authentication of that author in order to meet the accrediting standards.

Liability Issues

Any discussion of liability issues in the context of a computerized patient record can be broken down into two subcategories: (1) liability issues for which the patient record serves as proof in a lawsuit involving the quality of patient care and (2) liability issues that arise from unauthorized access to, or careless handling of, patient information (see Figure 11-3). For liability issues involving the patient record as proof in a lawsuit, the focus rests on whether the CPR may properly be admitted as evidence. For liability issues involving access or handling of patient information, the focus rests on the legal requirement to keep the CPR safe and secure. The following discussion addresses each of these focuses and offers practical advice to the health information manager who may face these issues in practice.

Admissible Evidence

As discussed in Chapters 4 and 7, medical records serve as the backbone of virtually every professional liability action. They are used to reconstruct an episode of patient care and establish whether the applicable standard of care was met. Other civil actions require the admissibility of medical records, including credentialing and disciplinary proceedings of physicians and other health professionals. Additionally, medical records may be used in criminal matters to establish the cause of the victim's death or an insanity defense.

In each lawsuit in which the medical record will be used to prove or disprove a fact, the issue of admissibility of the medical record will be present. **Admissibility** concerns pertinent and proper evidence that may be considered by the judge and/or jury when deciding the issues in a lawsuit. As a

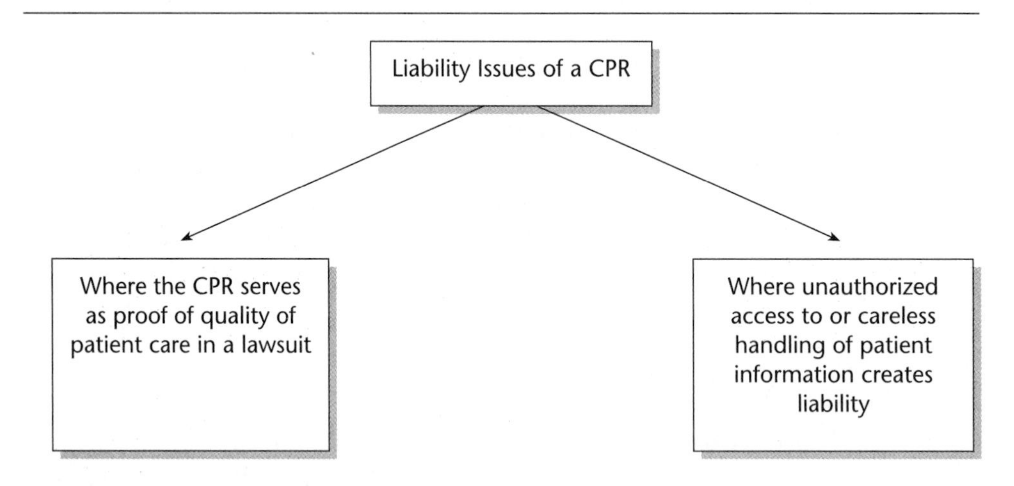

Figure 11-3. Categories of Liability Issues of a CPR

general matter, medical records are not admitted into evidence unless they overcome the hearsay rule. This rule prohibits the introduction into evidence of out-of-court statements that are offered to prove the truth of the matter asserted. This introduction into evidence is accomplished through the use of the business record exception to the hearsay rule or through a subset to that exception specifically governing medical records.[15] For more general information concerning the hearsay rule and the business record exception, see Chapter 7.

Under the **business record exception,** the party seeking to admit the medical record must first meet the foundation requirements of the exception. A foundation is made by establishing that the record was made (1) and kept in the ordinary course of business, (2) at or near the time of the event was recorded, and (3) by a person with knowledge of the acts, events, conditions, opinions, and diagnoses appearing in it.[16] After meeting these requirements, the party seeking to introduce the record must demonstrate the accuracy and trustworthiness of it. The party accomplishes these tasks by presenting the custodian of records as a witness to explain record-keeping procedures.

Just as with traditional paper-based records, health information managers must be able to testify as to both the foundation and trustworthiness and accuracy requirements of the business record exception. In addition to the knowledge that the health information manager possesses as to the paper-based system, the health information manager must possess knowledge of those aspects unique to a computerized system. First, the health information manager should be familiar with the manner in which the data are recorded: for example, who makes the entry, whether the entry is made by someone using a computer key or biometric identification,[17] what data entry procedures are routine, and so forth. This knowledge will be useful in meeting the foundation requirement. Second, the health information manager should be familiar with both the hardware and software used in the system, the quality control measures used to ensure the reliability and validity of the data, and the policies and rules governing access to the system and how to make corrections to the record. This knowledge will apply to meeting the accuracy and trustworthiness requirements.

Finally, the health information manager must possess knowledge of the end product that the party is trying to admit into evidence. Instead of admitting into evidence the paper record used by the health-care professional to record patient data, the party is admitting into evidence a computer printout of the data that the health-care professional recorded directly into the computer. This computer printout may serve either as the original record of care or its equivalent, depending on what that jurisdiction's statutes, rules, and regulations allow.[18] The health information manager should be familiar with the equipment used to produce the printout, the reliability of the software used to process the data, and the actual creation of the printout.

The use of a computer printout of a computerized patient record as evidence of patient care in court has not been widely tested because of the small number of health-care providers who have fully computerized their patient records. Federal courts have allowed the computer printout into evidence in instances where the foundation and trustworthiness and accuracy requirements have been met. One example is *United States v. Sanders.*[19] In *Sanders,* the government prosecuted a pharmacist for Medicaid fraud, relying in large measure on computer printouts kept by the state agency involved in administering Medicaid funds. The printout showed the number and type of reimbursement claims made by the pharmacist and paid by the state. The court admitted the printouts into evidence pursuant to Federal Rule of Evidence 803(6) after the custodian of records' testimony established the foundation and trustworthiness and accuracy requirements.

As the number of health-care providers using computerized patient records grows, the computer printout as evidence of the quality of patient care should become widely accepted by courts. Health information managers must be prepared to assist in the analysis and design process of computer-based patient record systems with the requirements of the business records exception in mind in order to facilitate the acceptance of computer printouts as evidence in court and advance the transformation to the computerized patient record.

Security Issues

Just as in a paper-based record system, the security of the patient record in a computer-based system is of immense importance. Health-care providers are charged under the Medicare Conditions of Participation, the standards of the Joint Commission on Accreditation of Healthcare Organizations, and most state licensing laws with the responsibility to safeguard patient information.[20] Health care providers are also charged under the Health Insurance Portability and Accountability Act with following security and privacy regulations issued by the Department of Health and Human Services.[21] The breach of this responsibility may result in legal liability: claims of breach of confidentiality, invasion of privacy, defamation, or negligence may result from unauthorized access to or careless handling of patient information.

Safeguarding access to the medical record is essential to maintaining the record's integrity and the confidentiality of the data contained in it. Computerized patient records pose many of the same security issues as paper-based patient records. Who has access to the record? How does that person use the data contained in the record? With a paper-based record, patient information is contained in a single physical file folder and access to this folder can be monitored and controlled. No matter how stringent security arrangements are, however, it is not always possible to know who has had access to a paper-based medical record. The same concerns are present in a computer-based system. The tracking capabilities available with computers offer the advantage of knowing who has had access to the patient record and when. Nonetheless, the presence of computer terminals throughout a health-care facility, combined with participation in computer networks, raises the possibility of larger numbers of individuals having unauthorized access to confidential patient information.

Whether the health-care provider chooses a traditional paper-based patient record or a computerized patient record, the same legal requirements apply: the record must be kept secure and guarded from unauthorized access. Special security issues are present with a computerized patient record, however, and these security issues may be subdivided into the following categories: physical security, personnel security, and risk prevention techniques.[21] The interrelationship of these categories is illustrated by Figure 11-4.

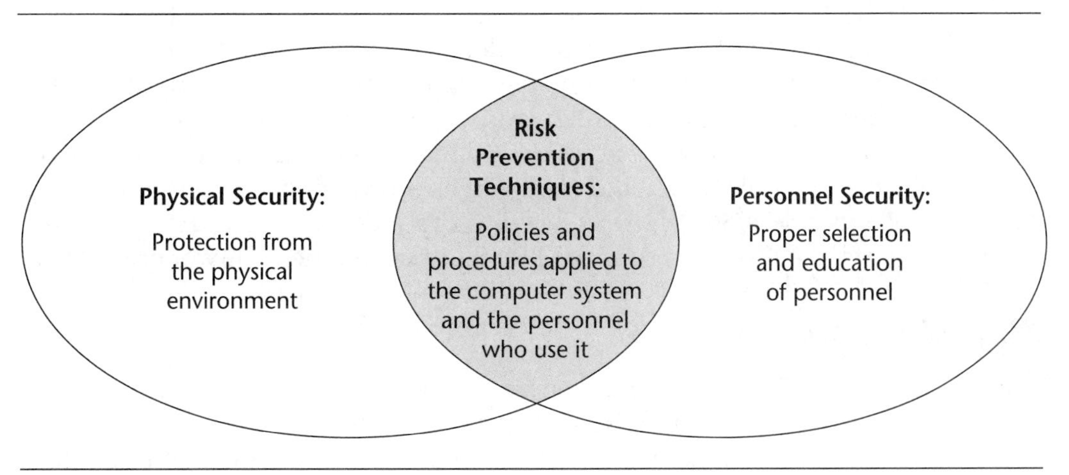

Figure 11-4. Interrelationship of Categories of Security Issues

Physical Security

As the health information manager may imagine, physical security concerns the nuts and bolts of the computer system. **Physical security** is best illustrated by a series of questions. What protections from the physical environment are in place? Do the protections include temperature and humidity controls, power surge and failure protection devices, and the like? Are fire alarms installed and magnetic media used for storage secured in a fireproof location? Are there rules limiting access to computer terminals and storage areas? Are terminals bolted to desks and disks stored in locked cabinets to prevent theft? Are maintenance requirements documented and maintenance logs maintained? These questions must be addressed to ensure physical security of the computerized patient record.

Personnel Security

Personnel security focuses on the human aspect of security. In addition to the normal reference checks associated with hiring of personnel, the health-care provider may wish to consider the following for personnel hired to work with the CPR: screening for past criminal history, work-related security problems, or a high school or college record of computer hacking. Once hired, the health-care provider should educate the employee about the provider's confidentiality policy and the employee's responsibility to keep data confidential. Further education should address how to access the computer system properly, the limits on access to information, and the consequences for violating the provider's policy. Furthermore, health-care providers should document this education of employees. For example, the health-care provider may require employees to sign a statement acknowledging that they understand and will abide by the provider's confidentiality policy and procedures. This statement should also address the consequences for violating the provider's confidentiality policy. The employer should maintain a record of employees' attendance at inservice sessions and the viewing of videotapes that are specifically designed to address the security, privacy, and confidentiality of health data.

Risk Prevention Techniques

Risk prevention techniques merge physical and personnel security concepts. Risk prevention techniques serve to protect the integrity and confidentiality of the data at issue. In practice, these techniques translate into policies and procedures to be applied to the computer system and the personnel who use it. The following discussion of risk prevention techniques, although not exhaustive, should serve health information managers evaluating a computerized patient record system. These risk prevention techniques are listed in Table 11-1.

One basic risk prevention technique involves determining who has access to what information for what purpose at which times. Different levels of access apply to different personnel and should be maintained by the system administrator. The highest level of health information manager in an organization should participate in assigning levels of access to various groups of personnel. Some need read-only access whereas others will need to also copy and/or edit data. Editing capabilities can range from adding data to the system to deleting data. Editing capabilities in a computerized patient record are similar to corrections being made to a paper-based medical record. Any policy that involves editing capabilities must address (1) how corrections to the record are made so that it is possible to compare the original data to the corrected data, (2) who is authorized to make corrections, and (3) what restrictions exist on editing another person's entry. The health-care provider should then create an audit trail to determine if the policy is being followed.

Another risk prevention technique involves the use of unique computer passwords, key cards, or biometric identification. Because computer passwords are widely used to access health information, this section focuses on them. The health-care provider should control issuing these passwords. Requiring the use of longer rather than shorter passwords or combinations

Table 11-1. Risk Prevention Techniques for a CPR

1. Restrict access.
2. Determine who has access, for what purpose.
3. Use computer passwords, key cards, or biometric ID.
4. Restrict copying functions.
5. Place security mechanisms in contracts with outside computer service bureaus.
6. Establish confidentiality agreements among network participants.
7. Address the potential for computer sabotage.
8. Safeguard the use of laptop computers and personal digital assistants.

of alpha and numeric characters are simple security efforts that can be used. The health-care provider should require employees not to disclose or share their password with others and should strictly enforce this requirement. Further, employees should be required to log off the system immediately after finishing a session so that no other person can access data using another's password. Failure to log off the system after use leaves confidential information unprotected. And when an employee ends employment with the health-care provider, the provider should expeditiously cancel that employee's access to the computerized patient record system.

Risk prevention techniques must also address the risk associated with one of the best benefits of a computerized patient record system: storage savings. As noted in the transformation section of this chapter, computerized patient record systems permit the storage of a tremendous amount of patient data. The converse to this benefit is the risk that data stored electronically may also be copied electronically, and the more data stored electronically, the more data that can be copied electronically. To decrease risk, the health-care provider should consider restricting the copying function to no more than one patient record at a time, and should run periodic security checks to determine who is copying what data, how often, and for what purpose.

One additional risk posed by computer storage involves the use of an outside computer service bureau to store patient data. Until recently, laws, regulations, and standards governing health information addressed the health-care provider's obligation to safeguard confidential patient data, but did not necessarily address the obligations of a third party, such as a computer service bureau, to safeguard these data. Because the business associate rule is now contained in the final privacy rule issued pursuant to the Health Insurance Portability and Accountability Act (HIPAA), computer service bureaus are required to safeguard these data.[23] To minimize the risk of unauthorized access to or mishandling of confidential patient information by a computer service bureau, a health-care provider should include the HIPAA provisions in the service contract. Such provisions cover the confidential nature of the data, the use to which the data will be put, the security mechanisms to be used to safeguard these data, and indemnification in the event data are improperly disclosed by the service bureau. Additional information about the HIPAA provisions governing business associates can be found in Chapter 5.

One often overlooked risk prevention technique involves the safeguarding of portable computers, sometimes known as laptop computers, and personal digital assistants (PDA). As portable computers and PDAs become more common in the health-care environment, they are being used to facilitate the collection of more complete and accurate information from the patient. Because of the portable nature of laptop computers and use of wireless technology for PDAs, the risks for breach of patient confidentiality are increased for these computers as compared to networked desktop computers.

To minimize these risks, the health-care provider should establish or improve control over portable computers and PDAs, provide employees with theft awareness instructions, and invest in certain computer accessories designed to make theft less profitable. The health-care provider should consider improved controls, including the establishment of written policies and procedures covering the loan and use of portable computers and PDAs and whether patient-specific health information should even be maintained on these devices at all. If this information is to be maintained on a portable computer or PDA, the health-care provider should institute standard practices for backing up the information on a secure computer network or disk stored separately from the computer carrying case or PDA. In addition, the health-care provider should instruct employees to avoid leaving a portable computer or PDA unattended for any length of time and to carry the device in something other than a readily identifiable computer carrying case. Furthermore, the health-care provider may wish to add an antitheft plaque or engraving on the portable computer or PDA to identify the health-care provider as owner. Many antitheft plaques contain a metallic bar code and registration number which when removed show the imprint of the words *stolen property*. Removal of these plaques may damage the computer casing, resulting in a lower retail value for the computer or PDA by the thief.

Risk prevention techniques should also address communications that are external to the provider. If the health-care provider agrees to network her computer system with other providers, she risks the confidentiality of her patient data because more users have access to those patient data. This risk can be minimized by establishing confidentiality agreements among the network participants. If the network involves public channels of communication such as telephone lines, radio waves, and microwaves, the health-care provider may consider encrypting patient data communicated over these public channels.

Furthermore, risk prevention techniques should address computer sabotage. Computer sabotage often arises as the act of a disgruntled employee or an outside user, such as those who participate with the health-care provider in a computer network. A common form of computer sabotage is the introduction of a computer virus into a computer system. Such viruses may destroy or alter data or cause a computer system to slow or crash. Health-care providers should recognize the potential for computer sabotage when considering whether to participate in a computer network and should consider the use of antivirus software and firewalls to combat this problem. Further, health-care providers can discourage the possibility of hackers' scanning for passwords by limiting the number of access attempts. For example, the user can be allowed three log-on attempts. Attempts to log on that exceed the maximum number of permitted log-ons can result in long delays that discourage hackers.

As this discussion indicates, the security issues involved with a computerized patient record are complex and multifaceted. This section has focused on identifying the risks that computerization poses to confidential patient data and the safeguards that can be crafted to minimize these risks. By addressing these issues, the health information manager lessens the possibility of legal liability for unauthorized access to or careless handling of patient information.

Electronic Health Issues

Electronic tools such as the Internet, electronic mail, digital imaging, and telemedicine are now indispensable tools for conducting business in the health-care field. While these tools open up a myriad of opportunities, they also raise legal concerns relating to privacy and security of patient-specific health information.

Internet

The use of the Internet in the health-care field can be viewed from more than one perspective. The health-care provider may visit sites on the World Wide Web to obtain information to deliver patient care better by reviewing the latest health-care news, accessing libraries of medical data and clinical alerts, scheduling continuing education, and researching poison center databases and the results of clinical studies. At the same time, patients may visit Web sites to seek answers to their health-care needs by researching their conditions, registering for clinical trials, learning about their prescriptions, scheduling participation in screening programs, and purchasing durable medical equipment.

In addition, some organizations actively engage in electronic health practice, known as e-health, to exchange health information between the patient and the health-care provider. These entities are known as e-health organizations, defined as organizations that collect and display individually identifiable health information over the Internet.[24] Patients who participate in e-health are known as e-health consumers, defined as individuals whose individually identifiable health information is collected, maintained, or displayed over the Internet.[25]

Certain security issues are associated with use of the Internet for e-health. Patient-specific health information may be obtained or used inappropriately by unauthorized persons or organizations. This information may be copied or altered without detection, resulting in financial or health-related harm to the consumer. Or the patient-specific health information may be incorrect, incomplete, or merely out of date.

Health-care providers who engage in e-health practice should remain aware that the same requirements for safeguarding the confidentiality of patient-specific health information in a traditional setting also applies to an e-health practice. Although a method of delivering care has changed, the application of statutes, rules, and regulations to the provision of care has not. For example, e-health organizations that treat Medicare patients are subject to the Medicare Conditions of Participation, just as they would be if they were treating the patient in a face-to-face setting.[26] Those that operate federally assisted alcohol and substance abuse programs are also subject to federal regulations governing the confidentiality of alcohol and substance abuse information.[27] And those that submit billing electronically to insurers for reimbursement are held to the privacy guidelines of the Health Insurance Portability and Accountability Act (HIPAA).[28] Finally, accrediting standards such as those issued by the Joint Commission on Accreditation of Healthcare Organizations and ethical tenets such as those issued by the American Health Information Management Association also apply to providers in an e-health setting.[29] Health information managers involved in an e-health practice should assist in the design and monitoring of technology safeguards in order to ensure that the use of new information technologies is not at the expense of consumers' privacy.

Electronic Mail

Over the past decade, **electronic mail** (e-mail) has become one of the most popular modes of communication in the United States. E-mail is a form of communication between parties or individuals using only electronic means. As with private industry, the health-care field has incorporated e-mail into its business methods. Health-care organizations using e-mail that contains patient-specific health information should carefully consider security precautions as part of their business practice.

Although seemingly private when created, e-mail should never be considered a private form of communication. Once sent, e-mail may be collected, stored and reviewed by people other than the intended recipient if that recipient forwards the e-mail on to others. Further, many organizations maintain a policy of the right to review any e-mail sent or received by any member of the organization. And with the use of daily backups to networked computer systems, e-mail may be stored even after the recipient or sender has deleted the e-mail from her personal computer.

Although the law has not kept up with the pace of technology to the extent that online privacy is specifically protected, it is evolving in that direction. Regardless of the scarcity of laws specifically addressing online privacy, it is important to note that the laws and regulations that apply to patient-specific health information stored in a paper-based medical record logically extend to the health information contained in an e-mail. The Medicare Conditions of Participation, federal regulations issued pursuant to HIPAA and those governing alcohol and substance abuse, and the accrediting standards of the Joint Commission on the Accreditation of Healthcare Organizations all apply to patient-specific health information contained in an e-mail. Further security regulations issued pursuant to HIPAA address the use of e-mail, as do HIPAA's privacy regulations in the context of notifying the patient of the health-care organization's information privacy practices.[30]

In addition to legal requirements, prudent business practice dictates that health-care organizations develop an action plan concerning the use of e-mail as a form of clinical documentation. Of foremost concern is to address patient confidentiality and informed consent policies, along with the instructions to patients on the proper structure, permissible content, and sensitivity needs of e-mail as a form of clinical communication. Technical security measures should also be taken to ensure the safe use of e-mail. For example, the use of encryption algorithms may protect the content of the e-mail while in transit and prevent unauthorized users from reading the e-mail.[31] Similarly, disclosure and redisclosure policies should define the circumstances under which e-mail should be forwarded and distributed to multiple recipients. Finally, organizations should establish processes to incorporate the e-mail into the existing medical record, whether paper based or electronic in format, so that the record is a true and correct reflection of the patient's care.[32] In creating this action plan, health-care organizations may look to emerging industry guidelines addressing each of these issues.[33]

Digital Imaging

One technology with the potential to save money for health-care organizations is digital imaging. **Digital imaging** permits a paper document to be scanned on a device that works similarly to a photocopier. The image is saved to an optical disc, a compact disk (CD), or magnetic tape and after electronic indexing can be viewed through a server or web browser. The image is then available to multiple users who need access to the data contained in the image. Advantages of a digital imaging system are listed in Figure 11-5.

Unlike e-health and e-mail, some states have enacted laws and regulations dealing directly with digital imaging.[34] These laws and regulations generally address digital imaging in the context of storage media for health information. In addition, digital imaging is subject to the same principles addressed in federal and state regulations governing confidentiality, record retention, and security of patient-specific information.

---

1. Simultaneous access by multiple users to the same medical record.

2. Easy accessibility compared to locating a paper-based medical record

3. Data integrity (the image cannot be altered)

4. Protection against disaster

5. Savings on storage space

6. Audit trail capabilities

Figure 11-5. Advantages of a Digital Imaging System

Telemedicine

One area of technology that has expanded the means of medical practice is the use of telemedicine. **Telemedicine** is defined as:

> the use of electronic communications and information technologies to provide or support clinical care at a distance. [35]

Often used in remote areas where access to health-care professionals may be limited, telemedicine serves to connect patients with a health-care professional through the use of multimedia communications and information systems. This connection allows the health-care professionals to diagnose, treat, and monitor patients. Examples of use include the transfer of diagnostic images such as CAT scans, MRIs, and x-rays to a specialist for a second opinion; the use of video visits for home-bound patients; and videoconferencing between a counselor and a patient located some distance apart.

Telemedicine technologies can include facsimile, audio capabilities including radio and telephone, still images, full-motion video, and color screens to facilitate face-to-face contact. Application packages can include image capture, blood pressure and pulse meters, analog-based audio stethoscopes, and digital dermascopes built into the video system. These technologies can be used as permanent features of the health-care facility or could be located on a rollabout system.

Telemedicine offers the opportunity for tremendous benefits to both patients and health-care professionals. A listing of such benefits may be found in Figure 11-6.

One of the reasons the field of telemedicine has not advanced more rapidly is the unresolved question of which state's laws apply to such issues as privacy, licensing, and medical reimbursement. The following examples illustrate how complicated the questions concerning telemedicine have become:

- Is the patient receiving care in the state in which she resides or the state in which the health-care professional is present?
- Has the physician created a physician-patient relationship through the use of telemedicine, thereby subjecting the physician to claims of medical malpractice?

1. Improved access to health care, such as obtaining second opinions

2. Improved continuity of care, patient education, and timely treatment (including monitoring the condition of chronically ill patients; reduced travel time for physicians, other health-care providers, and patients; and better access for patients in underserved areas)

3. Improved access to medical records and information (including promoting self-help by increasing the online availability of medical information, knowledge-based self-diagnosis programs, and distance learning programs)

4. Improved continuing medical education

5. Improved delivery of health care by bringing a wider range of services such as radiology, mental health services, and dermatology to underserved communities and individuals in urban and rural areas

6. Increased recruitment and retention of health professionals in rural areas by providing ongoing training and collaboration with other health professionals

7. The potential for improved control of health-care costs by helping to avoid unnecessary patient trips and allocation of resources to outlying areas

Figure 11-6. Benefits of Telemedicine

(Adapted from Telemedicine Report to Congress by the Joint Working Group on Telemedicine (1997); American Health Information Management Association, Practice Brief-Telemedicine Records (1997); J. Welch, *The Technology of Medicine*, 70 AM. HEALTH INFOR. MGMT. ASS'N. Vol. 2 (1999).)

- Is the physician practicing medicine in the state in which the patient resides or where the physician is present, thereby raising licensing and reimbursement concerns?
- In the event of technical failures, is there liability for injuries caused by the disconnection of the signal between the patient and the physician?
- In the event health information is lost while being transported across state lines, has there been a wrongful disclosure of a medical record? Complicating this situations, the law of which state would apply: the one from which the records were sent, the one to which the records were sent, the one in which the transmission became disconnected, or the one in which the company operating the transmission medium resides?

Settling these types of questions would lead to a determination of which state's law applies to any given situation, providing a more stable environment in which telemedicine could expand.

Very limited guidance concerning telemedicine is provided on the federal level. The Telecommunications Act of 1996 provides the general public with access to modern communication media, such as the Internet but addresses telemedicine in only two sections.[36] While promoting telemedicine, the act does not address any standards by which telemedicine should be governed. The Comprehensive Telehealth Act of 1996 addresses Medicare reimbursement payments but little else.[37]

It has therefore been up to the states to provide guidance through legislation and regulation. In most instances, states have defined telemedicine and allowed for its practice in the state, sometimes modifying licensure statutes to permit out-of-state physicians to treat patients within the state borders.[38] Some states have taken a more expansive approach to telemedicine regulation, imposing requirements for informed consent from the patient before treatment.[39] California has taken the lead in creating more comprehensive legislation governing consent requirements for consultation, physician licensure, unprofessional physician conduct, and payment for services.[40] In addition to these statutes, the American Health Information Management Association has developed recommended guidelines for health information practitioners to follow concerning the content of and security measures to be used in a telemedical record.[41] Although much work has been performed by state legislatures, much work remains to be done in order to answer the many questions referenced above.

Conclusion

The tranformation from a paper-based medical record to a computerized patient record is only a matter of time. To accomplish this transformation, the health information manager must be able to identify the legal issues that a computerized patient record presents that may affect accreditation, licensure, and liability. Knowledge of these legal requirements is essential to a proper evaluation, selection, and implementation of an information system that safeguards health information from unauthorized access or careless handling.

Health information managers owe to their employers, patients, and the public at large an obligation to prevent improper use of confidential data maintained in a computerized patient record. This chapter assists in providing a basis for the development of confidentiality standards for the computerized patient record.

Case Study

General Hospital has determined that within three years, the paper-based medical record it currently uses will be replaced with a computerized patient record. General Hospital prefers to have a vendor install a computer system that allows for some tailoring to its institutional needs. You are a member of a committee that will evaluate and select the computer system. What legal issues should you raise to the committee and hospital about possible barriers and problems to implementing a computerized patient record? Assuming those barriers and problems are resolved, what legal issues should you address with the committee and hospital in the evaluation and selection process?

Review Questions

1. What impact do licensing authorities and accrediting organizations have on a health-care provider's decision to adopt a computerized patient record system?
2. Define a computerized patient record.
3. How is authentication represented in a computerized patient record?
4. What is admissibility, and how does it apply to the computerized medical record?
5. What protections from the physical environment should be in place to protect a computerized patient record?
6. What steps should be taken to ensure personnel security in a computerized patient record environment?
7. How does the business associate rule apply to the computerized patient record?
8. What efforts should the health information manager take to safeguard portable computers and personal digital assistants?
9. Discuss the concept of computer sabotage and how the dangers posed by the concept can be minimized.

Enrichment Activities

1. Obtain several examples of policies governing the security of computerized health information from local health-care facilities. For each policy, examine its strengths and weaknesses. For example, were the categories of physical security, personnel security, and risk prevention techniques addressed? Are there any flaws in the policies?
2. Review articles in health-care journals concerning electronic health (e-health) information. Are the discussions comprehensive? Should additional analysis have been provided concerning legal issues associated with e-health?

Notes

1. During the 102nd Congress, several bills were introduced that would mandate computerization of patient records. H.R. Bill 5919, 102nd Cong., 2d Sess. (1992); S. Bill 2878 102nd Cong., 2d Sess. (1992). In 1996, Congress passed the Health Insurance Portability and Accountability Act, P.L. 104-191, addressing the electronic transmission of patient-specific health information. 42 U.S.C. § 1320d (2001).
2. INSTITUTE OF MEDICINE, *The Computer-Based Patient Record: An Essential Technology for Health Care,* (National Academy Press 1991).
3. *Id.* at 11-12.
4. *Id.*
5. HAW. REV. STATE. § 622-58 (2000); LA. REV. STAT. ANN § 40:2109 (1999).
6. IND. CODE ANN. § 34-43-1-1 (Burns 2000). Also, Indiana's administrative regulations expressly authorize the use of computerized hospital records that maintain confidentiality. IND. ADMIN. CODE tit. 410, r. 15-1-8(2) & 15-1-9(2) (b) (1).
7. NEV. REV. STAT. ANN. § 629.051 (2001).
8. The Medical Records Act of 1974, TENN. CODE ANN. § 68-11-302 (2000).
9. MONT. ADMIN. R. 16.32.308; OR. ADMIN. R. 333-505-050(8); and WASH. ADMIN. CODE § 248-18-440.
10. For example, Georgia regulations specify the use of original, microfilm or "other usable forms," GA. COMP. R. & REGS. r. 290-5-6.11(h), and Mississippi

allows storage of hospital records by microfilming, photographing, photocopying, optical disks, or "other acceptable form of medium, as determined by the licensing agency." MISS. CODE ANN. § 41-9-77 (1999).

11. For example, Idaho permits preservation of hospital records by microfilm or other photographically reproduced film. IDAHO CODE § 39-1394 (2000). Minnesota allows for the transfer of original files and records to photographic film of convenient size. MINN. STAT. § 145.30 (2000).
12. It is especially important to obtain the licensing authority's interpretation where state regulations are internally inconsistent. For example, while Missouri's regulations governing hospitals allow for authentication electronically, MO. CODE REGS. tit. 19, § 30-20.021(D) (2) (1993), they require hospitals to preserve medical records in a permanent file in the original or on microfilm. MO. CODE REGS. tit. 19, § 30-20.021(D) (15) (1993).
13. 15 U.S.C. § 7001-7031 (2001).
14. 42 C.F.R. § 482.24(c) (1) (ii) (2001); JOINT COMMISSION ON ACCREDITATION OF HEALTHCARE ORGANIZATIONS, COMPREHENSIVE ACCREDITATION MANUAL FOR HOSPITALS, Management of Information, IM 7 (1999).
15. Federal Business Records Act, 28 U.S.C. § 1732(a) (2000) (general business record exception); FED. R. EVID. 803(6) (general business record exception); GA. CODE ANN. § 24-7-8 (Michie 2000) (subset of the general business record exception applicable to medical records).
16. FED. R. EVID. 803(6).
17. Examples of biometric identification include voiceprint, thumbprint, and retinal scan.
18. For example, Indiana law requires its courts to treat printouts of electronically recorded hospital medical records as originals for purposes of admissibility into evidence. IND. CODE § 34-43-1-1 (Burns 2000).
19. 749 F.2d 195 (5th Cir. 1984).
20. *See, e.g.,* Medicare Conditions of Participation, 42 C.F.R. § 405.1722(a) (1992); JOINT COMMISSION, ACCREDITATION MANUAL FOR HOSPITALS, Management of Information IM 2 (2001).
21. 42 C.F.R. §§ 164.502-.528 (2001).
22. JONATHAN P. TOMES., JD, *Compliance Guide to Electronic Health Records,* Chap. 10 (Faulkner & Gray 1994).
23. 42 C.F.R. § 164.506
24. www.ahima.org/infocenter/guidelines/tenets.
25. www.ahima.org/infocenter/guidelines/tenets.

26. 42 C.F.R. §§ 483-484 (2000).
27. 42 C.F.R. Part 2 (2000).
28. 42 C.F.R. §§ 164.502-.528 (2001).
29. www.ahima.org/infocenter/guidelines/tenets.
30. 42 C.F.R. §§ 164.502 -.528 (privacy)(2001); 63 FED. REG. 55 (proposed Aug. 12, 1998) (security).
31. E.g., Standard E1869-97 of the American Society for Testing and Materials calls for encryption of electronic mail. STANDARD GUIDE FOR CONFIDENTIALITY, PRIVACY, ACCESS, AND DATA SECURITY PRINCIPLES FOR HEALTH INFORMATION INCLUDING COMPUTER-BASED PATIENT RECORDS, ASTM standard no. E1869-97. Available at www.astm.org. Encryption is also addressed by the HEALTH CARE FINANCING ADMINSTRATION, HCFA, INTERNET SECURITY POLICY. Available at www.hcfa.gov/security/isecplcy.
32. AMERICAN HEALTH INFORMATION MANAGEMENT ASSOCIATION, Practice Brief-E-mail Security (Updated) (2000).
33. CHITA-AGORA PROJECT PRIVACY TASK FORCE, DRAFT POLICY 1.2 (Sept. 1999); KAISER PERMANENTE, *Doctor Appointments and Advice Available Online*, www.kaiserpermanente.org; David Z. Sands, *Guidelines for the Use of Patient Centered E-Mail* (1999) www.mahealthdata.org; PARTNERS HEALTHCARE, GUIDELINES FOR CLINICAL ELECTRONIC MAIL COMMUNICATION, Draft Policy (May 1999); STANFORD MEDICAL GROUP, Electronic Mail Services (1999), www.med.stanford.edu.
34. FLA. ADMIN. CODE ANN., r 59A-3.213; MISS. CODE ANN. § 41-9-77 (1999); TENN. CODE ANN. § 68-11-307 (2000); WASH. REV. CODE § 5.46.010 (2001).
35. Telemedicine Report to Congress by the Joint Working Group on Telemedicine (1997). Available at www.ntia.doc.gov/reports/telemed.
36. Telecommunications Act of 1996, 47 U.S.C. §§ 254(b) & (h)(2001).
37. 42 U.S.C. § 1395i, mm (2001).
38. See ARK. CODE ANN. § 10-3-1702 (1999); CAL. BUS. & PROF. CODE § 2290.5 (West 2001); COLO. REV. STAT. § 12-36-106 (2000); GA CODE ANN. § 50-5-192 (2000); HAW. REV. STAT. § 453-2 (2000); 225 ILL. COMP. STAT. 60/49.5 (West 2000); MISS. CODE ANN. § 73-25-34 (2000); MONT. CODE ANN. §§ 87-3-301 & -342 (2000); OHIO REV. CODE ANN. § 4731-296 (2001); OKLA. STAT. tit. 36 § 6802 (2001); TENN. CODE ANN. § 63-6-209 (2000); TEX UTIL. CODE ANN. § 57.042 (West 2000); W. VA. CODE § 30-3-13 (2000).
39. See, e.g., ARIZ. REV. STAT. § 36-3602 (2000); CAL. BUS. & PROF. CODE § 2290.5 (West 2001).

40. California Telemedicine Development Act of 1996, S.B. 1665 (codified in scattered sections of the Health & Safety Code and the Business & Professions Code).
41. AMERICAN HEALTH INFORMATION MANAGEMENT ASSOCIATION, Practice Brief—Telemedical Records (1997).

Chapter 12

Health-Care Fraud and Abuse

Learning Objectives

After reading this chapter, the learner should be able to:

1. Define the meaning of fraud and abuse.
2. Compare and contrast the major laws supporting a prosecution for health-care fraud and abuse.
3. List and describe the roles of various law enforcement agencies in the prosecution of health-care fraud and abuse.
4. Define the meaning of compliance and compliance programs.
5. List the components of a compliance program.

Key Concepts

Antikickback statute
Civil money penalty
Compliance
Compliance programs
Fraud and abuse
Mail and wire fraud
Permissive and mandatory exclusion
Physician self-referral prohibitions
Qui tam actions
Relators
Unbundling
Upcoding
Whistle blowers

Introduction

During the past ten years, health-care fraud and abuse has become a front-burner issue. Federally funded health-care programs such as Medicare and Medicaid have lost of billions of dollars through fraud and abuse, as have private insurance companies. In response, the Congress and state legislatures have passed laws to address this problem, federal and state governments have increased their enforcement efforts of existing regulations and laws, and private insurance companies have escalated their efforts to expose fraudulent claims.

The increase in scrutiny has caused health-care providers and organizations to change their methods of operation and has called into being new jobs that did not exist a decade ago. Because health information management professionals manage many risk areas open to health-care fraud and abuse, such as accurate documentation, coding, and billing, it is important for these professionals to know and understand this area of law. This understanding can assist the organization in preventing the submission of false or inaccurate claims to the government or private payors.

Fraud and Abuse

Fraud and abuse is defined as a false misrepresentation of fact that is relied on by another to that person's detriment and is a departure from reasonable use. This false misrepresentation of fact may take the form of words or conduct, including false or misleading allegations or concealment of facts that should have been disclosed. This misrepresentation is done knowingly and is not the result of negligence. The departure from reasonable use means that the misrepresentation is contrary to the proper order established by usage in the industry.

In the health-care context, fraud and abuse means the efforts of a health-care provider or organization to misrepresent facts to a government entity or third-party payor so that the misrepresented facts appear legal and customary in the industry and results in some form of benefit, monetary or otherwise, to the health-care provider or organization. This misrepresentation is not a matter of mistake, but is rather a willful act or omission. In other words, fraud and abuse requires a willful and knowing action on behalf of the health-care provider or organization to misrepresent a fact, to the government's or third-party payor's detriment.

The most common forms of health-care fraud and abuse relate to the areas of false claims and billing practices—for example, billing for services not rendered such as submitting bills for physician examinations, x-rays, and laboratory tests that were never delivered. Other examples are upcoding and unbundling. **Upcoding** involves submitting a bill for a higher level of reimbursement than actually rendered in order to receive a higher reimbursement rate. **Unbundling** involves submitting separate bills for each component of a procedure instead of using the proper procedural code for the entire procedure, resulting in a higher reimbursement rate to the health-care provider—for example, billing separately for groups of laboratory tests performed together in order to receive a higher reimbursement.

Other common forms of health-care fraud and abuse include a health-care provider's referral of a patient to a facility in which the provider holds a financial interest (commonly referred to as a Stark violation)[1] or a provider's referral of a patient to another provider in exchange for compensation (commonly referred to as a kickback violation).[2] Additionally, the health-care provider may bill for services not considered medically necessary, double-bill for a service rendered, or bill for a covered service when the service provided was not in fact covered.

Major Laws Addressing Fraud and Abuse

The federal government has responded to the economic threat posed by health-care fraud and abuse by passing legislation specifically addressing the issue and by focusing prosecution efforts by using existing legislation originally intended for different purposes. A list of the major laws addressing health-care fraud and abuse is contained in Figure 12-1.

The linchpin for the prosecution of health-care fraud and abuse is the False Claims Act (FCA).[3] Originally used during the Civil War as a method

Figure 12-1. Major Laws Addressing Fraud and Abuse

1. False Claims Act.
2. Qui tam actions.
3. Antikick back statutes.
4. Physician self-referral prohibitions (Stark I & II).
5. Mail and wire fraud statutes.
6. Health Insurance Portability and Accountability Act (HIPAA).

to prosecute individuals and organizations that supplied the Union with inferior products or cheated the government outright, the FCA has taken on a new use over the past decade. It is used to protect the government against those who charge for services not rendered and is often used in the Medicare and Medicaid context. Typically, a health-care provider or organization violates the FCA by knowingly submitting a false or fraudulent claim to the government or by making a false statement in order to get the claim approved or paid.[4] This knowing submission may be proven by showing that the provider or organization actually intended to commit fraud. Or it may be proven by showing that the provider or organization actually knew the statement was false and was either deliberately ignorant of the truth or acted with reckless disregard of the truth when submitting the false statement.

FCA claims are typically brought as **qui tam actions**.[5] Qui tam actions allow private plaintiffs (technically referred to as **relators**) to sue on behalf of the U.S. government and receive a portion of the recovered funds if successful. The relator begins the lawsuit on his own initiative; however, the government may decide to intervene in the case and take over prosecution or may join in the prosecution with the relator. The government may decide to allow the relator to proceed with the case on his own without any form of government intervention.

Typically, a relator is a current or former employee of the health-care provider or organization who has learned of the fraud and abuse and wishes to expose the activity. These relators are called **whistle-blowers.** Whistle-blowers have included physicians who supervised laboratories and supervisors responsible for billing, coding and claims processing procedures.[6] Relators have even included persons whose insurance benefits were the subject of coverage and payment disputes between Medicare and third-party payors.[7]

Another potent weapon in the fight against health-care fraud and abuse is the federal **antikickback statute**.[8] This statute prohibits the offer or solicitation of remuneration, including kickbacks and rebates, in exchange for referrals of Medicare-payable services. Many states have followed Congress's lead, passing their own legislation prohibiting payment for referrals for services offered by managed care companies and private insurance companies. In the strictest sense, an instance where a physician is paid for referrals would be prohibited under antikickback statutes at both the federal and state levels. Health-care organizations have been prosecuted under this statute for, among other things, acting pursuant to the terms of a partnership agreement that allowed for profit sharing and below cost testing in exchange for test referrals that could be billed at full rates.[9] Because the anti-kickback statutes examine the relationships between health-care providers closely, it has now become customary to formalize business relationships through the use of written agreements. This formalization process has resulted in providers' engaging in more arm's-length transactions for goods and services, allowing for the avoidance of impropriety.

Physician self-referral prohibitions[10] have also been the subject of much litigation. In response to concerns that physicians were abusing the system by referring patients to their own services, Congress passed laws that prohibit self-referral for a number of services. Under the first law (commonly referred to as Stark I), a physician is barred from referring Medicare patients to a clinical laboratory in which the physician or an immediate family member possesses a financial interest. Congress later extended the prohibition to other services so that a physician is barred from referring Medicare patients to a designated health service in which the physician or immediate family member possesses a financial interest (commonly referred to as Stark II). The term *designated health service* is broad enough to include durable medical equipment, clinical laboratories, occupational therapy, physical therapy, hospital services, orthotics and prosthetics, radiology, parenteral and enteral nutrition services and supplies, home health services and outpatient prescription drugs. Under Stark II, a physician violates the law by referring a Medicare patient to any entity listed above if the physician or immediate family member holds any financial interest in the entity. By making such a referral, the physician taints the claim for reimbursement made by the referred entity.

Less frequently seen in the prosecution of a fraud and abuse case is the use of federal **mail and wire fraud** statutes.[11] These statutes prohibit the use of the U.S. Postal Service or commercial wire services for the advancement of a scheme relating to fraud. Because modern business practices routinely involve the use of the mail system or wire services, it would be fairly easy for a health-care provider or organization involved with fraud to violate these statutes. A violation of these statutes is a felony, punishable by a fine of $1000, a five-year term of imprisonment, or both.

Because of the significance of the remedies the federal government may wield in a fraud and abuse case, health-care providers and organizations have two additional incentives to obey the law. First, the federal government may apply the **civil money penalty** law to a violation.[12] Under this statute, the Department of Health and Human Services (HHS) is permitted to recover money damages for false or fraudulent claims. The health-care provider would be responsible to make restitution to the government for the fraud at issue and could also be fined up to three times the amount of damages plus an additional fine not to exceed $10,000.

An even more significant deterrent to health-care providers and organizations is the statute providing for **permissive and mandatory exclusion** from participation in Medicare and all other federally financed health-care programs.[13] This statute provides for the exclusion of a health-care provider or organization due to criminal or other program violations. For instance, a five-year to permanent mandatory exclusion applies to health-care providers and organizations that have received felony criminal convictions. For misdemeanor actions, debarment from participation for a minimum of one year may apply. Because it is not economically feasible for a health-care provider or organization to forgo service to Medicare beneficiaries, the exclusion provision is a powerful weapon for the government to exercise.

A recent development in the prosecution of health-care fraud and abuse is the Health Insurance Portability and Accountability Act (HIPAA).[14] HIPAA both modifies the civil money penalty law and provides enhanced resources for the federal government to combat health-care fraud. The civil money penalty law is modified to include penalties for actions specifically related to health-care fraud and abuse, such as unbundling and upcoding. A list of these actions is found in Figure 12-2. HIPAA also has established four programs to assist with fraud enforcement (see Figure 12-3).

Figure 12-2. HIPAA Enhancements

1. Engaging in upcoding.
2. Engaging in patterns of claiming medically unnecessary items of service.
3. Transferring remuneration to a Medicare beneficiary that may influence the beneficiary to order or receive items or services, to include the waiver of coinsurance and deductibles for service.
4. Submitting a claim when the provider has been excluded from the Medicare and Medicaid programs while retaining ownership or a controlling interest in an entity that still participates in Medicare or Medicaid.

Figure 12-3. Fraud Enforcement Programs:

1. Fraud and Abuse Control Program—operated jointly by the Department of Justice and the Office of Inspector General to control health-care fraud and abuse and conduct investigations relating to the delivery of health-care services.
2. Medicare Integrity Program—directs the Department of Health & Human Services to enter into agreements with private companies to carry out fraud and abuse protections.
3. Beneficiary Incentive Program—encourages Medicare beneficiaries to report suspected cases of fraud and abuse.
4. Health-care Fraud and Abuse Data Collection Program—designed to create a national health-care fraud and abuse database in coordination with the National Practitioner Data Bank.

Law Enforcement Agencies

Several law enforcement agencies share responsibility to prosecute health-care fraud and abuse. One of the most prominent agencies is the Office of Inspector General (OIG) of the Department of Health and Human Services. The OIG is authorized to conduct civil, administrative, and criminal investigations of fraud associated with the federal Medicare and Medicaid programs. In keeping with its responsibilities, the OIG provides guidance to health-care providers on how to comply with applicable local, state, and federal laws and regulations. Other law enforcement agencies and their areas of responsibility include the Postal Inspection Service, responsible for investigating fraud schemes involving the U.S. mail system, and the Defense Criminal Investigative Service (DCIS), responsible for investigating fraud schemes committed against the military's health insurance programs.

The law enforcement agency with the widest responsibility to investigate health-care fraud is the Federal Bureau of Investigation (FBI). In contrast to the agencies listed above, the FBI possesses authority that extends beyond the jurisdiction of a particular governmental program. The FBI may work jointly with the OIG, the DCIS, the Postal Inspection Service, or the Centers for Medicare and Medicaid Services (CMS), or it may act on its own based on complaints received through calls, letters, or visits from members of the public. Additionally, the FBI may investigate due to the efforts of a whistle-blower acting pursuant to the False Claims Act.

Investigations of health-care fraud typically extend over several years and may involve interviews with the whistle-blower, members of the public, and possibly the health-care provider or organization itself. Documentation may be obtained through the use of subpoenas and search warrants. Institutions other than the health-care provider, such as CMS and billing services, may be asked to supply further documentation.

In the event the health information manager is confronted by a law enforcement agent with a search warrant, the manager should remember that he has a duty to cooperate with the agent but at the same time has the obligation to notify the provider's or organization's legal counsel of the request presented by the agent. Although it may appear difficult to balance the duty and obligation, it is imperative that the manager do so. Upon notice, legal counsel will assist the manager in determining how to respond cooperatively to the agent's request, including what to say and what not to say. Until legal counsel has provided advice or has arrived on the premises, the health information manager should cooperate with the agent's request to gather specific records and information while not answering any additional questions.

Upon completion of the investigative process, the law enforcement agency works with the local U.S. attorney's office to pursue prosecution of health-care providers or organizations suspected of wrongdoing. Both government offices will determine whether to proceed with a lawsuit, including which statute forms the basis of the claim against the health-care provider or organization. To avoid going to trial, those same government agencies may craft a financial settlement agreement with those suspected of wrongdoing.

Compliance Programs

Compliance has been a part of health information management since the beginning of the profession. For decades, health information managers have worked to comply with voluntary accreditation standards, federal and state laws and regulations, institutional bylaws and rules, and professional codes of ethics. The effort to comply with these external forces has become even more complex with the advent of third-party payment systems and government reimbursement programs. With the focus on health-care fraud and abuse intensifying and the advent of implementing rules addressing privacy and security under the Health Insurance Portability and Accountability Act, compliance is now a formalized part of health information management.

Compliance is defined as the efforts to establish a culture that promotes prevention, detection, and resolution of instances of conduct that do not conform to applicable local, state, and federal laws and regulations. A **compliance program** ensures the establishment of effective internal controls that promote adherence to the applicable local, state, and federal laws and regulations and the program requirements of federal, state, and private health plans.

The establishment of compliance programs can be performed from an ethics-based or minimum legal requirements approach. Under the ethics-based approach, a health-care organization decides that it wishes to conform to local, state, and federal laws and regulations because it is the right thing to do or because a cost-benefit analysis reveals it would be a sound business practice. The ethics-based approach encourages good behavior and is in essence a voluntary form of improvement. This approach demonstrates to employees and the community at large that the health-care organization is committed to responsible corporate conduct. Under the minimum legal requirements approach, a health-care organization decides it will conform to local, state, and federal laws and regulations because of the fear of punishment in the event of nonconformance—the so-called fear of getting caught. Because the conformance standards are externally imposed, the motivation under this approach is to avoid or minimize penalties or punishment.

Under either approach, the result is that health-care providers that implement effective compliance programs reduce their exposure to civil damages and penalties, criminal sanctions, and administrative remedies. The provider also benefits through a greater ability to assess and improve the efficiency, effectiveness, and quality of patient services. The health-care provider develops a centralized internal mechanism for distributing information on health-care statutes, regulations, and other program directives.

Compliance programs take all shapes and sizes, mostly dependent on the type of health-care provider or organization. The Office of the Inspector General (OIG) of the Department of Health and Human Services has released compliance program guidelines for hospitals, clinical laboratories, long-term care facilities, hospices, home care organizations, and physician offices.[15] These guidelines are not actually compliance programs; rather, they provide basic procedural and structural information for health-care providers and organizations to use in tailoring a compliance program to fit their own culture, structure, and processes. These compliance program guidelines share the key elements listed in Figure 12-4.

Figure 12-4. Compliance Program Guidelines (Office of Inspector General, U.S. Department of Health and Human Services, http://www.dhhs.gov/poorg/oig.

1. Written standards of conduct and policies and procedures.
2. Designation of a chief compliance officer to oversee the compliance program.
3. Regular, effective education and training programs for all affected employees.
4. A process for receiving complaints of possible violations.
5. Development of a system to respond to allegations of improper or illegal activities and enforcement of appropriate disciplinary actions through well-publicized disciplinary directives.
6. Audits and other evaluation techniques to monitor compliance.
7. Investigation and corrective action of identified problems.

Compliance programs have also been imposed on health-care providers through financial settlement agreements. These agreements settle litigation brought by the government in the battle against fraud and abuse.[16] In some instances, the government has reduced the fines of those accused of fraud and abuse where an effective compliance program was in place. In other instances, the government has required the establishment of compliance programs as part of the financial settlement agreement.

In addition, health information managers may be guided by the U.S. Sentencing Guidelines for Organizations. These guidelines, listed in Figure 12-5, formed the basis for the compliance program guidelines and financial settlement agreements instituted by the federal government.[17]

Figure 12-5. U.S. Sentencing Guidelines for Organizations (U.S. Sentencing Guideline 8A1.2K)

1. Establish compliance standards and procedures for all employees to follow.
2. Assign specific individuals with overall responsibility to oversee compliance with Step 1.
3. Use due diligence not to delegate substantial discretionary authority to individuals who may have a propensity to engage in illegal activities.
4. Take steps to communicate effectively to all employees and other agents the standards and procedures.
5. Take reasonable steps to ensure compliance with the standards.
6. Use consistent enforcement of the standards to include disciplinary action.
7. If an offense has been detected, take all reasonable steps to respond to the offense and prevent further offenses.

Case Study

You are the head of the health information management department at General Hospital. An FBI agent has arrived at your office with a search warrant in hand. He asks to speak with you about the hospital's medical records. How should you respond?

Conclusion

In the face of increased scrutiny, health-care providers and organizations have responded to questions of health-care fraud and abuse by developing compliance programs to document that they are adhering to the rule of law. These compliance programs make good business sense and will likely not disappear in the future. Because health information professionals manage risk areas critical to an allegation of health-care fraud and abuse, they owe to their employers, third-party payors, and the government at large an obligation to assist in preventing the submission of false or inaccurate claims.

Review Questions

1. What forms of fraud and abuse may be present in a health-care setting?
2. What do the terms *upcoding* and *unbundling* mean?
3. What is the False Claims Act, and how does it apply to the health-care setting?
4. Name two remedies the federal government may use in a fraud and abuse case, and explain their application.
5. Name and explain the responsibility of the federal law enforcement agencies who share responsibility for prosecuting health-care fraud and abuse.
6. Compare and contrast the approaches to the establishment of a compliance program.

7. What are the benefits to a health-care provider that develops an effective compliance program?

Enrichment Activity

Imagine you are a health-care facility's chief compliance officer. Based on the contents of this chapter, draft an outline of the elements of your organization's compliance program. Following your outline, develop an inservice training program for staff concerning compliance standards, procedures, and policies.

Notes

1. 42 U.S.C. § 1395nn(b) (2001).
2. 42 U.S.C. §1320a-7b(b)(2001).
3. 31 U.S.C. § 3729-33(civil) and 42 U.S.C. § 1320a-7b(a)(criminal)(2001).
4. An example of a criminal prosecution of Medicare fraud is *United States v. Gieger*, 190 F.3d 661 (5th Cir. 1999) (conspiracy to submit false claims to Medicare concerning ambulance services).
5 Qui tam is part of the longer Latin phrase: "qui tam pro domino rege quam pro se ipso in hac parte sequitur," meaning he "who brings the action for the king as well as himself." *See United States ex rel. Stinson v. Prudential Ins.*, 944 F.2d 1149, 1152 n.2 (3d.Cir.1991).
6. *United States ex rel. Merena v. Smithkline Beecham Clinical Laboratories*, 114 F. Supp. 352 (E.D. Pa. 2000).
7. *United States ex rel. Cooper v. Blue Cross & Blue Shield of Florida*, 19 F.3d 562 (11th Cir. 1994).
8. 42 U.S.C. § 1320a-7b(b) (2001).
9. *United States ex rel. Kneepkins v. Gambro Healthcare Inc., et al.* 115 F. Supp. 2d 35 (D.Mass. 2000).
10. *42 U.S.C. § 1395nn; See also, United States ex rel. Thompson v. Columbia/ HCA Healthcare Corp.*, 125 F.3d 251 (5th Cir. 1997).
11. 18 U.S.C.§ 1341, 1343 (2001).
12. 42 U.S.C. § 1320a-7a (2001).
13. 42 U.S.C. § 1320a-7 (2001).

14. 42 U.S.C. §1320d (2001).
15. Http://www.hhs.gov/progorg/oig.
16. Examples of cases involving settlement agreements include: *Merena,* supra n. 6; *Assoc. Mutual Hosp. Serv. of Michigan v. Health Care Service Corp. of Illinois,* 71 F. Supp. 2d 750 (W.D. MI. 1999).
17. U.S. Sentencing Guideline 8A1.2/K.

Appendix

Case Studies: Things to Consider 253

Table of Cases 265

List of Common Acronyms 271

A Patient's Bill of Rights 277

Principles of Medical Record Documentation 281

Durable Power of Attorney for Health Care and Health-Care Directive (Sample Form) 287

Sample Living Will 293

Patient Self-Determination Act 297

Health Care Quality Improvement Act 309

Case Studies: Things to Consider

As stated in the Preface, no one right answer exists to the case study included at the end of a chapter. Learners should resolve each case study by using the knowledge gained from the chapter and critical thinking skills. To guide the learner in developing an answer to the case studies, this section provides an outline of points that should be addressed for each case study. Each outline is not meant to provide a comprehensive answer to the case study; rather, each serves as the basis for class discussion. The case studies and their corresponding outlines are listed in chapter order.

Chapter 1: Workings of the American Legal System

Case Study

You are the director of health information services for a medium-sized health-care facility. Like many of your peers, you have contracted with an outside copying service to handle all requests for release of patient health information at your facility. You have learned that a lobbying organization for trial attorneys in your state is promoting legislation to place a cap on photocopying costs, which is significantly below the actual cost incurred as part of the contract. Discuss the roles each branch of government will play in considering this legislation and how you and your professional organization may act to influence this process.

Things to Consider

Part One: Branches of Government

All three branches will be involved:

1. The lobbying organization will need to find a member of the legislature willing to sponsor its legislative proposal and shepherd it through the committee process.

2. Before the bill can become law, the state governor must sign it or veto it. Furthermore, the bill may direct the state department of health to issue regulations to implement the legislation.

3. Should a dispute arise and a lawsuit be filed, the judiciary may also be called upon to interpret the statute once it has been passed by the legislature and signed into law by the governor.

Part Two: Influencing the Process

Working within your professional association, and possibly in conjunction with other professional associations similarly affected, you may take the following steps:

1. Contact the lobbying organization and/or trial attorneys group directly to educate them about why and how photocopying fees are charged. Depending on the result, the lobbying organization or trial attorneys group may abandon its efforts or work with your association to modify its proposal.

2. Contact the sponsoring member of the legislature to educate him or her in the same manner. Additionally, appear before the appropriate legislative committee to testify about the consequences of the bill.

3. If it appears that momentum has already been built on the topic and a bill on the topic is ripe to pass, submit a counterproposal that your association can accept to a different legislative member for sponsorship.

4. Contact the governor with your association's views on the topic as part of the signature/veto process.

5. Write letters to the editor or op-ed pieces for publication in your local paper in an effort to educate the voting public. Send copies of the published pieces to those persons or groups listed in numbers 1–4.

Chapter 2: Court Systems and Legal Procedures

Case Study

You are the in-house counsel at General Hospital. You have been contacted by an attorney for a former patient of the hospital whose inpatient hospitalization resulted in some harm to the patient. That harm was memorialized in an incident report prepared by hospital staff. Your review of the incident report indicates that the harm described by the attorney is consistent with the harm described in the incident report. Based on your conversation with the attorney, you believe a lawsuit is imminent. Because you believe it is in the best interest of all concerned to avoid the cost of litigation, you wish to consider methods of alternative dispute resolution. Discuss the relative advantages and disadvantages of each methods.

Things to Consider

1. Mediation offers the assistance of a third party who has nothing to gain or lose by the outcome of the mediation. Therefore, the neutrality of the mediator is a positive aspect for both sides. Also, the mediator brings the parties together to resolve the dispute, increasing the possibility that both sides will be satisfied with the result and comply with any of the result's requirements. Additionally, privacy of both sides is respected because no documents are filed on the public record. Finally, the mediator does not need to be an expert in the health-care field, which could have caused delay and additional expense to the process.

A disadvantage is that if the parties cannot agree when choosing the mediator, the mediation fails before any substance is discussed.

2. Arbitration also involves a neutral third party, but this third party is generally an expert on the substantive matter in question and therefore will understand the issues involved at a higher level. The parties do not have to compromise to reach an agreement but can rely on the neutral third party to come to an equitable decision. An aggrieved party still possesses the right to pursue a lawsuit overturning the arbitrator's award.

A disadvantage is that the use of an expert may cause additional expense and delay to the process. Also, the arbitrator's award is binding on the parties, meaning the parties are obligated to comply with the terms of the award until such time as a court of general jurisdiction overturns the award.

3. Negotiation and settlement have the advantage of not involving a third party, allowing a maximum of confidentiality to all parties and less expense and delay. A disadvantage is that a settlement agreement often contains a release of claims, barring any future litigation concerning the subject of the dispute. And if the parties display animosity for each other, the need for a neutral third party may be so great as to destroy any chance for negotiation and settlement.

Chapter 3: Principles of Liability

Case Study

A surgeon performs elective surgery on John Smith. Smith later complains to his surgeon about pain resulting from the surgery. His surgeon dismisses his complaints as not credible and eventually withdraws from the case. Smith is then treated by another surgeon who determines that he developed complications from surgery and that the delay in treatment has made the complications worse. Smith sees an attorney about a possible lawsuit against the first surgeon. Describe the theories that could support a lawsuit under these circumstances.

Things to Consider

1. Negligence:

Given these facts, one can assume that the first surgeon owed a duty of care to John Smith. Whether a negligence theory will apply depends on the answer to the following questions: Did the first surgeon apply the standard of care that a reasonably prudent professional in the same or similar circumstances would have applied? Does the appropriate standard of care encompass both the surgery and the credibility determination? Was the first surgeon's actions the cause of John Smith's medical complications?

2. Medical abandonment:

Given the facts listed, it appears necessary that John Smith continue to receive care. Whether the theory of medical abandonment will apply depends on the answer to the following question: Was John Smith given a list of qualified substitute physicians? Was his need for treatment immediate? Did the first surgeon withdraw from treatment for economic rather than medical reasons? What type of follow-up treatment did the first surgeon arrange?

3. *Res ipsa loquitur:*

For this theory to apply, additional facts concerning the nature of the complications would be necessary. For example, if a surgical sponge was discovered inside John Smith's body at the surgical site, it may be the cause of the complications. Under such a scenario, John Smith would have little difficulty establishing the three elements of *res ipsa loquitur.*

4. Technical battery:

For this theory to apply, it would be necessary to review the consent to surgery form signed by John Smith. If the first surgeon acted beyond the scope of the consent John Smith gave and that action resulted in the complications, a technical battery has occurred.

Chapter 4: Patient Record Requirements

Case Study

You are the director of health information at a large medical center that offers inpatient, outpatient, and emergency care at several sites in one state. Your medical center has announced that it will acquire a facility offering similar services in a neighboring state. The laws and regulations governing the retention and destruction of medical records differ between these states. Discuss how the lack of a consistent set of laws and regulations on these two matters affects the institution you serve, and outline the steps you will now take to deal with the situation.

Things to Consider

Although decisions to retain and destroy medical records are influenced by many forces, the predominant force is a legal one. The statutes and regulations governing retention and destruction provide the basis for any decision: they establish the minimum amount of time medical records should be maintained and the legally acceptable methods of destruction. Where one state's requirements differ from another's, as in this case study, the health information manager is left with two options: (1) maintain separate policies for retention and destruction for each state's sites, or (2) adopt one uniform policy of retention and destruction that is measured by whichever state's requirements are longest. Each option has its weaknesses: the first may lead to confusion and mistakes in execution; the second may lead to maintaining records at some sites longer than otherwise necessary, leading to possible storage and fiscal problems. Steps to deal with this situation include: (1) consulting with legal counsel to assist in making the policy choice, (2) educating the staff in both states of the problem and the policy choice selected, (3) educating any commercial contractor of the differences between the two states and the policy choice selected, and (4) educating administration of the budget impact the policy choice will make.

Chapter 5: Access to Health Information

Case Study

You are the director of health information services at a tertiary-care hospital. You and the director of emergency room services are jointly responsible for reporting instances of communicable disease, child abuse, and cancer to the appropriate state authority. You have just completed an audit of your institution's reporting mechanism and discovered that the reporting requirements are not consistently met. The audit could not definitively establish whether the reporting never occurred or occurred but was not documented in the patient's medical record. Discuss what legal issues are present and what approaches you should take to resolve this problem.

Things to Consider

1. The law places a burden on the health-care provider to report public health threats because the health-care provider is on the front line, available to observe the threats firsthand.

2. State law establishing reporting requirements places a mandatory, not optional, burden on the health-care provider. Failure to comply with the reporting requirements may subject the health-care provider to sanction and in the instance of reporting injuries caused by deadly weapons, may impede law enforcement efforts.

3. Steps to improve reporting include reexamination and/or revision of documentation and reporting policies. Inservice education is in order for those health-care providers who document public health threats and those who report the threats to the state's department of health or similar agency. Increased auditing of the institution's reporting mechanism should occur until the health information manager is convinced that the reporting requirements are consistently met.

Chapter 6: Confidentiality and Informed Consent

Case Study

You are the director of health information services at a medium-size health-care facility providing general, emergency, and pediatric care. Because of downsizing and consolidation of managerial functions, you are also responsible for staff education in your facility. Discuss how you would structure and present an inservice program to staff members of various departments that addresses confidentiality policies and procedures of your facility and the legal bases underlying these policies and procedures.

Things to Consider

This problem assumes that the audience at the inservice program is a mix of the facility's staff, as opposed to separate inservice programs for emergency services, and so forth. Building on that assumption, the program must be structured to address confidentiality on both a broad basis and regarding those areas of the facility that pose unique confidentiality concerns. In particular, the program must address questions of confidentiality in (1) an emergency room, which by its nature lends itself to eavesdropping, and (2) a pediatric ward, where relatives other than the parents may be seeking information. The legal underpinnings of confidentiality are addressed in constitutional provisions, federal and state statutes, and common law decisions.

Chapter 7: Judicial Process of Health Information

Case Study

You supervise the correspondence unit of the health information services department of a medical center. Today, you received a subpoena duces tecum from an attorney, demanding either the originals or copies of all medical records concerning Mary Smith, who allegedly is or was a patient of the medical center. The subpoena lacks sufficient information for you to determine whether Mary Smith is or was a patient in your facility. The subpoena is not accompanied by a valid authorization to release information for Mary Smith, as required in your state. How should you respond to the subpoena?

Things to Consider

Among the available choices are: (1) seeking the advice of legal counsel, and where appropriate, delegating to legal counsel the obligation to respond to the subpoena; and (2) contacting requesting counsel with a noncommittal answer acknowledging the confidentiality restrictions under which the health-care provider operates and forwarding a predrafted release of information form for the patient Mary Smith to sign.

Chapter 8: Specialized Patient Records

Case Study

You are the director of health information services in a major medical center that maintains both a psychiatric unit and a substance abuse unit in addition to general medical and surgical units. Your facility plans to join a computer network with fifteen hospitals throughout the state, which will allow online access to laboratory data, regardless of which facility performed the lab work. None of the other fifteen facilities offer psychiatric or substance abuse treatment. Identify and discuss the confidentiality issues present with such a network in the light of the statutory, regulatory, and accrediting requirements governing patients treated in these units.

Things to Consider

The general confidentiality principles would apply: Who should have access to what data for what purpose? Should the full lab data be available or only an abstract of information? How do you track access to the lab data with computer terminals present throughout the network?

In addition to the general confidentiality principles, patients treated in psychiatric and substance abuse units are subject to strict confidentiality protections, including restrictions on patient identification. Access to lab data as described in the case study will undoubtedly violate both federal and state law concerning restrictions on patient identification because mere status as a member of the network will not automatically authorize a health-care provider at another facility access to otherwise restricted patient information. Under both state and federal regulations governing psychiatric and substance abuse units, the health-care provider seeking access to the data would need to demonstrate that he or she plays a role in the patient's care.

Chapter 9: Risk Management and Quality Management

Case Study

You are a health information manager closely involved with risk management at General Hospital, a teaching institution. Beginning this July, the hospital will incorporate presentations by hospital employees into its Grand Rounds series of lectures. You have been asked to present the lecture covering risk management. Compose a presentation addressing the legal aspects of risk management, particularly concentrating on patient record requirements and incident reports.

Things to Consider

Any presentation should include discussion about:

1. The growth and development of risk management in general and as applied to General Hospital.

2. Patient record requirements must address: (a) proper documentation, using examples of a properly documented medical record and a poorly documented medical record; (b) security concerns, including the active management of the availability of medical records; and (c) confidentiality, focusing in particular on the risk of talking about patients in inappropriate spots, such as hospital elevators.

3. Incident reports must address (a) what they are, (b) why they are necessary, (c) how to and how not to complete one, (d) how they are used; and (e) how to protect them from discovery.

4. An explanation of the attorney–client privilege in the context of incident reports.

Chapter 10: HIV Information

Case Study

You are the director of health information services at General Hospital, supervising several employees who release health information. As a community service, your facility recently launched a new HIV/AIDS outreach program. Because of the anticipated increase in patients with HIV/AIDS, you have decided to reexamine your policies and procedures governing release of information. Discuss what points should be included in the policies and procedures, particularly how employees should handle inadequate requests for release of information and subpoenas concerning HIV/AIDS information.

Things to Consider

Any revision of policies and procedures should include an examination of the relevant state statutes and regulations. These statutes and regulations will set the minimum standard on which to base policies and procedures. In addition, the health information manager should examine the guidelines established by the Centers for Disease Control and professional associations. Particular points to include: (a) issue of identification of HIV/AIDS patients and test results; (b) whether the law requires certain forms to be used for release of information or minimum data to be contained in the release of information form; and (c) whether the law requires patient notification of an HIV-positive health-care provider.

Responses to inadequate requests for release of information or subpoenas should be handled in a manner similar to that explained in the answer to the case study for Chapter 7.

Chapter 11: Computerized Patient Records

Case Study

General Hospital has determined that within three years, the paper-based medical record it currently uses will be replaced with a computerized patient record. General Hospital prefers to have a vendor install a computer system that allows for some tailoring to its institutional needs. You are a member of a committee that will evaluate and select the computer system. What legal issues should you raise to the committee and hospital about possible barriers and problems to implementing a computerized patient record? Assuming those barriers and problems are resolved, what legal issues should you address with the committee and hospital in the evaluation and selection process?

Things to Consider

Issues of possible barriers that should be raised to the committee include:

1. Does the state licensing authority permit the creation and storage of a computerized patient record?
2. Does the state licensing authority specify authentication of a certain type, such as a physician's written signature?
3. Does the court system governing the health-care provider accept a computer printout as evidence in a court case?

Issues in the selection process include:

1. Physical security concerns.
2. Personnel security concerns, including ongoing educational programs for health-care employees.

3. Risk prevention techniques, such as audit trails of in-house use, restrictions on access and use of patient health information by the vendor selling and servicing the computer system, and restrictions on computer networks.

Chapter 12: Health-Care Fraud and Abuse

Case Study

You are the head of the health information management department at General Hospital. An FBI agent has arrived at your office with a search warrant in hand. He asks to speak with you about the hospital's medical records. How should you respond?

Things to Consider

The first consideration is balancing the duty to cooperate with law enforcement officers with the obligation to the health-care provider's or organization's legal counsel. If this balance is addressed in a policy of the provider or organization, the health information manager should follow the steps contained in the policy. If no such policy exists or the existing policy is inadequate, the health information manager should notify legal counsel for the provider or organization and seek guidance on what to say and what not to say. Until legal counsel has arrived on the premises, the manager should cooperate with the agent's request to gather specific records and information while not answering any additional questions. The manager should determine whether the agent wishes to receive the original or copies of the records in question and act accordingly.

Table of Cases

Chapter 1: Workings of the American Legal System

Bartling v. Superior Court, 18
John Roe v. Jane Doe, 4
Marbury v. Madison, 16
Mordecai v. Blue Cross/Blue Shield of Alabama, 3
Prevost v. Coffee County Hospital Authority, 3

Chapter 3: Principles of Liability

Bernardi v. Community Hospital Association, 49
Bing v. Thunig, 57
Brooks v. Robinson, 55
Burditt v. U.S. Dept. of Health & Human Services, 41
Corn v. French, 52
Darling v. Charleston Community Memorial Hospital, 50
Dashiell v. Griffith, 54
Foran v. Carangelo, 55
Horowitz v. Bogart, 55
Johnson v. Misericordia Community Hospital, 51
Johnson v. Vaughn, 54
Katsetos v. Nolan, 54
Larrimore v. Homeopathic Hosp. Assoc., 46
McDonald v. Massachusetts General Hospital, 62
Mohr v. Williams, 52
Mucci v. Houghton, 54
Seymour v. Victory Memorial Hospital, 59
Tarasoff v. Regents of University of California, 51
Vann v. Harden, 54

Warwick v. Bliss, 54
Ybarra v. Spangard, 48

Chapter 4: *Patient Record Requirements*

Ahrens v. Katz, 74
Bondu v. Gurvich, 77
Carr v. St. Paul Fire & Marine Insurance, 79
Collins v. Westlake Community Hospital, 72
Henry by Henry v. St. John's Hospital, 74
Hurlock v. Park Lane Medical Center, 72
Ravenis v. Detroit General Hospital, 71

Chapter 5: *Access to Health Information*

Application of Romano, 109
Cannel v. Medical & Surgical Clinic, S.C., 102
Golan v. Louise Wise Services, 107
In re: *Wilson*, 107
Pyramid Life Insurance Co. v. Masonic Hospital Association, 90
Rabens v. Jackson Park Hospital Foundation, 90

Chapter 6: *Confidentiality and Informed Consent*

Baltzwell v. Baptist Medical Center, 126
Bly v. Rhoads, 126
Canterbury v. Spence, 126
Cobbs v. Grant, 126
Collins v. Itoh, 126
Conrad v. Imatani, 126
Cross v. Trapp, 126
Cruzan v. Director, Missouri Department of Health, 124
Halley v. Birbiglia, 126
Hook v. Rothstein, 126
Kohoutek v. Hafner, 126
Natanson v. Kline, 126
Pratt v. Davis, 122
Rice vs. Jaskolski, 126
Rolater v. Strain, 122

Scott v. Bradford, 126
Sard v. Hardy, 126
Schloendorff v. Society of New York Hospital, 122
Skripek v. Bergamo, 126
Weekly vs. Solomon, 126
Whalen v. Roe, 119
Wilkinson v. Vesey, 126

Chapter 7: Judicial Process of Health Information

Henry v. Lewis, 143
John Roe v. Jane Doe, 144
Pacheco v. Ortiz, 143
People v. Bickham, 143

Chapter 9: Risk Management and Quality Management

Bernardi v. Community Hospital Association, 183
Butterfield v. Okubo, 179
Clark v. Norris, 183
Community Hospitals of Indianapolis, Inc. v. Medtronic, 183
Darling v. Charleston Community Memorial Hospital, 177
Enke v. Anderson, 183
Estate of Behringer v. Medical Center at Princeton, 180
Kay Laboratories, Inc. v. District Court, 183
Sierra Vista Hospital v. Shaffer, 183
Sligar v. Tucker, 183
Weiner v. Memorial Hospital, 183

Chapter 10: HIV Information

Estate of Behringer v. Medical Center at Princeton, 203
Glover v. Eastern Nebraska Community Center, 202
Helman v. Sacred Heart Hospital, 202
In re: Milton Hershey Medical Center, 204
John Roe v. Jane Doe, 200
Kapuschinsky v. United States, 202
Leckelt v. Board of Commissioners, 202
Taaje v. St. Olaf Hospital, 202

Chapter 11: Computerized Patient Records

United States v. Sanders, 218

Chapter 12: Health-Care Fraud and Abuse

Assoc. Mutual Hosp. Serv. of Michigan v. Health Care Service Corp of Illinois, 246
U.S. v. Gieger, 240
U.S. ex rel. Cooper v. Blue Cross & Blue Shield of Florida, 240
U.S. ex rel. Merena v. Smithkine Beecham Clinical Laboratories, 240
U.S. ex rel. Stinson v. Prudential Ins., 240
U.S. ex rel. Kneepkins v. Gambro Healthcare Inc., 241
U.S. ex rel. Thompson v. Columbia/HCA Healthcare Corp., 241

Case Name	*Chapter*
Assoc. Mutual Hosp. Serv. of Michigan v. Health Care Service Corp of Illinois, 246	12
Ahrens v. Katz, 74	4
Application of Romano, 107	5
Baltzwell v. Baptist Medical Center, 126	6
Bartling v. Superior Court, 18	1
Bernardi v. Community Hospital Association, 49	3
Bing v. Thunig, 57	3
Bly v. Rhoads, 126	6
Bondu v. Gurvich, 77	4
Brooks v. Robinson, 55	3
Butterfield v. Okubo, 179	9
Burditt v. U.S. Dept. of Health & Human Services, 41	3
Cannel v. Medical & Surgical Clinic, S.C., 102	5
Canterbury v. Spence, 126	6
Carr v. St. Paul Fire & Marine Insurance, 79	4
Clark v. Norris, 183	9
Cobbs v. Grant, 126	6
Collins v. Itoh, 126	6
Collins v. Westlake Community Hospital, 72	4
Community Hospitals of Indianapolis, Inc. v. Medtronic, 183	9
Conrad v. Imatani, 126	6
Corn v. French, 52	3

Case Name	Chapter
Cross v. Trapp, 126	6
Cruzan v. Director, Missouri Department of Health, 124	6
Darling v. Charleston Community Memorial Hospital, 50	3
Dashiell v. Griffith, 54	3
Enke v. Anderson, 183	9
Estate of Behringer v. Medical Center at Princeton, 180	9
Foran v. Carangelo, 55	3
Glover v. Eastern Nebraska Community Center, 202	10
Golan v. Louise Wise Services, 107	5
Halley v. Birbiglia, 126	6
Helman v. Sacred Heart Hospital, 202	10
Henry by Henry v. St. John's Hospital, 74	4
Henry v. Lewis, 143	7
Hook v. Rothstein, 126	6
Horowitz v. Bogart, 55	3
Hurlock v. Park Lane Medical Center, 72	4
In re: *Milton Hershey Medical Center*, 204	10
In re: *Wilson*, 107	5
John Roe v. Jane Doe, 144, 200	7, 10
Johnson v. Misericordia Community Hospital, 51	3
Johnson v. Vaughn, 54	3
Kapuschinsky v. United States, 202	10
Katsetos v. Nolan, 54	3
Kay Laboratories, Inc. v. District Court, 183	9
Kohoutek v. Hafner, 126	6
Larrimore v. Homeopathic Hosp. Assoc., 46	3
Leckelt v. Board of Commissioners, 202	10
Marbury v. Madison, 16	11
McDonald v. Massachusetts General Hospital, 57	3
Mordecai v. Blue Cross/Blue Shield of Alabama, 3	1
Mohr v. Williams, 52	3
Mucci v. Houghton, 54	3
Natanson v. Kline, 126	6
Pacheco v. Ortiz, 143	7
People v. Bickham, 143	7
Pratt v. Davis, 122	6
Prevost v. Coffee County Hospital Authority, 3	1

Case Name	*Chapter*
Pyramid Life Insurance Co. v. Masonic Hospital Association, 90	5
Rabens v. Jackson Park Hospital Foundation, 90	5
Ravenis v. Detroit General Hospital, 71	4
Rice vs. Jaskolski, 126	6
Rolater v. Strain, 122	6
Scott v. Bradford, 126	6
Sard v. Hardy, 126	6
Schloendorff v. Society of New York Hospital, 122	6
Seymour v. Victory Memorial Hospital, 59	3
Sierra Vista Hospital v. Shaffer, 183	9
Skripek v. Bergamo, 126	6
Sligar v. Tucker, 183	9
Taaje v. St. Olaf Hospital, 202	10
Tarasoff v. Regents of University of California, 51	3
U.S. ex rel. Cooper v. Blue Cross & Blue Shield of Florida, 240	12
U.S. ex rel. Merena v. Smithkine Beecham Clinical Laboratories, 240	12
U.S. ex rel. Stinson v. Prudential Ins., 240	12
U.S. ex rel. Kneepkins v. Gambro Healthcare Inc., 241	12
U.S. ex rel. Thompson v. Columbia/HCA Healthcare Corp., 241	12
United States v. Sanders, 218	11
Vann v. Harden, 54	3
Warwick v. Bliss, 54	3
Weekly vs. Solomon, 126	6
Weiner v. Memorial Hospital, 183	7
Whalen v. Roe, 119	6
Wilkinson v. Vesey, 126	6
Ybarra v. Spangard, 48	3

List of Common Acronyms

Many of these acronyms may also be found in the text.

ACP	American College of Physicians
ACS	American College of Surgeons
ADA	American Dental Association; American Dietetic Association; American Diabetes Association
AHA	American Hospital Association
AHIMA	American Health Information Management Association
AIDS	Acquired Immunodeficiency Syndrome
AJPH	*American Journal of Public Health*
AMA	American Medical Association
ANA	American Nurses Association
AOA	American Osteopathic Association
APHA	American Public Health Association
ART	Accredited Record Technician
BC	Blue Cross
BS	Blue Shield
BSN	Bachelor of Science in Nursing
CAHEA	Committee on Allied Health Education and Accreditation
CAT	Computerized Axial Tomography
CBO	Congressional Budget Office
CCS	Clinical Coding Specialist
CDC	Centers for Disease Control (formerly, Communicable Disease Center)
CFR	Code of Federal Regulations

CHAMPUS	Civilian Health and Medical Program of the Uniformed Services
CHAMPVA	Civilian Health and Medical Program of the Veterans Administration
CHAP	Community Health Accreditation Program
CME	Council on Medical Education; Continuing Medical Education
CMS	Center for Medicare and Medicaid Services
COBRA	Consolidated Omnibus Budget Reconciliation Act
CON	Certificate of Need
CPR	Computerized Patient Record
CPT	Current Procedural Terminology
CSR	Code of State Regulations
CT	Computed Tomography
DC	Doctor of Chiropractic
DCIS	Defense Criminal Investigative Services
DDS	Doctor of Dental Surgery
DHEW	Department of Health, Education and Welfare; succeeded by the DHHS
DHHS	Department of Health and Human Services
DMD	Doctor of Dental Medicine
DO	Doctor of Osteopathy
DPM	Doctor of Podiatric Medicine
DRG	Diagnostic-Related Group(s)
EENT	Eye, Ear, Nose and Throat
ELISA	Enzyme-linked Immunosorbent Assay
EMS	Emergency Medical Services
ENT	Ear, Nose, and Throat
EPA	Environmental Protection Agency
FBI	Federal Bureau of Investigation
FCA	False Claims Act
FDA	Food and Drug Administration
FOIA	Freedom of Information Act
FTC	Federal Trade Commission

FTCA	Federal Tort Claims Act
FY	Fiscal Year
GAO	General Accounting Office
GDP	Gross Domestic Product
GNP	Gross National Product
GP	General Practitioner
GYN	Gynecology
H-B	Hill Burton Act
HCFA	Health Care Financing Administration
HCPCS	Health Care Financing Administration Common Procedure Coding System
HEW	Health, Education and Welfare; succeeded by HHS
HFMA	Healthcare Financial Management Association
HHA	Home Health Agency
HHS	Health and Human Services
HIAA	Health Insurance Association of America
HIM	Health Information Management
HIPAA	Health Insurance Portability and Accountability Act
HIV	Human Immunodeficiency Virus
HMO	Health Maintenance Organization
HSA	Health Services Administration
ICD-9-CM	International Classification of Diseases 9th Revision Clinical Modification
ICF	Intermediate Care Facility
IFA	Indirect Immunofluoroescence Assay
IOM	Institute of Medicine
IPA	Individual Practice Association
IRB	Institutional Review Board
JAHIMA	*Journal of the American Health Information Management Association*
JAMA	*Journal of the American Medical Association*
JCAH	Joint Commission on Accreditation of Hospitals; succeeded by JCAHO

JCAHO Joint Commission on Accreditation of Healthcare Organizations
JME *Journal of Medical Education*

LPN Licensed Practical Nurse
LVN Licensed Vocational Nurse

MCAT Medical College Admission Test
MCH Maternal and Child Health
MD Doctor of Medicine
Med Medicine
MEDLARS Medical Literature and Analysis Retrieval System
MH Mental Health; Mental Hygiene
MPP Medicare Participating Physician
MR Mental Retardation
MRA Medical Record Administration
MRI Magnetic Resonance Imaging
MRT Medical Record Technology

NBME National Board of Medical Examiners
NCHS National Center for Health Statistics
NCI National Cancer Institute
NEI National Eye Institute
NEJM *New England Journal of Medicine*
NIH National Institutes of Health
NIMH National Institutes of Mental Health
NLM National Library of Medicine
NLN National League of Nursing
NLRB National Labor Relations Board
NMR Nuclear Magnetic Resonance

OB Obstetrics
OD Doctor of Optometry
OIG Office of Inspector General
OMB Office of Management and Budget
OR Operating Room
OSHA Occupational Safety and Health Administration

OTA	Office of Technology Assessment
PA	Physical Assistant
PL	Public Law
PPO	Preferred Provider Organization
PPS	Prospective Payment or Pricing System
PRO	Professional Review Organization
PRRB	Provider Reimbursement Review Board
PSDA	Patient Self-Determination Act
PSRO	Professional Standards Review Organization
QA	Quality Assurance
RFP	Request for Proposal
RM	Risk Management
RN	Registered Nurse
RRA	Registered Record Administrator
SNF	Skilled Nursing Facility
SSA	Social Security Administration
SSI	Supplementary Security Income
STD	Sexually Transmitted Disease
TB	Tuberculosis
UCR	Usual, Customary and Reasonable
UR	Utilization Review
VA	Veterans Affairs
VD	Venereal Disease
VNA	Visiting Nurse Association
WHO	World Health Organization
WIC	Women, Infants and Children

(Adapted in part from Raffel and Barsukiewicz, *The U.S. Health System: Origins and Functions, 5th edition.* Clifton Park, NY: Delmar Learning, 2002).

A Patient's Bill of Rights

Patient and Community Relations

Introduction

Effective health care requires collaboration between patients and physicians and other health care professionals. Open and honest communication, respect for personal and professional values, and sensitivity to differences are integral to optimal patient care. As the setting for the provision of health services, hospitals must provide a foundation for understanding and respecting the rights and responsibilities of patients, their families, physicians, and other caregivers. Hospitals must ensure a health care ethic that respects the role of patients in decision making about treatment choices and other aspects of their care. Hospitals must be sensitive to cultural, racial, linguistic, religious, age, gender, and other differences as well as the needs of persons with disabilities.

The American Hospital Association presents *A Patient's Bill of Rights* with the expectation that it will contribute to more effective patient care and be supported by the hospital on behalf of the institution, its medical staff, employees, and patients. The American Hospital Association encourages health care institutions to tailor this bill of rights to their patient community by translating and/or simplifying the language of this bill of rights as may be necessary to ensure that patients and their families understand their rights and responsibilities.

*Bill of Rights**

1. The patient has the right to considerate and respectful care.

2. The patient has the right to and is encouraged to obtain from physicians and other direct caregivers relevant, current, and understandable information concerning diagnosis, treatment, and prognosis.

Except in emergencies when the patient lacks decision-making capacity and the need for treatment is urgent, the patient is entitled to the opportunity to discuss and request information related to the specific procedures and/or treatments, the risks involved, the possible length of recuperation, and the medically reasonable alternatives and their accompanying risks and benefits.

Patients have the right to know the identity of physicians, nurses, and others involved in their care, as well as when those involved are students, residents, or other trainees. The patient also has the right to know the immediate and long-term financial implications of treatment choices, insofar as they are known.

3. The patient has the right to make decisions about the plan of care prior to and during the course of treatment and to refuse a recommended treatment or plan of care to the extent permitted by law and hospital policy and to be informed of the medical consequences of this action. In case of such refusal, the patient is entitled to other appropriate care and services that the hospital provides or transfer to another hospital. The hospital should notify patients of any policy that might affect patient choice within the institution.

4. The patient has the right to have an advance directive (such as living will, health care proxy, or durable power of attorney for health care) concerning treatment or designing a surrogate decision maker with the expectation that the hospital will honor the intent of that directive to the extent permitted by law and hospital policy.

Health care institutions must advise patients of their rights under state law and hospital policy to make informed medical choices, ask if the patient has an advance directive, and include that information in patient records. The patient has the right to timely information about hospital policy that may limit its ability to implement fully a legally valid advance directive.

*These rights can be exercised on the patient's behalf by a designated surrogate or proxy decision maker if the patient lacks decision-making capacity, is legally incompetent, or is a minor.

5. The patient has the right to every consideration of privacy. Case discussion, consultation, examination, and treatment should be conducted so as to protect each patient's privacy.

6. The patient has the right to expect that all communications and records pertaining to his/her care will be treated as confidential by the hospital, except in cases such as suspected abuse and public health hazards when reporting is permitted or required by law. The patient has the right to expect that the hospital will emphasize the confidentiality of this information when it releases it to any other parties entitled to review information in these records.

7. The patient has the right to review the records pertaining to his/her medical care and to have the information explained or interpreted as necessary, except when restricted by law.

8. The patient has the right to expect that, within its capacity and policies, a hospital will make reasonable response to the request of a patient for appropriate and medically indicated care and services. The hospital must provide evaluation, service, and/or referral as indicated by the urgency of the case. When medically appropriate and legally permissible, or when a patient has so requested, a patient may be transferred to another facility. The institution to which the patient is to be transferred must first have accepted the patient for transfer. The patient must also have the benefit of complete information and explanation concerning the need for, risks, benefits, and alternatives to such a transfer.

9. The patient has the right to ask and be informed of the existence of business relationships among the hospital, educational institutions, other health care providers, or payers that may influence the patient's treatment and care.

10. The patient has the right to consent to or decline to participate in proposed research studies or human experimentation affecting care and treatment or requiring direct patient involvement, and to have those studies fully explained prior to consent. A patient who declines to participate in research or experimentation is entitled to the most effective care that the hospital can otherwise provide.

11. The patient has the right to expect reasonable continuity of care when appropriate and to be informed by physicians and other caregivers of available and realistic patient care options when hospital care is no longer appropriate.

12. The patient has the right to be informed of hospital policies and practices that relate to patient care, treatment, and responsibilities. The patient has the right to be informed of available resources for resolving disputes, grievances, and conflicts, such as ethics committees, patient representatives, or other mechanisms available in the institution. The patient has the right to be informed of the hospital's charges for services and available payment methods.

The collaborative nature of health care requires that patients, or their families/surrogates, participate in their care. The effectiveness of care and patient satisfaction with the course of treatment depend, in part, on the patient fulfilling certain responsibilities. Patients are responsible for providing information about past illnesses, hospitalizations, medications, and other matters related to health status. To participate effectively in decision making, patients must be encouraged to take responsibility for requesting additional information or clarification about their health status or treatment when they do not fully understand information and instructions. Patients are also responsible for ensuring that the health care institution has a copy of their written advance directive if they have one. Patients are responsible for informing their physicians and other caregivers if they anticipate problems in following prescribed treatment.

Patients should also be aware of the hospital's obligation to be reasonably efficient and equitable in providing care to other patients and the community. The hospital's rules and regulations are designed to help the hospital meet this obligation. Patients and their families are responsible for making reasonable accommodations to the needs of the hospital, other patients, medical staff, and hospital employees. Patients are responsible for providing necessary information for insurance claims and for working with the hospital to make payment arrangements, when necessary.

A person's health depends on much more than health care services. Patients are responsible for recognizing the impact of their life-style on their personal health.

Conclusion

Hospitals have many functions to perform, including the enhancement of health status, health promotion, and the prevention and treatment of injury and disease; the immediate and ongoing care and rehabilitation of patients; the education of health professionals, patients, and the community; and research. All these activities must be conducted with an overriding concern for the values and dignity of patients.

Principles of Medical Record Documentation

The following is an excerpt from a brochure titled *Principles of Medical Record Documentation* developed jointly by representatives of the American Health Information Management Association, the American Hospital Association, the American Managed Care and Review Association, the American Medical Association, the American Medical Peer Review Association, the Blue Cross and Blue Shield Association, and the Health Insurance Association of America. Although their joint development of this brochure is not intended to imply either endorsement of, or opposition to, specific documentation requirements, all seven groups share the belief that the fundamental reason to maintain an adequate medical record is its contribution to the high quality of medical care. (Reprinted with permission of the American Health Information Management Association, Chicago, Illinois)

What Is Documentation and Why Is It Important?

Documentation is the recording of pertinent facts and observations about an individual's health history including past and present illnesses, tests, treatment, and outcomes. The medical record chronologically documents the care of the patient in order to:

- enable the physician and other healthcare professionals to plan and evaluate the patient's treatment,
- enhance communication and promote continuity of care among physicians and other healthcare professionals involved in the patient's care.

- facilitate claims review and payment,
- assist in utilization review and quality of care evaluations,
- reduce hassles related to medical review,
- provide clinical data for research and education, and
- serve as a legal document to verify the care provided (for example, in defense of an alleged professional liability claim).

What Do Payers Want and Why?

Payers want to know that they are getting value for their healthcare dollars.

Because payers have a contractual obligation to enrollees, they may request additional documentation to validate that services provided were:

- appropriate to the treatment of the patient's condition,
- medically necessary for the diagnosis and/or treatment of an illness or injury, and
- coded correctly.

What Are Covered Services?

Covered services are those services that are payable in accordance with the terms of the benefit plan contract by the insurer. Such services must be documented and medically necessary in order for payment to be made.

What Are Medically Necessary Services?

Typically, payers define medically necessary services as those services or supplies that are:

- in accordance with standards of good medical practice,
- consistent with the diagnosis, and
- the most appropriate level of care provided in the most appropriate setting.

Note that the definition of medical necessity may differ among insurers. Medically necessary services may or may not be covered depending on the benefit plan.

How Does the Documentation in Your Medical Record Measure Up?

1. Is the reason for the patient encounter documented in the medical record?
2. Are all services that were provided documented?
3. Does the medical record clearly explain why support services, procedures, and supplies were provided?
4. Is the assessment of the patient's condition apparent in the medical record?
5. Does the medical record contain information on the patient's progress and on the results of treatment?
6. Does the medical record include the patient's plan for care?
7. Does the information in the medical record describing the patient's condition provide reasonable medical rationale for the services and the choice of setting that are to be billed?
8. Does the information in the medical record support the care given in the case where another healthcare professional must assume care or perform medical review?

Principles of Documentation

1. The medical record should be complete and legible.
2. The documentation of each patient encounter should include: the date; the reason for the encounter; appropriate history and physical exam; review of lab, x-ray data, and other ancillary services, where appropriate; assessment; and plan for care (including discharge plan, if appropriate).
3. Past and present diagnoses should be accessible to the treating and/or consulting physician.

4. The reasons for, and results of, x-rays, lab tests, and other ancillary services should be documented or included in the medical record.
5. Relevant health risk factors should be identified.
6. The patient's progress including response to treatment, change in treatment, change in diagnosis, and patient non-compliance should be documented.
7. The written plan for care should include, when appropriate: treatments and medications, specifying frequency and dosage; any referrals and consultations; patient/family education; and specific instructions for follow-up.
8. The documentation should support the intensity of the patient evaluation and/or the treatment, including thought processes and the complexity of medical decision making.
9. All entries to the medical record should be dated and authenticated.
10. The CPT/ICD-9 codes reported on the health insurance claim form or billing statement should reflect the documentation in the medical record.

Developed by representatives from:

American Health Information Management Association
232 North Michigan Avenue, Suite 2150
Chicago, IL 60601-5800
(312) 233-1100
www.ahima.org

American Hospital Association
1 North Franklin
Chicago, IL 60606
(312) 422-3000
www.aha.org

American Managed Care and Review Association
1227 25th Street, NW, Suite 610
Washington, DC 20037
(202) 728-0506

American Medical Association
515 North State Street
Chicago, IL 60610
(312) 464-5000
www.ama-assn.org

American Medical Peer Review Association
810 First Street, NE, Suite 410
Washington, DC 20002
(202) 371-5610

Blue Cross and Blue Shield Association
676 North St. Clair Street
Chicago, IL 60610
(312) 440-5526
www.bcbsa.com

Health Insurance Association of America
1201 F Street, NW, Suite 500
Washington, DC 20004
(202) 824-1600

Durable Power of Attorney for Health Care and Health-Care Directive

---

Sample Form

(Developed and printed by the Missouri Bar)

Part I. Durable Power of Attorney for Health Care

- If you do *NOT* wish to name an agent to make health care decisions for you, write your initials in the box to the right and go to Part II.

______ Initials

This form has been prepared to comply with the "Durable Power of Attorney for Health Care Act" of Missouri.

It is suggested that only one Agent be named. However, if more than one Agent is named, any one may act individually unless you specify otherwise.

1. Selection of Agent. I appoint:

Name: ______________________________

Address: ______________________________

____

Telephone: ______________________________

as my Agent.

2. Alternate Agents. Only an Agent named by me may act under this Durable Power of Attorney. If my Agent resigns or is not able or available to make health care decisions for me, or if an Agent named by me is divorced from me or is my spouse and legally separated from me, I appoint the person(s) named below (in the order named if more than one):

First Alternate Agent

Name: ______________________________

Address: ______________________________

____

Telephone: ______________________________

Second Alternate Agent

Name: ______________________________

Address: ______________________________

____

Telephone: ______________________________

This is a Durable Power of Attorney, and the authority of my Agent shall not terminate if I become disabled or incapacitated.

Part I. Durable Power of Attorney for Health Care (Continued)

3. Effective Date and Durability. This Durable Power of Attorney is effective when two physicians decide and certify that I am incapacitated and unable to make and communicate a health-care decision.

- If you want ONE physician, instead of TWO, to decide whether you are incapacitated, write your initials in the box to the right.

  ______ Initials

4. Agent's Powers. I grant to my Agent full authority to:

A. Give consent to, prohibit or withdraw any type of health-care, medical care, treatment or procedure, even if my death may result;

- If you wish to AUTHORIZE your Agent to direct a health care provider to withhold or withdraw artificially supplied nutrition and hydration (including tube feeding of food and water), write your initials in the box to the right.

  ______ Initials

- If you DO NOT WISH TO AUTHORIZE your Agent to direct a health-care provider to withhold or withdraw artificially supplied nutrition and hydration (including tube feeding of food and water), write your initials in the box to the right.

  ______ Initials

B. Make all necessary arrangements for health care services on my behalf, and to hire and fire medical personnel responsible for my care;

C. Move me into or out of any health-care facility (even if against medical advice) to obtain compliance with the decisions of my Agent; and

D. Take any other action necessary to do what I authorize here, including (but not limited to) granting any waiver or release from liability required by any health-care provider, and taking any legal action at the expense of my estate to enforce this Durable Power of Attorney.

5. Agent's Financial Liability and Compensation. My Agent acting under this Durable Power of Attorney will incur no personal financial liability. My Agent shall not be entitled to compensation for services performed under this Durable Power of Attorney, but my Agent shall be entitled to reimbursement for all reasonable expenses incurred as a result of carrying out any provision hereof.

Part II. Health-Care Directive

- If you DO NOT WISH to make a health-care directive, write your initials in the box to the right, and go to Part III. ______ Initials

I make this HEALTH-CARE DIRECTIVE ("Directive") to exercise my right to determine the course of my health care and to provide clear and convincing proof of my wishes and instructions about my treatment.

If I am persistently unconscious or there is no reasonable expectation of my recovery from a seriously incapacitating or terminal illness or condition, I direct that all of the life-prolonging procedures which I have initialed below be withheld or withdrawn.

I want the following life-prolonging procedures to be withheld or withdrawn:

- artificially supplied nutrition and hydration (including tube feeding of food and water) . . . . ______ Initials
- surgery or other invasive procedures . . . . ______ Initials
- heart-lung resuscitation (CPR) . . . . ______ Initials
- antibiotic . . . . ______ Initials
- dialysis . . . . ______ Initials
- mechanical ventilator (respirator) . . . . ______ Initials
- chemotherapy . . . . ______ Initials
- radiation therapy . . . . ______ Initials
- all other "life-prolonging" medical or surgical procedures that are merely intended to keep me alive without reasonable hope of improving my condition or curing my illness or injury . . . . ______ Initials

However, if my physician believes that any life-prolonging procedure may lead to significant recovery, I direct my physician to try the treatment for a reasonable period of time. If it does not improve my condition, I direct the treatment be withdrawn even if it shortens my life. I also direct that I be given medical treatment to relieve pain or to provide comfort, even if such treatment might shorten my life, suppress my appetite or my breathing, or be habit-forming.

IF I HAVE NOT DESIGNATED AN AGENT IN THE DURABLE POWER OF ATTORNEY, THIS DOCUMENT IS MEANT TO BE IN FULL FORCE AND EFFECT AS MY HEALTH-CARE DIRECTIVE.

Part III. General Provisions Included in the Directive and Durable Power of Attorney

YOU MUST SIGN THIS DOCUMENT IN THE PRESENCE OF TWO WITNESSES.

IN WITNESS WHEREOF, I have executed this document this __________ day of __________, 19_____.

____
Signature

Print Name ______________________________

Address ______________________________

The person who signed this document is of sound mind and voluntarily signed this document in our presence. Each of the undersigned witnesses is at least eighteen years of age.

Signature ______________________________ Signature ______________________________

Print Name ______________________________ Print Name ______________________________

Address ______________________________ Address ______________________________

ONLY REQUIRED FOR PART I — DURABLE POWER OF ATTORNEY

STATE OF MISSOURI)

) as

_________ OF _________)

On this __________ day of __________, 19_____, before me personally appeared ____________________, to me known to be the person described in and who executed the foregoing instrument and acknowledged that he/she executed the same as his/her free act and deed.

IN WITNESS WHEREOF, I have hereunto set my hand and affixed my official seal in the County of ____________________, State of Missouri, the day and year first above written.

____
Notary Public

My Commission Expires:

Sample Living Will

Declaration made this _____ day of __________, 19_____.

I, ____________________, willfully and voluntarily make known my desire that my dying not be artificially prolonged under the circumstances set forth below, and I do hereby declare:

If at any time I have a terminal condition and if my attending or treating physician and another consulting physician have determined that there is no medical probability of my recovery from such condition, I direct that life-prolonging procedures be withheld or withdrawn when the application of such procedures would serve only to prolong artificially the process of dying, and that I be permitted to die naturally with only the administration of medication or the performance of any medical procedure deemed necessary to provide me with comfort care or to alleviate pain.

It is my intention that this declaration be honored by my family and physician as the final expression of my legal right to refuse medical or surgical treatment and to accept the consequences for such refusal.

In the event that I have been determined to be unable to provide express and informed consent regarding the withholding, withdrawal, or continuation of life-prolonging procedures, I wish to designate, as my surrogate to carry out the provisions of this declaration:

Name: ____

Address: ____

____ Zip Code: _______________

Phone: ____

I wish to designate the following person as my alternate surrogate, to carry out the provisions of this declaration should my surrogate be unwilling or unable to act on my behalf:

Name: ____

Address: ____

__________________________________ Zip Code: ____________

Phone: ____

Additional instructions (optional):

I understand the full importance of this declaration, and I am emotionally and mentally competent to make this declaration.

Signed: ____

Witness 1:

Signed: ____

Address: ____

Witness 2:

Signed: ____

Address: ____

Sample Designation of Health-Care Surrogate

Name: ____
(Last) *(First)* *(Middle Initial)*

In the event that I have been determined to be incapacitated to provide informed consent for medical treatment and surgical and diagnostic procedures, I wish to designate as my surrogate for health-care decisions:

Name: ____

Address: ____

______________________________ Zip Code: ______________

Phone: ____

If my surrogate is unwilling or unable to perform his duties, I wish to designate as my alternate surrogate:

Name: ____

Address: ____

______________________________ Zip Code: ______________

Phone: ____

I fully understand that this designation will permit my designee to make health care decisions and to provide, withhold, or withdraw consent on my behalf; to apply for public benefits to defray the cost of health care; and to authorize my admission to or transfer from a health care facility.

Additional instructions (optional):

I further affirm that this designation is not being made as a condition of treatment or admission to a health-care facility. I will notify and send a copy of this document to the following persons other than my surrogate, so they may know who my surrogate is:

Name: ______________________________

Address: ______________________________

Name: ______________________________

Address: ______________________________

Signed: ______________________________

Date: ______________________________

Witness 1:

Signed ______________________________

Address ______________________________

Witness 2:

Signed: ______________________________

Address: ______________________________

Courtesy of *Choice in Dying*, 200 Varick Street, New York, NY 10014.

Patient Self-Determination Act

UNITED STATES CODE
TITLE 42. THE PUBLIC HEALTH AND WELFARE
CHAPTER 7—SOCIAL SECURITY
SUBCHAPTER XVIII—HEALTH INSURANCE FOR AGED AND DISABLED
PART C—MISCELLANEOUS PROVISIONS

§ 1395cc. Agreements with providers of services

(a) Filing of agreements; eligibility for payment; charges with respect to items and services

(1) Any provider of services (except a fund designated for purposes of section 1395f(g) and section 1395n(e) of this title) shall be qualified to participate under this subchapter and shall be eligible for payments under this subchapter if it files with the Secretary an agreement—

(A) not to charge, except as provided in paragraph (2), any individual or any other person for items or services for which such individual is entitled to have payment made under this subchapter (or for which he would be so entitled if such provider of services had complied with the procedural and other requirements under or pursuant to this subchapter or for which such provider is paid pursuant to the provisions of section 1395f(e) of this title),

(B) not to charge any individual or any other person for items or services for which such individual is not entitled to have payment made under this subchapter because payment for expenses incurred for such items or services may not be made by reason of the provisions of paragraph (1) or (9) of section 1395y(a) of this title, but only if (i) such individual was without fault in incurring such expenses and (ii) the Secretary's determination that such payment may not be made for such items and services was made after the third year following the year in which notice of such payment was sent to such individual; except that the Secretary may reduce such three-year period to not less than one year if he finds such reduction is consistent with the objectives of this subchapter,

(C) to make adequate provision for return (or other disposition, in accordance with regulations) of any moneys incorrectly collected from such individual or other person,

(D) to promptly notify the Secretary of its employment of an individual who, at any time during the year preceding such employment, was employed in a managerial, accounting, auditing, or similar capacity (as determined by the Secretary by regulation) by an agency or organization which serves as a fiscal intermediary or carrier (for purposes of part A or part B, or both, of this subchapter) with respect to the provider.

(E) to release data with respect to patients of such provider upon request to an organization having a contract with the Secretary under part B of subchapter XI of this chapter as may be necessary (i) to allow such organization to carry out its functions under such contract, or (ii) to allow such organization to carry out similar review functions under any contract the organization may have with a private or public agency paying for health care in the same area with respect to patients who authorize release of such data for such purposes,

(F)(i) in the case of hospitals which provide inpatient hospital services for which payment may be made under subsection (b), (c), or (d) of section 1395ww of this title, to maintain an agreement with a professional standards review organization (if there is such an organization in existence in the area in which the hospital is located) or with a utilization and quality control peer review organization which has a contract with the Secretary under part B of subchapter XI of this chapter for the area in which the hospital is located, under which the organization will perform functions under that part with respect to the review of the validity of diagnostic information provided by such hospital, the completeness, adequacy, and quality of care provided, the appropriateness of admissions and discharges, and the appropriateness of care provided for which additional payments are sought under section 1395ww(d)(5) of this title, with respect to inpatient hospital services for which payment may be made under part A of this subchapter (and for purposes of payment under this subchapter, the cost of such agreement to the hospital shall be considered a cost incurred by such hospital in providing inpatient services under part A of this subchapter, and (I) shall be paid directly by the Secretary to such organization on behalf of such hospital in accordance with a rate per review established by the Secretary, (II) shall be transferred from the Federal Hospital Insurance Trust Fund, without regard to amounts appropriated in advance in appropriation Acts, in the same manner as transfers are made for payment for services provided directly to beneficiaries, and (III) shall not be less in the aggregate for a fiscal year than the aggregate amount expended in fiscal year 1988 for direct and administrative costs (adjusted for inflation and for any direct or administrative costs incurred as a result of review functions added with respect to a subsequent fiscal year) of such reviews),

(ii) in the case of hospitals, rural primary care hospitals, skilled nursing facilities, and home health agencies, to maintain an agreement with a utilization and quality control peer review organization (which has a contract with the Secretary under part B of subchapter XI of this chapter for the area in which the hospital, facility, or agency is located) to perform the functions described in paragraph (3)(A),

(G) in the case of hospitals which provide inpatient hospital services for which payment may be made under subsection (b) or (d) of section 1395ww of this title, not to charge any individual or any other person for inpatient hospital services for which such individual would be entitled to have payment made under part A of this subchapter but for a denial or reduction of payments under section 1395ww(f)(2) of this title,

(H) in the case of hospitals which provide services for which payment may be made under this subchapter and in the case of rural primary care hospitals which provide rural primary care hospital services, to have all items and services (other than physicians' services as defined in regulations for purposes of section 1395y(a)(14) of this title, and other than services described by section 1395x(s)(2)(K)(i) of this title or 1395x(s)(2)(K)(iii) of this title, certified nurse-midwife services, qualified psychologist services, and services of a certified registered nurse anesthetist) (i) that are furnished to an individual who is a patient of the hospital, and (ii) for which the individual is entitled to have payment made under this subchapter, furnished by the hospital or otherwise under arrangements (as defined in section 1395x(w)(1) of this title) made by the hospital,

(I) in the case of a hospital or rural primary care hospital—

(i) to adopt and enforce a policy to ensure compliance with the requirements of section 1395dd of this title and to meet the requirements of such section,

(ii) to maintain medical and other records related to individuals transferred to or from the hospital for a period of five years from the date of the transfer, and

(iii) to maintain a list of physicians who are on call for duty after the initial examination to provide treatment necessary to stabilize an individual with an emergency medical condition; [FN1]

(J) in the case of hospitals which provide inpatient hospital services for which payment may be made under this subchapter, to be a participating provider of medical care under any health plan contracted for under section 1079 or 1086 of Title 10, or under section 1713 of Title 38, in accordance with admission practices, payment methodology, and amounts as prescribed under joint regulations issued by the Secretary and by the Secretaries of Defense and Transportation, in implementation of sections 1079 and 1086 of Title 10,

(K) not to charge any individual or any other person for items or services for which payment under this subchapter is denied under section 1320c-3(a)(2) of this title by reason of a determination under section 1320c-3(a)(1)(B) of this title,

(L) in the case of hospitals which provide inpatient hospital services for which payment may be made under this subchapter, to be a participating provider of medical care under section 1703 of Title 38, in accordance with such admission practices, and such payment methodology and amounts, as are prescribed under joint regulations issued by the Secretary and by the Secretary of Veterans Affairs in implementation of such section,

(M) in the case of hospitals, to provide to each individual who is entitled to benefits under part A of this subchapter (or to a person acting on the individual's behalf), at or about the time of the individual's admission as an inpatient to the hospital, a written statement (containing such language as the Secretary prescribes consistent with this paragraph) which explains—

(i) the individual's rights to benefits for inpatient hospital services and for post-hospital services under this subchapter,

(ii) the circumstances under which such an individual will and will not be liable for charges for continued stay in the hospital,

(iii) the individual's right to appeal denials of benefits for continued inpatient hospital services, including the practical steps to initiate such an appeal, and

(iv) the individual's liability for payment for services if such a denial of benefits is upheld on appeal, and which provides such additional information as the Secretary may specify,

(N) in the case of hospitals and rural primary care hospitals—

(i) to make available to its patients the directory or directories of participating physicians (published under section 1395u(h)(4) of this title) for the area served by the hospital or rural primary care hospital,

(ii) if hospital personnel (including staff of any emergency or outpatient department) refer a patient to a nonparticipating physician for further medical care on an outpatient basis, the personnel must inform the patient that the physician is a nonparticipating physician and, whenever practicable, must identify at least one qualified participating physician who is listed in such a directory and from whom the patient may receive the necessary services,

(iii) to post conspicuously in any emergency department a sign (in a form specified by the Secretary) specifying rights of individuals under section 1395dd of this title with respect to examination and treatment for emergency medical conditions and women in labor, and

(iv) to post conspicuously (in a form specified by the Secretary) information indicating whether or not the hospital participates in the medicaid program under a State plan approved under subchapter XIX of this chapter, and

(O) in the case of hospitals and skilled nursing facilities, to accept as payment in full for inpatient hospital and extended care services that are covered under this subchapter and are furnished to any individual enrolled with an eligible organization (i) with a risk-sharing contract under section 1395mm of this title, under section 1395mm(i)(2)(A) of this title (as in effect before February 1, 1985), under section 1395b-1(a) of this title, or under section 222(a) of the Social Security Amendments of 1972, and (ii) which does not have a contract establishing payment amounts for services furnished to members of the organization the amounts (in the case of hospitals) or limits (in the case of skilled nursing facilities) that would be made as a payment in full under this subchapter if the individuals were not so enrolled;

(P) in the case of home health agencies which provide home health services to individuals entitled to benefits under this subchapter who require catheters, catheter supplies, ostomy bags, and supplies related to ostomy care (described in section 1395x(m)(5) of this title), to offer to furnish such supplies to such an individual as part of their furnishing of home health services, and (Q) in the case of hospitals, skilled nursing facilities, home health agencies, and hospice programs, to comply with the requirement of subsection (f) of this section (relating to maintaining written policies and procedures respecting advance directives).

In the case of a hospital which has an agreement in effect with an organization described in subparagraph (F), which organization's contract with the Secretary under part B of subchapter XI of this chapter is terminated on or after October 1, 1984, the hospital shall not be determined to be out of compliance with the requirement of such subparagraph during the six month period beginning on the date of the termination of that contract.

(2)(A) A provider of services may charge such individual or other person (i) the amount of any deduction or coinsurance amount imposed pursuant to section 1395e(a)(1), (a)(3), or (a)(4), section 1395l(b), or section 1395x(y)(3) of this title with respect to such items and services (not in excess of the amount customarily charged for such items and services by such provider), and (ii) an amount equal to 20 per centum of the reasonable charges for such items and services (not in excess of 20 per centum of the amount customarily charged for such items and services by such provider) for which payment is made under part B of this subchapter or which are durable medical equipment furnished as home health services (but in the case of items and services furnished to individuals with end-stage renal disease, an amount equal to 20 percent of the estimated amounts for such items and services calculated on the basis established by the Secretary). In the case of items and services described in section 1395l(c) of this title, clause (ii) of the preceding sentence shall be applied by substituting for 20 percent the proportion which is appropriate under such section. A provider of services may not impose a charge under clause (ii) of the first sentence of this subparagraph with respect to items and services described in section 1395x(s)(10)(A) of this title, and with respect to clinical diagnostic laboratory tests for which payment is made under part B of this subchapter. Notwithstanding the first sentence of this subparagraph, a home health agency may charge such an individual or person, with respect to covered items subject to payment under section 1395m(a) of this title, the amount of any deduction imposed under section 1395l(b) of this title and 20 percent of the payment basis described in section 1395m(a)(1)(B) of this title.

(B) Where a provider of services has furnished, at the request of such individual, items or services which are in excess of or more expensive than the items or services with respect to which payment may be made under this subchapter, such provider of services may also charge such individual or other person for such more expensive items or services to the extent that the amount customarily charged by it for the items or services furnished at such request exceeds the amount customarily charged by it for the items or services with respect to which payment may be made under this subchapter.

(C) A provider of services may in accordance with its customary practice also appropriately charge any such individual for any whole blood (or equivalent quantities of packed red blood cells, as defined under regulations) furnished him with respect to which a deductible is imposed under section 1395e(a)(2) of this title, except that (i) any excess of such charge over the cost to such provider for the blood (or equivalent quantities of packed red blood cells, as so defined) shall be deducted from any payment to such provider under this subchapter, (ii) no such charge may be imposed for the cost of administration of such blood (or equivalent quantities of packed red blood cells, as so defined), and (iii) such charge may not be made to the extent such blood (or equivalent quantities of packed red blood cells, as so defined) has been replaced on behalf of such individual or arrangements have been made for its replacement on his behalf. For purposes of this subparagraph, whole blood (or equivalent quantities of packed red blood cells, as so defined) furnished an individual shall be deemed replaced when the provider of services is given one pint of blood for each pint of blood (or equivalent quantities of packed red blood cells, as so defined) furnished such individual with respect to which a deduction is imposed under section 1395e(a)(2) of this title.

(D) Where a provider of services customarily furnishes items or services which are in excess of or more expensive than the items or services with respect to which payment may be made under this subchapter, such provider, notwithstanding the preceding provisions of this paragraph, may not, under the authority of subparagraph (B)(ii) of this paragraph, charge any individual or other person any amount for such items or services in excess of the amount of the payment which may otherwise be made for such items or services under this subchapter if the admitting physician has a direct or indirect financial interest in such provider.

(3)(A) Under the agreement required under paragraph (1)(F)(ii), the peer review organization must perform functions (other than those covered under an agreement under paragraph (1)(F)(i)) under the third sentence of section 1320c-3(a)(4)(A) of this title and under section 1320c-3(a)(14) of this title with respect to services, furnished by the hospital, rural primary care hospital, facility, or agency involved, for which payment may be made under this subchapter.

(B) For purposes of payment under this subchapter, the cost of such an agreement to the hospital, rural primary care hospital, facility, or agency shall be considered a cost incurred by such hospital, rural primary care hospital, facility, or agency in providing covered services under this subchapter and shall be paid directly by the Secretary to the peer review organization on behalf of such hospital, rural primary care hospital, facility, or agency in accordance with a schedule established by the Secretary.

(C) Such payments—

(i) shall be transferred in appropriate proportions from the Federal Hospital Insurance Trust Fund and from the Federal Supplementary Medical Insurance Trust Fund, without regard to amounts appropriated in advance in appropriation Acts, in the same manner as transfers are made for payment for services provided directly to beneficiaries, and

(ii) shall not be less in the aggregate for a fiscal year—

(I) in the case of hospitals, than the amount specified in paragraph(1)(F)(i)(III), and

(II) in the case of facilities, rural primary care hospitals, and agencies, than the amounts the Secretary determines to be sufficient to cover the costs of such organizations' conducting the activities described in subparagraph (A) with respect to such facilities, rural primary care hospitals, or agencies under part B of subchapter XI of this chapter.

(b) Termination or nonrenewal of agreements

(1) A provider of services may terminate an agreement with the Secretary under this section at such time and upon such notice to the Secretary and the public as may be provided in regulations, except that notice of more than six months shall not be required.

(2) The Secretary may refuse to enter into an agreement under this section or, upon such reasonable notice to the provider and the public as may be specified in regulations, may refuse to renew or may terminate such an agreement after the Secretary—

(A) has determined that the provider fails to comply substantially with the provisions of the agreement, with the provisions of this subchapter and regulations thereunder, or with a corrective action required under section 1395ww(f)(2)(B) of this title,

(B) has determined that the provider fails substantially to meet the applicable provisions of section 1395x of this title, or

(C) has excluded the provider from participation in a program under this subchapter pursuant to section 1320a-7 or section 1320a-7a of this title.

(3) A termination of an agreement or a refusal to renew an agreement under this subsection shall become effective on the same date and in the same manner as an exclusion from participation under the programs under this subchapter becomes effective under section 1320a-7(c) of this title.

(c) Refiling after termination or nonrenewal; notice of termination or nonrenewal

(1) Where the Secretary has terminated or has refused to renew an agreement under this subchapter with a provider of services, such provider may not file another agreement under this subchapter unless the Secretary finds that the reason for the termination or nonrenewal has been removed and that there is reasonable assurance that it will not recur.

(2) Where the Secretary has terminated or has refused to renew an agreement under this subchapter with a provider of services, the Secretary shall promptly notify each State agency which administers or supervises the administration of a State plan approved under subchapter XIX of this chapter of such termination or nonrenewal.

(d) Decision to withhold payment for failure to review long-stay cases

If the Secretary finds that there is a substantial failure to make timely review in accordance with section 1395x(k) of this title of long-stay cases in a hospital, he may, in lieu of terminating his agreement with such hospital, decide that, with respect to any individual admitted to such hospital after a subsequent date specified by him, no payment shall be made under this subchapter for inpatient hospital services (including inpatient psychiatric hospital services) after the 20th day of a continuous period of such services. Such decision may be made effective only after such notice to the hospital and to the public, as may be prescribed by regulations, and its effectiveness shall terminate when the Secretary finds that the reason therefor has been removed and that there is reasonable assurance that it will not recur. The Secretary shall not make any such decision except after reasonable notice and opportunity for hearing to the institution or agency affected thereby.

(e) "Provider of services" defined

For purposes of this section, the term "provider of services" shall include—

(1) a clinic, rehabilitation agency, or public health agency if, in the case of a clinic or rehabilitation agency, such clinic or agency meets the require-

ments of section 1395x(p)(4)(A) of this title (or meets the requirements of such section through the operation of section (1395x(g) of this title), or if, in the case of a public health agency, such agency meets the requirements of section 1395x(p)(4)(B) of this title (or meets the requirements of such section through the operation of section 1395x(g) of this title), but only with respect to the furnishing of outpatient physical therapy services (as therein defined) or (through the operation of section 1395x(g) of this title) with respect to the furnishing of outpatient occupational therapy services; and

(2) a community mental health center (as defined in section 1395x(ff)(3)(B) of this title), but only with respect to the furnishing of partial hospitalization services (as described in section 1395x(ff)(1) of this title).

(f) Maintenance of written policies and procedures

(1) For purposes of subsection (a)(1)(Q) of this section and sections 1395i-3(c)(2)(E), 1395l(s), 1395mm(c)(8), and 1395bb(a)(6) of this title, the requirement of this subsection is that a provider of services or prepaid or eligible organization (as the case may be) maintain written policies and procedures with respect to all adult individuals receiving medical care by or through the provider or organization—

(A) to provide written information to each such individual concerning—

(i) an individual's rights under State law (whether statutory or as recognized by the courts of the State) to make decisions concerning such medical care, including the right to accept or refuse medical or surgical treatment and the right to formulate advance directives (as defined in paragraph (3)), and

(ii) the written policies of the provider or organization respecting the implementation of such rights;

(B) to document in the individual's medical record whether or not the individual has executed an advance directive;

(C) not to condition the provision of care or otherwise discriminate against an individual based on whether or not the individual has executed an advance directive;

(D) to ensure compliance with requirements of State law (whether statutory of as recognized by the courts of the State) respecting advance directives at facilities of the provider or organization; and

(E) to provide (individually or with others) for education for staff and the community on issues concerning advance directives.

Subparagraph (C) shall not be construed as requiring the provision of care which conflicts with an advance directive.

(2) The written information described in paragraph (1)(A) shall be provided to an adult individual—

(A) in the case of a hospital, at the time of the individual's admission as an inpatient,

(B) in the case of a skilled nursing facility, at the time of the individual's admission as a resident,

(C) in the case of a home health agency, in advance of the individual coming under the care of the agency,

(D) in the case of a hospice program, at the time of initial receipt of hospice care by the individual from the program, and

(E) in the case of an eligible organization (as defined in section 1395 mm(b) of this title) or an organization provided payments under section 1395l(a)(1)(A) of this title, at the time of enrollment of the individual with the organization.

(3) In this subsection, the term "advance directive" means a written instruction, such as a living will or durable power of attorney for health care, recognized under State law (whether statutory or as recognized by the courts of the State) and relating to the provision of such care when the individual is incapacitated.

(g) Penalties for improper billing

Except as permitted under subsection (a)(2) of this section, any person who knowingly and willfully presents, or causes to be presented, a bill or request for payment inconsistent with an arrangement under subsection (a)(1)(H) of this section or in violation of the requirement for such an arrangement, is subject to a civil money penalty of not to exceed $2,000. The provisions of section 1320a-7a of this title (other than subsections (a) and (b)) shall apply to a civil money penalty under the previous sentence in the same manner as such provisions apply to a penalty or proceeding under section 1320a-7a(a) of this title.

(h) Dissatisfaction with determination of Secretary; appeal by institutions or agencies; single notice and hearing

(1) Except as provided in paragraph (2), an institution or agency dissatisfied with a determination by the Secretary that it is not a provider of services or with a determination described in subsection (b)(2) of this section shall be entitled to a hearing thereon by the Secretary (after reasonable notice) to the same extent as is provided in section 405(b) of this title, and to judicial review of the Secretary's final decision after such hearing as is provided in section 405(g) of this title, except that, in so applying such sections and in applying section 405(l) of this title thereto, any reference

therein to the Commissioner of Social Security or the Social Security Administration shall be considered a reference to the Secretary or the Department of Health and Human Services respectively".

(2) An institution or agency is not entitled to separate notice and opportunity for a hearing under both section 1320a-7 of this title and this section with respect to a determination or determinations based on the same underlying facts and issues.

(i) Intermediate sanctions for psychiatric hospitals

(1) If the Secretary determines that a psychiatric hospital which has an agreement in effect under this section no longer meets the requirements for a psychiatric hospital under this subchapter and further finds that the hospital's deficiencies—

(A) immediately jeopardize the health and safety of its patients, the Secretary shall terminate such agreement; or

(B) do not immediately jeopardize the health and safety of its patients, the Secretary may terminate such agreement, or provide that no payment will be made under this subchapter with respect to any individual admitted to such hospital after the effective date of the finding, or both.

(2) If a psychiatric hospital, found to have deficiencies described in paragraph (1)(B), has not complied with the requirements of this subchapter—

(A) within 3 months after the date the hospital is found to be out of compliance with such requirements, the Secretary shall provide that no payment will be made under this subchapter with respect to any individual admitted to such hospital after the end of such 3-month period, or

(B) within 6 months after the date the hospital is found to be out of compliance with such requirements, no payment may be made under this subchapter with respect to any individual in the hospital until the Secretary finds that the hospital is in compliance with the requirements of this subchapter.

Health Care Quality Improvement Act

UNITED STATES CODE ANNOTATED
TITLE 42. THE PUBLIC HEALTH AND WELFARE
CHAPTER 117—ENCOURAGING GOOD FAITH PROFESSIONAL REVIEW ACTIVITIES
Current through P.L. 104-37, approved 10-21-95

§ 11101. Findings

The Congress finds the following:
(1) The increasing occurrence of medical malpractice and the need to improve the quality of medical care have become nationwide problems that warrant greater efforts than those that can be undertaken by any individual State.
(2) There is a national need to restrict the ability of incompetent physicians to move from State to State without disclosure or discovery of the physician's previous damaging or incompetent performance.
(3) This nationwide problem can be remedied through effective professional peer review.
(4) The threat of private money damage liability under Federal laws, including treble damage liability under Federal antitrust law, unreasonably discourages physicians from participating in effective professional peer review.
(5) There is an overriding national need to provide incentive and protection for physicians engaging in effective professional peer review.

SUBCHAPTER I—PROMOTION OF PROFESSIONAL REVIEW ACTIVITIES

§ 11111. Professional review

(a) In general

(1) Limitation on damages for professional review actions

If a professional review action (as defined in section 11151(9) of this title) of a professional review body meets all the standards specified in section 11112(a) of this title, except as provided in subsection (b) of this section—

(A) the professional review body,

(B) any person acting as a member or staff to the body,

(C) any person under a contract or other formal agreement with the body, and

(D) any person who participates with or assists the body with respect to the action.

shall not be liable in damages under any law of the United States or of any State (or political subdivision thereof) with respect to the action. The preceding sentence shall not apply to damages under any law of the United States or any State relating to the civil rights of any person or persons, including the Civil Rights Act of 1964, 42 U.S.C. 2000e, et seq. and the Civil Rights Acts, 42 U.S.C. 1981, et seq. Nothing in this paragraph shall prevent the United States or any Attorney General of a State from bringing an action, including an action under section 15c of Title 15, where such an action is otherwise authorized.

(2) Protection for those providing information to professional review bodies

Notwithstanding any other provision of law, no person (whether as a witness or otherwise) providing information to a professional review body regarding the competence or professional conduct of a physician shall be held, by reason of having provided such information, to be liable in damages under any law of the United States or of any State (or political subdivision thereof) unless such information is false and the person providing it knew that such information was false.

(b) Exception

If the Secretary has reason to believe that a health care entity has failed to report information in accordance with section 11133(a) of this title, the Secretary shall conduct an investigation. If, after providing notice of noncompliance, an opportunity to correct the noncompliance, and an opportunity for a hearing, the Secretary determines that a health care entity has failed substantially to report information in accordance with section 11133(a) of this title, the Secretary shall publish the name of the entity in the Federal Register. The protections of subsection (a)(1) of this section shall not apply to an entity the name of which is published in the Federal Register under the previous sentence with respect to professional review actions of the entity commenced during the 3-year period beginning 30 days after the date of publication of the name.

(c) Treatment under State laws

(1) Professional review actions taken on or after October 14, 1989

Except as provided in paragraph (2), subsection (a) of this section shall apply to State laws in a State only for professional review actions commenced on or after October 14, 1989.

(2) Exceptions

(A) State early opt-in

Subsection (a) of this section shall apply to State laws in a State for actions commenced before October 14, 1989, if the State by legislation elects such treatment.

(B) Effective date of election

An election under State law is not effective, for purposes of, for actions commenced before the effective date of the State law, which may not be earlier than the date of the enactment of that law.

§ 11112. Standards for professional review actions

(a) In general

For purposes of the protection set forth in section 11111(a) of this title, a professional review action must be taken—

(1) in the reasonable belief that the action was in the furtherance of quality health care,

(2) after a reasonable effort to obtain the facts of the matter,

(3) after adequate notice and hearing procedures are afforded to the physician involved or after such other procedures as are fair to the physician under the circumstances, and

(4) in the reasonable belief that the action was warranted by the facts known after such reasonable effort to obtain facts and after meeting the requirement of paragraph (3).

A professional review action shall be presumed to have met the preceding standards necessary for the protection set out in section 11111(a) of this title unless the presumption is rebutted by a preponderance of the evidence.

(b) Adequate notice and hearing

A health care entity is deemed to have met the adequate notice and hearing requirement of subsection (a)(3) of this section with respect to a physician if the following conditions are met (or are waived voluntarily by the physician):

(1) Notice of proposed action

The physician has been given notice stating—

(A)(i) that a professional review action has been proposed to be taken against the physician,

(ii) reasons for the proposed action,

(B)(i) that the physician has the right to request a hearing on the proposed action,

(ii) any time limit (of not less than 30 days) within which to request such a hearing, and

(C) a summary of the rights in the hearing under paragraph (3).

(2) Notice of hearing

If a hearing is requested on a timely basis under paragraph (1)(B), the physician involved must be given notice stating—

(A) the place, time, and date, of the hearing, which date shall not be less than 30 days after the date of the notice, and

(B) a list of the witnesses (if any) expected to testify at the hearing on behalf of the professional review body.

(3) Conduct of hearing and notice

If a hearing is requested on a timely basis under paragraph (1)(B)—

(A) subject to subparagraph (B), the hearing shall be held (as determined by the health care entity)—

(i) before an arbitrator mutually acceptable to the physician and the health care entity,

(ii) before a hearing officer who is appointed by the entity and who is not in direct economic competition with the physician involved, or

(iii) before a panel of individuals who are appointed by the entity and are not in direct economic competition with the physician involved;

(B) the right to the hearing may be forfeited if the physician fails, without good cause, to appear;

(C) in the hearing the physician involved has the right—

(i) to representation by an attorney or other person of the physician's choice,

(ii) to have a record made of the proceedings, copies of which may be obtained by the physician upon payment of any reasonable charges associated with the preparation thereof,

(iii) to call, examine, and cross-examine witnesses,

(iv) to present evidence determined to be relevant by the hearing officer, regardless of its admissibility in a court of law, and

(v) to submit a written statement at the close of the hearing; and

(D) upon completion of the hearing, the physician involved has the right—

(i) to receive the written recommendation of the arbitrator, officer, or panel, including a statement of the basis for the recommendations, and

(ii) to receive a written decision of the health care entity, including a statement of the basis for the decision.

A professional review body's failure to meet the conditions described in this subsection shall not, in itself, constitute failure to meet the standards of subsection (a)(3) of this section.

(c) Adequate procedures in investigations or health emergencies

For purposes of section 11111(a) of this title, nothing in this section shall be construed as—

(1) requiring the procedures referred to in subsection (a)(3) of this section—

(A) where there is no adverse professional review action taken, or

(B) in the case of a suspension or restriction of clinical privileges, for a period of not longer than 14 days, during which an investigation is being conducted to determine the need for a professional review action; or

(2) precluding an immediate suspension or restriction of clinical privileges, subject to subsequent notice and hearing or other adequate proce-

dures, where the failure to take such an action may result in an imminent danger to the health of any individual.

§ 11113. Payment of reasonable attorneys' fees and costs in defense of suit

In any suit brought against a defendant, to the extent that a defendant has met the standards set forth under section 11112(a) of this title and the defendant substantially prevails, the court shall, at the conclusion of the action, award to a substantially prevailing party defending against any such claim the cost of the suit attributable to such claim, including a reasonable attorney's fee, if the claim, or the claimant's conduct during the litigation of the claim, was frivolous, unreasonable, without foundation, or in bad faith. For the purposes of this section, a defendant shall not be considered to have substantially prevailed when the plaintiff obtains an award for damages or permanent injunctive or declaratory relief.

§ 11114. Guidelines of the Secretary

The Secretary may establish, after notice and opportunity for comment, such voluntary guidelines as may assist the professional review bodies in meeting the standards described in section 11112(a) of this title.

§ 11115. Construction

(a) In general

Except as specifically provided in this subchapter, nothing in this subchapter shall be construed as changing the liabilities or immunities under law or as preempting or overriding any State law which provides incentives, immunities, or protection for those engaged in a professional review action that is in addition to or greater than that provided by this subchapter

(b) Scope of clinical privileges

Nothing in this subchapter shall be construed as requiring health care entities to provide clinical privileges to any or all classes or types of physicians or other licensed health care practitioners.

(c) Treatment of nurses and other practitioners

Nothing in this subchapter shall be construed as affecting, or modifying any provision of Federal or State law, with respect to activities of professional review bodies regarding nurses, other licensed health care practitioners, or other health professionals who are not physicians.

(d) Treatment of patient malpractice claims

Nothing in this chapter shall be construed as affecting in any manner the rights and remedies afforded patients under any provision of Federal or State law to seek redress for any harm or injury suffered as a result of negligent treatment or care by any physician, health care practitioner, or health care entity, or as limiting any defenses or immunities available to any physician, health care practitioner, or health care entity.

SUBCHAPTER II—REPORTING OF INFORMATION

§ 11131. Requiring reports on medical malpractice payments

(a) In general

Each entity (including an insurance company) which makes payment under a policy of insurance, self-insurance, or otherwise in settlement (or partial settlement) of, or in satisfaction of a judgment in, a medical malpractice action or claim shall report, in accordance with section 11134 of this title, information respecting the payment and circumstances thereof.

(b) Information to be reported

The information to be reported under subsection (a) of this section includes—

(1) the name of any physician or licensed health care practitioner for whose benefit the payment is made,

(2) the amount of the payment,

(3) the name (if known) of any hospital with which the physician or practitioner is affiliated or associated,

(4) a description of the acts or omissions and injuries or illnesses upon which the action or claim was based, and

(5) such other information as the Secretary determines is required for appropriate interpretation of information reported under this section.

(c) Sanctions for failure to report

Any entity that fails to report information on a payment required to be reported under this section shall be subject to a civil money penalty of not more than $10,000 for each such payment involved. Such penalty shall be imposed and collected in the same manner as civil money penalties under subsection (a) of section 1320a-7a of this title are imposed and collected under that section.

(d) Report on treatment of small payments

The Secretary shall study and report to Congress, not later than two years after November 14, 1986, on whether information respecting small payments should continue to be required to be reported under subsection (a) of this section and whether information respecting all claims made concerning a medical malpractice action should be required to be reported under such subsection.

§ 11132. Reporting of sanctions taken by Boards of Medical Examiners

(a) In general

(1) Actions subject to reporting

Each Board of Medical Examiners—

(A) which revokes or suspends (or otherwise restricts) a physician's license or censures, reprimands, or places on probation a physician, for reasons relating to the physician's professional competence or professional conduct, or

(B) to which a physician's license is surrendered,

shall report, in accordance with section 11134 of this title, the information described in paragraph (2).

(2) Information to be reported

The information to be reported under paragraph (1) is—

(A) the name of the physician involved,

(B) a description of the acts or omissions or other reasons (if known) for the revocation, suspension, or surrender of license, and

(C) such other information respecting the circumstances of the action or surrender as the Secretary deems appropriate.

(b) Failure to report

If, after notice of noncompliance and providing opportunity to correct noncompliance, the Secretary determines that a Board of Medical Examiners has failed to report information in accordance with subsection (a) of this section, the Secretary shall designate another qualified entity for the reporting of information under section 11133 of this title.

§ 11133. Reporting of certain professional review actions taken by health care entities

(a) Reporting by health care entities

(1) On physicians

Each health care entity which—

(A) takes a professional review action that adversely affects the clinical privileges of a physician for a period longer than 30 days;

(B) accepts the surrender of clinical privileges of a physician—

(i) while the physician is under an investigation by the entity relating to possible incompetence or improper professional conduct, or

(ii) in return for not conducting such an investigation or proceeding; or

(C) in the case of such an entity which is a professional society, takes a professional review action which adversely affects the membership of a physician in the society,

shall report to the Board of Medical Examiners, in accordance with section 11134(a) of this title, the information described in paragraph (3).

(2) Permissive reporting on other licensed health care practitioners

A health care entity may report to the Board of Medical Examiners, in accordance with section 11134(a) of this title, the information described in paragraph (3) in the case of a licensed health care practitioner who is not a physician, if the entity would be required to report such information under paragraph (1) with respect to the practitioner if the practitioner were a physician.

(3) Information to be reported

The information to be reported under this subsection is—

(A) the name of the physician or practitioner involved,

(B) a description of the acts or omissions or other reasons for the action or, if known, for the surrender, and

(C) such other information respecting the circumstances of the action or surrender as the Secretary deems appropriate.

(b) Reporting by Board of Medical Examiners

Each Board of Medical Examiners shall report, in accordance with section 11134 of this title, the information reported to it under subsection (a) of this section and known instances of a health care entity's failure to report information under subsection (a)(1) of this section.

(c) Sanctions

(1) Health care entities

A health care entity that fails substantially to meet the requirement of subsection (a)(1) of this section shall lose the protections of section 11111(a)(1) of this title if the Secretary publishes the name of the entity under section 11111(b) of this title.

(2) Board of Medical Examiners

If, after notice of noncompliance and providing an opportunity to correct noncompliance, the Secretary determines that a Board of Medical Examiners has failed to report information in accordance with subsection (b) of this section, the Secretary shall designate another qualified entity for the reporting of information under subsection (b) of this section.

(d) References to Board of Medical Examiners

Any reference in this subchapter to a Board of Medical Examiners includes, in the case of a Board in a State that fails to meet the reporting requirements of section 11132(a) of this title or subsection (b) of this section, a reference to such other qualified entity as the Secretary designates.

§ 11134. Form of reporting

(a) Timing and form

The information required to be reported under sections 11131, 11132(a), and 11133 of this title shall be reported regularly (but not less often than monthly) and in such form and manner as the Secretary prescribes. Such information shall first be required to be reported on a date (not later than one year after November 14, 1986) specified by the Secretary.

(b) To whom reported

The information required to be reported under sections 11131, 11132(a), and 11133(b) of this title shall be reported to the Secretary, or, in the Secretary's discretion, to an appropriate private or public agency which has made suitable arrangements with the Secretary with respect to receipt, storage, protection of confidentiality, and dissemination of the information under this subchapter.

(c) Reporting to State licensing boards

(1) Malpractice payments

Information required to be reported under section 11131 of this title shall also be reported to the appropriate State licensing board (or boards) in the State in which the medical malpractice claim arose.

(2) Reporting to other licensing boards

Information required to be reported under section 11133(b) of this title shall also be reported to the appropriate State licensing board in the State in which the health care entity is located if it is not otherwise reported to such board under subsection (b) of this section.

§ 11135. Duty of hospitals to obtain information

(a) In general

It is the duty of each hospital to request from the Secretary (or the agency designated under section 11134(b) of this title), on and after the date information is first required to be reported under section 11134(a) of this title)—

(1) at the time a physician or licensed health care practitioner applies to be on the medical staff (courtesy or otherwise) of, or for clinical privileges at, the hospital, information reported under this subchapter concerning the physician or practitioner, and

(2) once every 2 years information reported under this subchapter concerning any physician or such practitioner who is on the medical staff (courtesy or otherwise) of, or has been granted clinical privileges at, the hospital.

A hospital may request such information at other times.

(b) Failure to obtain information

With respect to a medical malpractice action, a hospital which does not request information respecting a physician or practitioner as required under subsection (a) of this section is presumed to have knowledge of any information reported under this subchapter to the Secretary with respect to the physician or practitioner.

(c) Reliance on information provided

Each hospital may rely upon information provided to the hospital under this chapter and shall not be held liable for such reliance in the absence of the hospital's knowledge that the information provided was false.

§ 11136. Disclosure and correction of information

With respect to the information reported to the Secretary (or the agency designated under section 11134(b) of this title) under this subchapter respecting a physician or other licensed health care practitioner, the Secretary shall, by regulation, provide for—

(1) disclosure of the information, upon request, to the physician or practitioner, and

(2) procedures in the case of disputed accuracy of the information.

§ 11137. Miscellaneous provisions

(a) Providing licensing boards and other health care entities with access to information

The Secretary (or the agency designated under section 11134(b) of this title) shall, upon request, provide information reported under this subchapter with respect to a physician or other licensed health care practitioner to State licensing boards, to hospitals, and to other health care entities (including health maintenance organizations) that have entered (or may be entering) into an employment or affiliation relationship with the physician or practitioner or to which the physician or practitioner has applied for clinical privileges or appointment to the medical staff.

(b) Confidentiality of information

(1) In general

Information reported under this subchapter is considered confidential and shall not be disclosed (other than to the physician or practitioner involved) except with respect to professional review activity, as necessary to carry out subsections (b) and (c) of section 11135 of this title (as specified in regulations by the Secretary), or in accordance with regulations of the Secretary promulgated pursuant to subsection (a) of this section. Nothing in this subsection shall prevent the disclosure of such information by a party which is otherwise authorized, under applicable State law, to make such disclosure. Information reported under this subchapter that is in a form that does not permit the identification of any particular health care entity, physician, other health care practitioner, or patient shall not be considered confidential. The Secretary (or the agency designated under section 11134(b) of this title), on application by any person, shall prepare such information in such form and shall disclose such information in such form.

(2) Penalty for violations

Any person who violates paragraph (1) shall be subject to a civil money penalty of not more than $10,000 for each such violation involved. Such penalty shall be imposed and collected in the same manner as civil money penalties under subsection (a) of section 1320a-7a of this title are imposed and collected under that section.

(3) Use of information

Subject to paragraph (1), information provided under section 11135 of this title and subsection (a) of this section is intended to be used solely with respect to activities in the furtherance of the quality of health care.

(4) Fees

The Secretary may establish or approve reasonable fees for the disclosure of information under this section or section 11136 of this title. The amount of such a fee may not exceed the costs of processing the requests for disclosure and of providing such information. Such fees shall be available to the Secretary (or, in the Secretary's discretion, to the agency designated under section 11134(b) of this title) to cover such costs.

(c) Relief from liability for reporting

No person or entity (including the agency designated under section 11134(b) of this title) shall be held liable in any civil action with respect to any report made under this subchapter (including information provided under subsection (a) of this section without knowledge of the falsity of the information contained in the report.

(d) Interpretation of information

In interpreting information reported under this subchapter, a payment in settlement of a medical malpractice action or claim shall not be construed as creating a presumption that medical malpractice has occurred.

SUBCHAPTER III—DEFINITIONS AND REPORTS

§ 11151. Definitions

In this chapter:

(1) The term "adversely affecting" includes reducing, restricting, suspending, revoking, denying, or failing to renew clinical privileges or membership in a health care entity.

(2) The term "Board of Medical Examiners" includes a body comparable to such a Board (as determined by the State) with responsibility for the licensing of physicians and also includes a subdivision of such a Board or body.

(3) The term "clinical privileges" includes privileges, membership on the medical staff, and the other circumstances pertaining to the furnishing of medical care under which a physician or other licensed health care practitioner is permitted to furnish such care by a health care entity.

(4)(A) The term "health care entity" means—

(i) a hospital that is licensed to provide health care services by the State in which it is located,

(ii) an entity (including a health maintenance organization or group medical practice) that provides health care services and that follows a formal peer review process for the purpose of furthering quality health care (as determined under regulations of the Secretary), and

(iii) subject to subparagraph (B), a professional society (or committee thereof) of physicians or other licensed health care practitioners that follows a formal peer review process for the purpose of furthering quality health care (as determined under regulations of the Secretary).

(B) The term "health care entity" does not include a professional society (or committee thereof) if, within the previous 5 years, the society has been found by the Federal Trade Commission or any court to have engaged in any anticompetitive practice which had the effect of restricting the practice of licensed health care practitioners.

(5) The term "hospital" means an entity described in paragraphs (1) and (7) of section 1395x(e) of this title.

(6) The terms "licensed health care practitioner" and "practitioner" mean, with respect to a State, an individual (other than a physician) who is licensed or otherwise authorized by the State to provide health care services.

(7) The term "medical malpractice action or claim" means a written claim or demand for payment based on a health care provider's furnishing (or failure to furnish) health care services, and includes the filing of a cause of action, based on the law of tort, brought in any court of any State or the United States seeking monetary damages.

(8) The term "physician" means a doctor of medicine or osteopathy or a doctor of dental surgery or medical dentistry legally authorized to practice medicine and surgery or dentistry by a State (or any individual who, without authority holds himself or herself out to be so authorized).

(9) The term "professional review action" means an action or recommendation of a professional review body which is taken or made in the conduct of professional review activity, which is based on the competence or professional conduct of an individual physician (which conduct affects or could affect adversely the health or welfare of a patient or patients), and which affects (or may affect) adversely the clinical privileges, or membership in a professional society, of the physician. Such term includes a formal decision of a professional review body not to take an action or make a recommendation described in the previous sentence and also includes professional review activities relating to a professional review action. In this chapter, an action is not considered to be based on the competence or professional conduct of a physician if the action is primarily based on—

(A) the physician's association, or lack of association, with a professional society or association,

(B) the physician's fees or the physician's advertising or engaging in other competitive acts intended to solicit or retain business,

(C) the physician's participation in prepaid group health plans, salaried employment, or any other manner of delivering health services whether on a fee-for-service or other basis,

(D) a physician's association with, supervision of, delegation of authority to, support for, training of, or participation in a private group practice with, a member or members of a particular class of health care practitioner or professional, or

(E) any other matter that does not relate to the competence or professional conduct of a physician.

(10) The term "professional review activity" means an activity of a health care entity with respect to an individual physician—

(A) to determine whether the physician may have clinical privileges with respect to, or membership in, the entity,

(B) to determine the scope or conditions of such privileges or membership, or

(C) to change or modify such privileges or membership.

(11) The term "professional review body" means a health care entity and the governing body or any committee of a health care entity which conducts professional review activity, and includes any committee of the

medical staff of such an entity when assisting the governing body in a professional review activity.

(12) The term "Secretary" means the Secretary of Health and Human Services.

(13) The term "State" means the 50 States, the District of Columbia, Puerto Rico, the Virgin Islands, Guam, American Samoa, and the Northern Mariana Islands.

(14) The term "State licensing board" means, with respect to a physician or health care provider in a State, the agency of the State which is primarily responsible for the licensing of the physician or provider to furnish health care services.

§ 11152. Reports and memoranda of understanding

(a) Annual reports to Congress

The Secretary shall report to Congress, annually during the three years after November 14, 1986, on the implementation of this chapter.

(b) Memoranda of understanding

The Secretary of Health and Human Services shall seek to enter into memoranda of understanding with the Secretary of Defense and the Administrator of Veterans' Affairs to apply the provisions of subchapter II of this chapter to hospitals and other facilities and health care providers under the jurisdiction of the Secretary or Administrator, respectively. The Secretary shall report to Congress, not later than two years after November 14, 1986, on any such memoranda and on the cooperation among such officials in establishing such memoranda.

(c) Memorandum of understanding with Drug Enforcement Administration

The Secretary of Health and Human Services shall seek to enter into a memorandum of understanding with the Administrator of Drug Enforcement relating to providing for the reporting by the Administrator to the Secretary of information respecting physicians and other practitioners whose registration to dispense controlled substances has been suspended or revoked under section 824 of Title 21. The Secretary shall report to Congress, not later than two years after November 14, 1986, on any such memorandum and on the cooperation between the Secretary and the Administrator in establishing such a memorandum.

Glossary

Action A judicial or administrative proceeding for the enforcement or protection of a right; a lawsuit.

Adjudication The final decision of a court, usually made after the trial of the case; the court's final judgment.

Admissibility Information is considered admissible into evidence at trial if the applicable rules establish that the information is both pertinent and proper for the judge and/or jury to consider when deciding the issues involved in the lawsuit.

Admissible Pertinent and proper evidence. Rules of evidence determine if evidence is pertinent and proper. For example, in the context of medical records, the applicable rule of evidence is the hearsay rule.

Adoption records Records of the individual placed for adoption. Access to adoption records is controversial. The competing issues involved in access are the interests of the biological parent(s) in placing the child up for adoption, often with the promise of confidentiality, and the interests of the adoptee for genetic information and information about his or her natural identity.

Advance directive Written instructions recognized under state law, such as living wills or durable powers of attorney for health care, which relate to the kind of health care the patient wishes to have or not have if he or she becomes incapacitated.

Alternative dispute resolution A practice involving several methods of resolving conflicts and disagreements to the satisfaction of all parties without using the court system.

Anonymous testing A system that assigns a unique identifier to the individual tested, thereby protecting his or her identity.

Antikickback statute A law prohibiting the offer or solicitation of remuneration, including kickbacks and rebates, in exchange for referrals of Medicare-payable services.

Appeal The process by which a higher court is requested by a party to a lawsuit to review the decision of a lower court. Such reconsideration is normally confined to a review of the record from the lower court, with no new testimony taken and no new issues raised. Review by the higher court may result in affirmation, reversal, or modification of the lower court's decision.

Appellant A party who appeals from a lower court to a higher court.

Appellee A party against whom a case is appealed from a lower court to a higher court.

Arbitration The use of a neutral third party to hear both sides of a dispute and render a written decision, called an award. The award is imposed on the parties following consideration of each side's position.

Assault An act of force or threat of force intended to inflict harm upon a person or to put the person in fear that such harm is imminent; an attempt to commit a battery. The perpetrator must have or appear to have the present ability to carry out the act.

Assumption of risk A doctrine stating that a plaintiff who voluntarily exposes himself or herself to a known and appreciated danger may not recover damages caused by incurring that risk.

Attorney-client privilege The legal protection of communications between a client and his or her attorney, made in confidence for the purpose of obtaining legal advice.

Authentication Confirms the content and accuracy of an entry into the medical record by written signature, initials, or computer-generated signature code.

Authorization Permission given to the health-care provider by the patient allowing the provider to disclose patient-specific health information.

Authorship Identifies the health-care provider who has made an entry in the patient record, in writing or by dictation, keyboard, or keyless data entry.

Battery The unconsented-to touching or striking of one person by another or by an object put in motion by him or her, with the intention of doing harm or giving offense. Battery is both a crime and a tort.

Breach of contract The failure to perform according to the terms of the parties' agreement.

Breach of duty of care The failure to conform to a particular standard of care toward another. Such failure to conform will result in liability for harm sustained by another person.

Business associate One who performs or assists in performing a function or activity involving the use or disclosure of individually identifiable health information on behalf of a health-care provider.

Business record exception An exception to the hearsay rule that permits business records to be admitted into evidence even though they are hearsay. Medical records admitted as evidence under this exception must first meet the foundation requirements of the exception.

Business records rule An exception to the hearsay rule that permits business records to be admitted into evidence even though they are hearsay.

Causation A causing; the producing of a result.

Cause of action An action; a lawsuit; a case.

Certiorari A writ issued by a higher court to a lower court requiring the certification of the record in a particular case so that the higher court can review the record and correct any actions taken in the case that are not in accordance with the law. The Supreme Court of the United States uses the writ of certiorari to select the lower federal court and the state court cases it is willing to review.

Charitable immunity A defense that shields a charitable institution from liability for any torts committed on its property or by its employees.

Civil money penalty A fine imposed on a health-care provider who files false or fraudulent claims.

Clinical information system System with a central focus of clinical data, not financial or billing information.

Common law (1) A law found in the decisions of the courts rather than in statutes; judge-made law. (2) English law adopted by the early American colonists, which is part of the U.S. judicial heritage and forms the basis of much of its law today.

Comparative negligence The doctrine adopted by most states that requires a comparison of the negligence of the defendant with the negligence of the plaintiff; the greater the negligence of the defendant, the lesser the level of care required of the plaintiff to permit her to recover. In other words, the plaintiff's negligence does not defeat her cause of action, but it does reduce the damages she is entitled to recover.

Complaint (1) The initial pleading in a civil action, in which the plaintiff alleges a cause of action and asks that the wrong done to him or her be remedied by the court. (2) A formal charge of a crime.

Compliance The efforts to establish a culture that promotes prevention, detection, and resolution of instances of conduct that do not conform to applicable local, state, and federal laws and regulations.

Compliance program A program ensuring the use of effective internal controls that promote adherence to the applicable local, state, and federal laws and regulations the program requirements of federal, state, and private health plans.

Computerized patient record Records created, authenticated, stored, and retrieved by computers.

Confidentiality The obligation of the health-care provider to maintain patient information in a manner that will not permit dissemination beyond the health-care provider. The origin of confidentiality is found in the Hippocratic Oath.

Confidentiality statutes Statutes that place restrictions on identifying both the patient tested and the test results.

Consent A concurrence of wills. An agreement by a person in the possession and exercise of sufficient mental capacity to make an intelligent choice to do something proposed by another.

Constitution (1) The system of fundamental principles by which a nation, state, or corporation is governed. A nation's constitution may be written (example: the U.S. Constitution) or unwritten (example: the British Constitution). A nation's laws must conform to its constitution. A law that violates a nation's constitution is unconstitutional and therefore unenforceable. (2) The document setting forth the fundamental principles of governance. (3) The constitution of the United States.

Continuum of ownership Questions of ownership of health information range from the traditional view of the health-care provider having sole ownership of the medical record, to a joint patient–health-care provider having sole ownership of the medical record, toward a trend placing health information in a trust capacity.

Contract An agreement entered into, for adequate consideration, to do, or refrain from doing, a particular thing. The Uniform Commercial Code defines a contract as the total legal obligation resulting from the parties' agreement. In addition to adequate consideration, the transaction must involve an undertaking that is legal to perform, and there must be mutuality of agreement and obligation between at least two competent parties.

Contributory negligence In the law of negligence, a failure by the plaintiff to exercise reasonable care that, in part at least, is the cause of an injury. Contributory negligence defeats a plaintiff's cause of action for negligence in states that have not adopted the doctrine of comparative negligence.

Corporate negligence A doctrine defined as the failure of a hospital, entrusted with the task of providing the accommodations necessary to carry out its purpose, to follow the established standard of conduct to which it should conform.

Court order (1) An adjudication by a court. (2) The ruling by a court with respect to a motion or any other question before it for determination during the course of a proceeding.

Court structure A multitiered structure consisting of trial courts, intermediate courts of appeal, and supreme courts. The multitiered structure is the same at both state and federal levels.

Damages The sum of money that may be recovered in the courts as financial reparation for an injury or wrong suffered as a result of breach of contract or tort. Divided into three types: nominal, actual, punitive.

Defamation Libel or slander; the written or oral publication, false or intentional, of anything that is injurious to the good name or reputation of another person.

Defendant The person against whom an action is brought.

Digital imaging A system by which paper documents are scanned on devices that work similar to a photocopier, allowing the image to be saved and viewed through a server or web browser.

Disclosure of information Disclosure of health information is governed by two principles: (1) medical records remain within the provider's control and safekeeping and may be removed only in accordance with a court order or subpoena; (2) the health-care provider may not disclose or withhold health information at will.

Disclosure with patient authorization Health information may be disclosed to third parties on written authorization of the patient. Certain components must be present for the written authorization form to be valid.

Disclosure without patient authorization Health information may be disclosed to third parties without written patient authorization in limited circumstances such as medical emergencies, scientific research activities, and audits.

Discoverability Information is considered discoverable if the applicable rules require disclosure of the information upon the formal request of a party.

Discovery A means for providing a party, in advance of trial, with access to facts that are within the knowledge of the other side, to enable the party to better try his or her case. Examples include depositions, written interrogatories, production of documents or things, physical and mental examinations, and requests for admission.

Diversity jurisdiction The jurisdiction of a federal court arising from diversity of citizenship when the jurisdictional amount has been met.

Durable power of attorney for health care Allows a competent individual to name someone else to exercise health-care-related decisions on his or her behalf, in the event the individual becomes incapacitated or unable to make personal decisions.

Duty of care An obligation, enforced by law, to conform to a particular standard of care toward another. Failure to conform to this standard will result in liability for any harm sustained by another person.

Electronic mail A form of communication between parties or individuals using only electronic means.

Emancipation The legal ability of a minor to act as an adult when she has moved away from home and receives no support from her parents.

Employment challenges Lawsuits brought by employees of health-care providers asserting the employee's legal right to refuse to undertake or undergo certain actions required by employer.

Equitable relief A remedy available in equity rather than at law; generally relief other than money damages.

Ethical guidelines Standards of conduct issued by professional organizations to guide their members' future course of action. These standards are sometimes used to establish the standard of care in a negligence action.

Evidence The means by which any matter of fact may be established or disproved. Such means may include testimony, documents, and physical objects. The law of evidence is made up of rules that determine what evidence is to be admitted or rejected in the trial of a civil action or a criminal prosecution and what weight is to be given to admitted evidence. Medical records may be used as evidence in civil or criminal court actions or in administrative agency proceedings.

Failure to warn A negligence theory that applies to a psychotherapist's failure to take steps to protect an innocent third party from a dangerous patient. Also known as failure to protect.

Federal question jurisdiction Refers to cases that question or involve a U.S. constitutional principle, treaty, federal statute, or federal rule or regulation. It also includes cases that would normally proceed in state court but did not because they occurred on federal land.

Felony A crime of a grave or serious nature punishable by a term of imprisonment exceeding one year.

Foundation requirements Foundation requirements of the business record exception must be established during testimony by the health information manager. The manager must possess knowledge of the requirements to create and maintain a medical record issued by governmental entities, accrediting agencies, and internal policies and procedures of the health-care provider, along with knowledge of the manner in which data are recorded.

Fraud and abuse A false misrepresentation of fact that is relied on by another to that person's detriment and is a departure from reasonable use. This false misrepresentation of fact may take the form of words or conduct.

Garnishment A proceeding by a creditor to obtain satisfaction of a debt from money or property of the debtor that is in the possession of a third person or is owed by such a person to the debtor.

Genetic information Information about an individual or family obtained from a genetic test or an individual's DNA sample. Genetic information relates to a person's future, not past, health.

Good Samaritan statutes Statutes that protect physicians and other rescuers from civil liability as a result of their acts or omissions in rendering emergency care, unless their actions or omissions were grossly negligent or intentionally injuring to the patient.

Governmental immunity A doctrine that precludes a plaintiff from asserting a meritorious lawsuit against a governmental entity unless the governmental entity consents to the lawsuit.

Health-care relationship A connection between a health-care provider, patient, and/or hospital that serves as the basis of a lawsuit.

Hearsay rule The rule that hearsay testimony is not admissible unless it falls within an exception to the hearsay rule.

Hospital-patient relationship Begins when the patient is voluntarily admitted to the hospital and agrees to pay for the treatment to be rendered. The relationship ends when the patient leaves the hospital through discharge or against medical advice.

Hospital-physician relationship A contractual agreement between the physician and the hospital allowing the physician to bring patients to the hospital to receive treatment.

Improper disclosure The disclosure of test results or other health information to a third party without the consent of the individual treated.

Incident report The documentation of an adverse incident, whether done on a paper form or through a computerized database with access controls. It describes the incident itself, including the time, date, and place of occurrence, along with the condition of the subject of the incident, statements or observations of witnesses, and any responsive action taken.

Incompetent A person who is unable or unfit to make decisions.

Informed consent The legal doctrine that requires the health-care provider to disclose information to the patient about treatment options and risks so that the patient may knowledgeably consent to treatment.

Injunction A court order that commands or prohibits some act or course of conduct. It is preventive in nature and designed to protect a plaintiff from irreparable injury to his or her property or property rights by prohibiting or commanding the doing of certain acts. An injunction is a form of equitable relief.

Institutional review board A group formally designated by an institution to safeguard the rights and welfare of human subjects by reviewing, approving, and monitoring medical research.

Intellectual property Property (examples: copyrights; patents; trade secrets) that is the physical or tangible result of original thought. Modern technology has brought about widespread infringement of intellectual property rights. (Examples: the unauthorized reproduction and sale of videotapes, audiotapes, and computer software).

Intentional torts Torts committed by persons with the intent to do something wrong.

Invasion of privacy The dissemination of information about another person's private, personal matters.

Jurisdiction (1) In a general sense, the right of a court to adjudicate lawsuits of a certain kind. (2) In a specific sense, the right of a court to determine a particular case; in other words, the power of the court over the subject matter of, or property involved in, the case at bar. (3) In a geographical sense, the power of a court to hear cases only within a specific territorial area. (4) Authority; control; power. (5) District; area; locality. The term also applies to the authority of an administrative agency to hear and determine a case brought before it.

Jury instructions Directions given to the jury by the judge before he or she sends the jurors out to deliberate and return a verdict, explaining the law that applies in the case and spelling out what must be proven and by whom.

Laches The equitable doctrine that a plaintiff's neglect or failure to assert a right may cause the court to deny him or her relief if, as a result, the defendant has changed position so that the defendant's rights are at risk.

Legal process Stages through which a lawsuit passes.

Legal remedy A remedy available through legal action.

Living will A document, executed while a patient is competent, that provides direction as to medical care in the event the patient is incapacitated or unable to make personal decisions. A form of advance directive; each state must determine the legal rights of the patient to use a living will.

Mail and wire fraud The use of the U.S. Postal Service or commercial wire services for the advancement of a scheme relating to fraud.

Malpractice Misconduct involving a professional who fails to follow a standard of care prevalent for his or her profession that results in harm to another person.

Mandatory testing A decision by the legislature or court that forces an individual to receive testing for some health reason, without granting the individual the right to refuse.

Mediation The use of a neutral third party to assist both sides of a dispute in resolving their differences and reducing their resolution to writing. The resolution is based on the parties' agreement.

Medical abandonment The unilateral severing, by the physician, of the physician-patient relationship without providing the patient with reasonable notice at a time when there is a necessity for continuing care.

Medical malpractice The failure of a medical professional to follow a standard of care prevalent for his or her profession that results in harm to the patient. Legal theories supporting a medical malpractice lawsuit include negligence, *res ipsa loquitur*, failure to warn, vicarious liability, and corporate negligence.

Medical record content The characteristics that are essential to constitute an adequate medical record.

Medical staff privileges The scope and limit of a physician's practice in a medical institution as defined by the institution's governing board.

Minimum necessary standard This standard requires the health-care provider to make reasonable efforts to limit the patient-specific health information to the minimum necessary to accomplish the intended purpose of the use, disclosure, or request.

Misdemeanor A crime of a less serious nature punishable by a fine or a term of imprisonment of less than a year.

Negligence The failure to do something that a reasonable person would do in the same circumstances, or the doing of something a reasonable person would not do. Negligence is a wrong generally characterized by carelessness, inattentiveness, and neglectfulness rather than by positive intent to cause injury.

Negotiation and settlement The parties to a dispute work without the help of a third party neutral to reach resolution of a dispute and memorialize the resolution.

Nonintentional torts Torts committed by persons who lack the intent to do something wrong.

Notice of information practices A notice required by law that requires the health-care provider to notify the patient of the uses of patient-specific health information and an opportunity to consent, reject, or request restriction of the information for any of the uses contained in the notice.

Official record A record containing that information necessary to document the patient's care and treatment: history and mental status exam, consent forms, treatment plans, physician orders, laboratory results, etc. This record is required to be maintained by law.

Open record statutes Statutory provisions that address confidentiality requirements using a presumption of disclosure of information upon request, absent statutory exemption.

Patient identification Federal regulations restrict identification of a patient who is in a facility publicly identified as providing substance abuse treatment. Written consent of the patient or a court order is required for disclosure.

Patient notice Patients must be given notice of federal confidentiality requirements upon admission to a substance abuse treatment program or soon thereafter.

Patient record system Set of components that form the mechanism by which patient records are created, used, stored, and retrieved.

Peer review privileges State statutes that protect peer review deliberations and records from subpoena, discovery, or introduction into evidence. These statutes may also protect participants in peer review deliberations from civil liability.

Permissive and mandatory exclusion A deterrent to fraud and abuse where the health-care provider is barred from participation in the Medicare program and all other federally financed health-care programs.

Personal record A record, separate from the official medical record, maintained by the clinician in the mental health or developmental disability context that gives the clinician's viewpoint of the patient and their communications.

Personnel security In addition to standard considerations involved in employee hiring, personnel security related to the computerized patient record also involves comprehensive knowledge of the computer system and a continual, documented updating of education relating to it.

Physical security The physical protection of the medical record.

Physician-patient privilege The legal doctrine that prevents forced disclosure of, or testimony about, information obtained by the health-care provider during the course of treatment.

Physician-patient relationship Traditionally, the cornerstone of U.S. health care. Begins when the patient requests treatment and the physician agrees to render the treatment. Exists as an express or implied contract.

Physician self-referral prohibitions Laws that prohibit physicians from referring patients to services where the physician possesses a financial interest or will receive payment in return for the referral.

Plaintiff A person who brings a lawsuit.

Pleadings Formal statements by the parties setting forth their claims or defenses (examples: a complaint, a cross-complaint, an answer, a counterclaim). The various kinds of pleadings in civil cases, and the rules governing them, are set forth in detail in the Federal Rules of Civil Procedure and, with respect to pleading in state courts, by the rules of civil procedure of several states. These rules of procedure abolished common law pleading.

Preemption A doctrine adopted by the U.S. Supreme Court that certain matters are of such a national, as opposed to local, character that federal laws preempt or take precedence over state laws. As such, a state law inconsistent with that of the federal law will be held invalid.

Privacy The right to be let alone or the right to control personal information. The patient's right to privacy is the underpinning to legal protections for patient-specific health information.

Privacy statutes Laws that generally correspond with the principles found in the federal Privacy Act: a presumption of confidentiality which may be rebutted with evidence of patient authorization to disclose information.

Private law A law that regulates conflicts between private parties, (examples: contract law, tort law).

Procedural law That portion of law that focuses on the steps through which a case passes. Criminal procedural law ranges from the initial investigation of a crime through trial, sentencing, and the eventual release of the criminal offender.

Professional disclosure standard A standard used in the negligence context to determine liability. It is measured according to the level of information a reasonable health-care provider would disclose under the same or similar circumstances.

Proper documentation Timely and complete, meaning that all entries in the record are authored and authenticated and reflect the total care actually rendered to the patient.

Public health threat A wide variety of health-care problems that potentially endanger the public health and must be reported to a public health agency. Common public health threats include communicable diseases, child abuse, fetal deaths, and cancer.

Public law The body of rules and principles governing the rights and duties between government and a private party, or between two parts or agencies of government. It defines appropriate behavior between citizens, organizations, and government. Examples include criminal law, constitutional law, substantive law, and procedural law.

Quality management An improvement technique that examines patterns of activity to define optimum performance and determine how to achieve that performance. It is a clinical function that is process oriented and focuses on the improvement of patient care.

Qui tam actions Lawsuits that allow private plaintiffs to sue on behalf of the U.S. government and receive a portion of the recovered funds if successful.

Reasonable fees A fee charged by the health-care provider for the reproduction of the medical record. Individual facilities have policies determining what a reasonable fee should be. The amount of the fee is a controversial national issue.

Reasonable patient standard A standard used in the negligence context to determine liability. It is measured as the level of care that would be exercised by a reasonably prudent person under the same or similar circumstances.

Record destruction policy The general principles determining the length of time medical records must be maintained before being destroyed. The length of time is determined by state statutes and state and federal regulations.

Record retention policy The general principles determining the length of time medical records must be maintained by the health-care provider. The length of time is influenced by the needs of continuing patient care, education, research, and the law, to name a few.

Release of information The written consent form that permits the dissemination of confidential health information to third parties. The components of a valid release of information are determined by state law and federal and state regulation.

Relators The technical term used to describe the private plaintiffs who bring qui tam actions.

Remedy The means by which a right is enforced, an injury is redressed, and relief is obtained. Examples: damages; an injunction. (1) To redress; to make right; to correct; to rectify. (2) To compensate; to indemnify; to make whole.

Remittitur A reduction by the judge of the amount of a verdict because of the excessiveness of the award.

Res ipsa loquitur Means " the thing speaks for itself." Used only when a plaintiff cannot prove negligence with the direct evidence available to him or her.

Res judicata Means "the thing [i.e., the matter] has been adjudicated"; the thing has been decided. The principle that a final judgment rendered on the merits by a court of competent jurisdiction is conclusive of the rights of the parties and is an absolute bar in other actions based on the same claim, demand, or cause of action.

Respondeat superior Means "let the master respond." The doctrine under which liability is imposed on an employer for the acts of its employees committed in the course and scope of their employment.

Reversed and remanded An expression used in appellate court opinions to indicate that the court has reversed the judgment of the trial court and that the case has been returned to the trial court for a new trial.

Risk management An improvement technique designed to achieve two purposes: (1) identify areas of operational and financial risk or loss to a health-care facility and its patients, visitors, and employees; and (2) implement measures to lessen the effects of unavoidable risks and losses, prevent recurrences of these risks or losses, and cover inevitable losses, at the lowest cost. It is a management function that is outcome oriented.

Risk prevention techniques Policies and procedures that serve to protect the integrity and confidentiality of the data at issue. These policies and procedures merge physical and personnel security concepts and apply to the computer system and the personnel who use it.

Satisfying the judgment A method used by the winning party in a lawsuit to collect the amount of judgment awarded (in cases involving money or property).

Show cause order A court decree directing a person or organization to appear in court and explain why the court should not take a proposed action. If the person or organization fails to appear or sufficiently persuade the court to take no action, the court will take the action originally proposed.

Specialized patient records Health records of patients undergoing treatment for certain illnesses, such as substance abuse or mental illness, or in nonacute-care settings, such as the patient's home. These records are subject to different legal requirements from those in an acute-care setting.

Stare decisis Means "standing by the decision." Stare decisis is the doctrine that judicial decisions stand as precedent for cases arising in the future. It is a fundamental policy of our law that, except in unusual circumstances, a court's determination on a point of law will be followed by courts of the same or lower rank in later cases presenting the same legal issue, even though different parties are involved and many years have elapsed.

Statutes Laws written by federal and state legislatures. They become effective upon signature of the president (federal) or governor (state).

Statutes of limitations Federal and state laws prescribing the maximum period of time during which various types of civil actions and criminal prosecutions can be brought after the occurrence of the injury or offense.

Subpoena A command in the form of written process requiring a witness to come to court to testify; short for *subpoena ad testificandum.*

Subpoena ad testificandum *Ad testificandum* means "testify under penalty." A subpoena ad testificandum is a subpoena to testify.

Subpoena duces tecum *Duces tecum* means "bring with you under penalty." A subpoena duces tecum is a written command requiring a witness to come to court to testify and at that time to produce for use as evidence the papers, documents, books, or records listed in the subpoena. It is often used in the context of health information management to command the custodian of the records to produce a particular record at trial or deposition and provide testimony to the authenticity of the record produced.

Substantive law That portion of law that creates, defines, and regulates rights and duties. Criminal substantive law defines specific offenses, the general principles of liability, and the specific punishment.

Substituted consent The legal doctrine that allows an authorized person to consent to or forgo treatment on the patient's behalf when the patient is not legally competent to provide consent.

Summons (1) In a civil case, the process by which an action is commenced and the defendant is brought within the jurisdiction of the court. (2) In a criminal case involving a petty offense or infraction, process issued for the purpose of compelling the defendant to appear in court. In such a case, a summons is used as an alternative to arrest.

Telemedicine The delivery of health-care services over a distance with the use of interactive telecommunications and computer technology.

Tort A wrong involving a breach of duty and resulting in an injury to the person or property of another. A tort is distinguished from a breach of contract in that a tort is a violation of a duty established by law, whereas a breach of contract results from a failure to meet an obligation created by the agreement of the parties. Examples of activities considered a tort include medical malpractice, defamation, and invasion of privacy.

Treatment program Entities whose sole purpose is to provide alcohol or drug abuse diagnosis and treatment.

Trial A hearing or determination by a court of the issues existing between parties to an action; an examination by a court of competent jurisdiction, according to the law of the land, of the facts or law at issue in either a civil case or a criminal prosecution, for the purpose of adjudicating the matters in controversy.

Trustworthiness One of the requirements of the business record exception to the hearsay rule. It must be established through testimony of the health information manager. To assist in establishing trustworthiness, the manager must possess knowledge of internal policies and procedures governing access to the medical record and quality control techniques, such as approved methods to make corrections to and use abbreviations in the record.

Unbundling Submitting separate bills for each component of a procedure instead of using the proper procedural code for the entire procedure, resulting in a higher reimbursement rate to the health-care provider.

Upcoding Submitting a bill for a higher level of reimbursement than actually rendered in order to receive a higher reimbursement.

Verdict The final decision of a jury concerning questions of fact submitted to it by the court for determination in the trial of a case.

Vicarious liability A doctrine that makes a health-care organization responsible for the negligent acts of its employees committed within the course and scope of their employment. Also known as respondeat superior.

Voluntary testing Testing with patient consent. Voluntary testing for HIV encompasses three areas: consent for testing, delivery of pretest information, and disclosure of test results.

Whistle-blower Generally a current or former employee of a health-care provider or organization who has learned of fraud and abuse and wishes to expose the activity.

Index

Access to health information
  adoption, 107–108
  AIDS information, 106
  alcohol and drug abuse, 151–163
  business associates, 104–105
  cancer, 106
  child abuse, 106
  clinical data, 88
  communicable diseases, 106
  demographic data, 88
  fetal deaths, 106
  FOIA and, 120–121
  general principles, 96–100
  notice of information practices, 90–92
  ownership, 89–90
  patient's right, 96–103
  preemption, 95–96
  provider acting as trustee, 89
  reporting laws, 106
  researcher's, 103–104
  reasonable fees, 102–103
  third parties, 96, 101–102
Accreditation and licensure issues of CPR, 212–215
  authentication, 214–215
  creation and storage, 213–214
  security issues, 218–224
Accrediting standards, 16, 69, 168
Administrative agencies
  decisions and regulations, 8–10
  defined, 8
  quasi-judicial powers, 9–10
Administrative procedure acts, 9
Admissibility, 216–218
Admissible evidence, 135, 183
Admissions,
  requests for, 27, 29
Adoption records,
  access to, 107–108
Advance directives, 124
Ahrens v. Katz, 74
AIDS, *see* HIV/AIDS
Alcohol and drug abuse
  confidentiality, 152–153
    patient identification, 152
    patient notice, 153
    sample patient notice, 154
  miscellaneous issues, 161–163
  record destruction, 80–81, 162
  release of information, 153–161
    components of a valid authorization, 155
  emergency situations, 158
    form requirements, 153–157
    redisclosure notice, 157
    sample authorization form, 156
Alternative dispute resolution, 33–34
American Health Information Management Association (AHIMA), 70, 77, 97, 225
American Hospital Association (AHA), 77
American legal system, workings of, 1–18
  branches of government, 13–16
  private law, 2–4
  public law, 2, 4–5
  quasi-legal requirements, 16
  sources of law, 5–13
American Medical Association, 182
American Psychological Association, 51
Annotations, 9

Anonymous testing, (HIV/AIDS) 199
Answer, 26
Antikickback statute, 240–241
Appeal,
  courts, 20
  defined, 23–24, 32
Arbitration, 33–34
Assault, 2, 52
Assoc. Mutual Hosp. Serv. of Michigan v. Health Care Service Corp. of Illinois, 246
Assumption of risk, 60
Audit activities, 159
Authentication, 70–71, 214–215
Authorization, 93, 101–102
Authorship, 70–71, 214–215
Automation, *see* Computerized patient record
Autopsy results
  HIV and, 201

Bankruptcy, 81
Bartling v. Superior Court, 18
Battery, 2, 52
Bernardi v. Community Hospital Association, 49
Bill
  legislation, 14
  of Rights, 6–7
Bing v. Thunig, 57
Black's Law Dictionary, 62, 147
Blatzwell v. Baptist Medical Center, 131
Bly v. Rhoads, 131
Bondu v. Gurvich, 77
Branches of government
  defined, 13–16
  executive, 15
  illustrated, 5
  judicial, 15–16
  legislative, 14
Breach
  of confidentiality, 4
  of contract, 3, 43, 55
  of duty of care, 44, 45–46
Brooks v. Robinson, 55
Burditt v. U.S. Department of Health and Human Services, 41
Business associate, 104–105
Business record exception, 136, 217
Butterfield v. Okubo, 192
Canterbury v. Spence, 132
Carr v. St. Paul Fire & Marine Insurance, 79–80
Case studies: things to consider, 253–264
Cases, table of, 265–270
Causation, 47
Center for Disease Control, 106, 203, 206
Centers for Medicare and Medicaid Services (CMS), 10, 243–244
CFR, *see* Code of Federal Regulations
Charitable immunity, 57, 177
Civil law
  defined, 3
  characteristics of lawsuit, 24–35
Civil money penalty, 241–242
Clark v. Norris, 193
Clinical information system, 213
CMS, *see* Centers for Medicare and Medical Services
Cobbs v. Grant, 132
Code of Federal Regulations (C.F.R.), 9
Code of State Regulations (C.S.R.), 9
Collins v. Itoh, 131
Collins v. Westlake Community Hospital, 72
Common acronyms, 271–275
Common law, 10, 57, 121
Community Health Accreditation Program (CHAP), 168
Community Hospitals of Indianapolis, Inc. v. Medtronic, 193
Comparative negligence, 59
Complaint, 22, 25–26
Completeness of the record, 71–73
Compliance, 245
Compliance programs, 244–246
Comprehensive Alcohol Abuse and Alcoholism Prevention, Treatment and Rehabilitation Act, 151–152
Comprehensive Telehealth Act, 230
Computerized patient record (CPR)
  accreditation and licensure issues, 212–215
    authentication, 214–215
    authorship, 214–215
    creation and storage, 213–214
    correction of information, 73
  electronic health issues, 224–230

liability issues, 215–224
admissibility, 216–218
security issues, 218–224
transformation to, 210–212
Confidentiality
autopsy results & HIV, 201
common law basis, 121
constitutional basis, 119–120
general principles, 116–118
HIV/AIDS, 200–201
medical research, 103–104
mental health and developmental disability care, 163–167
patient identification, 152–153
patient notice, 153
record destruction and, 79
release of information and, 88–108
risk management, 180, 186
statutes, 200
statutory basis, 120–121
Conrad v. Imatani, 131
Consent, *see* Informed consent
Consolidated Omnibus Budget Reconciliation Act of 1985 (COBRA), 41
Content requirements, *see* Medical record content requirements
Constitution
defined, 5–7
state, 7
United States, 5–6
Continuum of ownership, 100
Contract,
breach of, 3, 43, 55
express, 40
implied, 40
law, 3
Contributory negligence, 26, 59
Corn v. French, 62
Corporate negligence, 50–51
Corrections to the record, 73–75
Court(s)
appeal, 23–24
jurisdiction, 20–22
orders, 142–143
disclosure of substance abuse records, 159–161
generally, 142–143
procedures for applying for, 160
response methods, 143–145
show cause, 142
systems, 20–24
structures, 22–24
trial, 20, 22–23
CPR, *see* Computerized patient record
Credibility, 31
Criminal law
defined, 4
types, 4
Cross v. Trapp, 132
Cruzan v. Director, Missouri Department of Health, 124
CSR *see* Code of State Regulations

Damages,
actual, 47
nominal, 47
punitive, 47
Darling v. Charleston Community Memorial Hospital, 50, 177
Dashiell v. Griffith, 62
Defamation, 4
defined, 52–53
defenses, 53
Defendant, 25
Defense Criminal Investigative Service (DCIS), 243
Department of Health and Human Services (HHS), 9, 10, 15, 69, 103, 105, 120, 125, 187, 218, 241–242
Department of Labor, 15
Dependent, *see* Minor
Depositions, 26
Destruction due to closure, 80–81
Destruction in the ordinary course, 78–80
Diagnostic Related Group (DRG), 54
Digital imageing, 227
Disclosure of information, 96–100
medical research, 104
minimum necessary standard, 98–99
principles, 96–100
professional disclosure standard, 126
pursuant to court order, 159–161, 166–167
reasonable patient standard, 126
release of information, 96–100

Disclosure of information (*cont.*)
with patient authorization, 152, 153–157, 165–166
without patient authorization, 158–159, 166
Discovery,
defined, 26, 182
process, 22
types, 26–29
Diversity jurisdiction, 21
Documentation
to support defense, 59–60
Drug Abuse Prevention, Treatment and Rehabilitation Act, 151–152
Drug and alcohol abuse, *see* Alcohol and drug abuse
Durable powers of attorney, 124–125
sample, 287–291
Duty of care
defined, 44–45
breach of, 44, 45–46

Edelstein, L., 129
Electronic mail, 226–227
Electronic Signatures in Global and National Commerce Act, 215
Emancipated minor, *see* Minor patients
Emergency
release of information, 158
setting, 58
treatment, 41, 58, 125–126
Emergency Medical Treatment and Active Labor Act (EMTALA), 41
Employment challenges, 201–203
Enke v. Anderson, 193
Estate of Behringer v. Medical Center at Princeton, 180, 203–204,
Ethical guidelines, 201
Evidence, 135
Examination,
cross, 30
direct, 30
physical and/or mental, 27–29
Experimental, *see* medical research
Express contract, 40

Failure to warn, 51
False Claims Act (FCA), 239–240
FDA, *see* Food & Drug Administration
Federal Bureau of Investigation (FBI), 243
Federal Register, 9, 15
Federal Rules of Civil Procedure, 21, 24
Federal Rules of Evidence, 218
Federal Tort Claims Act, 58
Felony, 4
Florida Home Health Services Act, 167
FOIA, *see* Freedom of Information Act
Follow-up care, *see* medical abandonment
Food & Drug Administration (FDA)
generally, 103, 158, 163
medical research rules, 103
Foran v. Carangelo, 55
Foundation requirement, 136
Fraud and abuse, 238–244
law enforcement agencies, 243–244
major laws addressing, 239–242
Freedom of Information Act (FOIA), 120
Functions and uses of medical record, 65–66, 135
Furrow, Barry R. et al., 131, 192

Genetic information, 168–170
Glossary, 325–339
Glover v. Eastern Nebraska Community Center, 202
Goldstein, Louis, 62
Good Samaritan statutes, 58, 126
Government, branches of, 13–16
executive, 15
judicial, 15–16
legislative, 14
Governmental immunity, 57–58
Graham, Kenneth W., Jr., 147, 192

Halley v. Birbiglia, 132
Health Care Financing Administration (HCFA), 10
Health-care fraud and abuse, 237–249
compliance programs, 244–246
fraud and abuse, 238–244
Health Care Quality Improvement Act, 42, 187, 309–324
Health-care relationships, 39–43
hospital-patient, 40–42
hospital-physician, 42–43
illustrated, 39

physician-patient, 39–41
provider-patient, 117
Health information, *see* Access to health information
Health Insurance and Portability and Accountability Act (HIPAA), 9, 89, 218
and compliance, 245
and health-care fraud, 242–243
final privacy rule, 74–75, 90, 93, 95–105, 222, 225, 226
genetic information, 169–170
Hearsay, 135–137, 183, 217
Helman v. Sacred Heart Hospital, 208
Henry by Henry v. St. John's Hospital, 74
Henry v. Lewis, 147
HHS, *see* Department of Health and Human Services
HIPAA final privacy rule, 74–75, 90, 93, 95–102, 104–105, 222, 225, 226
minimum necessary standard, 98–99
HIPAA *see* Health Insurance Portability and Accountability Act
Hippocratic Oath, 117–118, 129
HIV/AIDS
anonymous testing, 199
autopsy results, 201
commonly used tests, 197
confidentiality, 180, 200–201
improper disclosure of information, 203–204
infection control, 202–203
legal challenges, 201–204
mandatory testing, 198–199
overview, 196–197
subpoenas, 144
voluntary testing, 197–198
HIV Health Care Services Program, 197
Home health care, 167–168
Hook v. Rothstein, 131
Horowitz v. Bogart, 55
Hurlock v. Park Lane Medical Center, 72–73

Illinois Mental Health and Developmental Disabilities Confidentiality Act, 165–166
Immunity
charitable, 57, 177
governmental, 57–58
peer review privilege, 185–186
Implied contract, 40
Improper disclosure of HIV/AIDS information, 203–204
Incident reports
definition and purpose, 181–182
discoverability and admissibility, 182–184
Incompetent patient, 124–125
Indian Health Services clinics, 100
Informed consent, 116
consent (agreement), 90
emergency situations, 125–126
express, 127
history, 121–122
implied, 127
legally incompetent patient, 124–125
medical research, 127
minor patients, 123–124
scope, 122–127
situations requiring informed consent, 127
who may consent, 123–126
In re: Milton Hershey Medical Center, 204
Institute of Medicine, 210, 212
Institutional review board (IRB), 104
Intellectual property, 4
Intentional tort, *see* Tort
Internet, 224–225
Interrogatories, 26–28
Invasion of privacy, 4, 53–54
IRB, *see* Institutional Review Board

John Roe v. Jane Doe, 4, 144, 200–201, 203
Johnson v. Misericordia Community Hospital, 51, 62
Johnson v. Vaughn, 62
Joint Commission on Accreditation of Healthcare Organizations (JCAHO),41, 69, 125, 164, 168, 177, 215, 218, 225, 226
Judgment
default, 26
satisfying, 32
Judicial process of health information, 133–147
medical records as evidence, 135–138
responses to legal process, 138–145
Judicial review, 10
Jurisdiction
concurrent, 22
diversity, 21
exclusive, 22

Jurisdiction (*cont.*)
federal question, 21
illustrated, 21
personal, 20, 22
subject matter, 20–21
Jury, 30

Kahoutek v. Hafner, 132
Kapuschinsky v. United States, 208
Katsetos v. Nolan, 62

Larrimore v. Homeopathic Hospital Association, 46
Law enforcement agencies, 243–244
Law(s)
generally, 2
major laws addressing fraud and abuse, 239–242
sources, 5–13
steps in lawsuit, 25–32
Leckelt v. Board of Commissioners, 202
Legal challenge (HIV/AIDS), 201–204
employment challenges, 201–203
improper disclosure challenges, 203–204
Legally incompetent patients
informed consent, 124–125
Legal process
appeal, 32
beginning the lawsuit, 25–26
court orders, 142–143
defined, 24
discovery, 26–29
pretrial conference, 29
responses to, 138–145
satisfying the judgment, 32–33
subpoena, 139–142
trial, 30–32
Liability
computerized patient record and, 215–223
defenses and limitations on, 55–60
assumption of risk, 60
charitable immunity, 57, 177
comparative negligence, 59–60
contributory negligence, 59–60
Good Samaritan statutes, 58
governmental immunity, 57–58
statutes of limitations, 55–57
general principles, 37–62
health-care relationships, 39–43
theories, 43–55
breach of contract, 55
intentional torts, 52–54
nonintentional torts, 43–51
Living will, 124
sample, 293–296
Locality rule, 46

Mail and wire fraud, 241
Malpractice, 44
Mandatory testing (HIV/AIDS) 198–199
Marbury v. Madison, 16
McDonald v. Massachusetts General Hospital, 62
Mediation, 33
Medicaid, 120, 124, 159, 218
fraud and abuse, 238
Medical abandonment, 54
Medical malpractice, 4, 22, 44
Medical record content, 64, 67–70
Medical record content, legal requirements, 8, 67–75
accrediting standards, 69
authentication and timeliness, 70–71, 214–215
authorization, 93
completeness, 71–73
consent form, 92–93
corrections to the record, 73–75
institutional standards, 69–70
mental health and developmental disability care, 163–167
professional guidelines, 70
proper documentation, 178
regulations, 68–69
risk management and, 178–180
statutory provisions, 68
Medical record destruction
alcohol and drug abuse records, 80–81, 162
due to closure, 80–81
in the ordinary course, 78–80
Medical record as evidence, 135–138
computerized record, 215–218
hearsay, 135–137
privilege, 137–138

Medical record, function and use of, 65–66, 135, 216
Medical record retention,
custodian of records, 137
generally, 75–78
risk management and, 179–180
Medical research, 103–104, 127
Medical staff privileges, 42, 187–188
Medicare
and False Claims Act, 240
amd Federal Privacy Act, 101
Comprehensive Telehealth Act, 230
Conditions of Participation, 69, 77, 163, 167, 215, 218, 225, 226
CMS, 10, 243–244
emergency care, 41
fraud and abuse, 238, 241–243
peer review, 159
permission and mandatory exclusion, 242
PSDA and, 124
Mental health and developmental disability care, 163–167
content requirements, 163–164
privacy restrictions, 165–167
release of information, 165–167
Minimum necessary standard, 98–99
Minor patients
release of information, 99
substituted consent, 123–124
Misdemeanor, 4
Missouri Register, 9
Monagle, John F., 192
Morbidity and Mortality Weekly Report, 106
Mordecai v. Blue Cross-Blue Shield of Alabama, 3
Mohr v. Williams, 62
Mucci v. Houghton, 62

Natanson v. Kline, 131
National Practitioner Data Bank, 187–190
Negligence
breach of duty of care, 45–46
causation, 47
comparative, 59
contributory, 59
corporate, 50–51
damages, 47–48
definition, 44
duty of care, 44
elements, 44
failure to warn, 51
informed consent, 122
Negotiation and settlement, 34
Notice of information practices, 90–92

Official record, 164
Open record statutes, 121
Ordinances, 8

Pacheco v. Ortiz, 147
Patent, 4, 11
Patient identification, 152–153
Patient notice, 153
Patient record system, 212
Patient record requirements, 63–85, 178–180
correction requests, 75
destruction requirements, 78–81
function and use of the medical record, 65–66
legal requirements for content, 67–75
retention requirements, 75–78
Patient's Bill of Rights, 277–280
Patient Self-Determination Act (PSDA), 124–125, 297–308
Peer review privileges, 185–186
People v. Bickham, 147
Permission and mandatory exclusion, 242
Personal record, 164
Personnel security, 219, 220
Physical security, 219–220
Physician
hospital relationship, 42–43
patient privileges, 121, 138
patient relationship, 39–40
self referral prohibitions, 241
Plaintiff, 25
Postal Inspection Service, 243
Pratt v. Davis, 130
Preemption, 95–96
Pretrial conference, 29
Prevost v. Coffee County Hospital Authority, 3

Principles of Medical Record Documentation, 70, 281–285
Privacy Act of 1974, 100–101, 120
Privacy, right to, 7, 89, 118–119
  common law basis, 121
  constitutional basis, 119–120
  rule incorporated into CFR, 9
  statutory basis, 120
Privacy restrictions in mental health, 165–167
Privacy standards established by HHS, 9
Privacy statutes, 121
Private law, 2–4
Privilege,
  attorney-client, 138, 183
  attorney work product, 138, 183
  generally, 137–138
  medical staff, 42, 187–188
  peer review, 185–186
  physician-patient, 121, 138
Procedural law, 4
Production of documents, 27, 28
Professional disclosure standard, 126
Proper documentation, *see* Medical record content requirements
Provider Reimbursement Review Board, 10, 22
Psychiatric, *see* Mental health and developmental disability care
Public health threats, 106
Public law, 2, 4–5
Punitive damages, *see* Damages

Qui tam actions, 240
Quality management,
  defined, 184–185
  National Practitioner Data Bank, 186–190
  peer review privileges, 185–186
Quasi-legal requirements, 16

Ravenis v. Detroit General Hospital, 71–72
Reasonable
  fee, 8, 102–103
  patient standard, 126
  prudent person standard, 45
Record destruction policies, 78–81, 162
Record retention policies, 75–78, 179–180
Regulations, 4, 68–69
  administrative, 8–10
  interplay with healthcare, 2, 161–162, 167–168
Realtors, 240
Release of information, 96–100
  alcohol and drug abuse, 152, 153–161
  audit activities, 159
  elements of valid release, 97
  HIV/AIDS, 200
  invalid release of information form, 98
  medical research, 106, 158
  mental health and developmental disability care, 165–167
  risk management, 179
  to the patient, 100–101
  to third parties, 101–102
  valid release of information form, 97
Research
  informed consent, 127
  proposal review, 104
Res ipsa loquitur, 48–49
Res judicata, 11, 15
Respondeat superior, see Vicarious liability
Restraints, patient, 164
Retention requirements, *see* Medical record retention
Risk management
  general principles, 176–178
  patient record requirements, 178
    proper documentation, 178–179
    security issues, 179–180
Risk prevention techniques, 219, 220–224
Rolater v. Strain, 130

Sard v. Hardy, 132
Schloendorff v. Society of New York Hospital, 130
Scott v. Bradford, 132
Security,
  computerized patient record and, 218–224
  personnel security, 219
  physical security, 219–220
  risk management and, 179–180
  risk prevention techniques, 219, 220–224
Service of process, 26
Seymour v. Victory Memorial Hospital, 59
Show cause order, 142
Sierra Vista Hospital v. Shaffer, 193
Skripek v. Bergamo, 131

Sligar v. Tucker, 193
Social Security Administration (SSA), 120
Sources of law, 5–13
Specialized patient records, 150
  drug and alcohol abuse, 151–163
  home health care, 167–168
  mental health and developmental disability care, 163–167
Standard of care, 16, 46
  locality rule, 46
Stare decisis, 10–11, 13, 15
Stark I and II, 241
Statutes, 4, 8, 68
  concerning an electronic medium, 213–214
  of limitation, 55–57, 77
  on telemedicine, 230
  privacy, 121
Subpoena, 138–142
  ad testificandum, 139
  AIDS/HIV and, 144
  duces tecum, 28, 137, 139, 159–160
  elements of valid, 142
  sample, 140–141
Substantive law, 4
  felonies, 4
  misdemeanors, 4
Substituted consent, 123
Supreme Court,
  state, 24
  United States, 10, 24, 32, 119–120, 124

Taaje v. St. Olaf Hospital, 208
Tarasoff v. Regents of University of California, 51
Technology, 4
  computerized patient record, 210–212
  record retention and, 77–78
Telecommunications Act, 230
Telemedicine, 228–230
Tennessee Medical Records Act, 68
Timeliness, 71, 194
Testing, *see* HIV/AIDS
Tomes, Jonathan P., 85, 199
Tort(s)
  generally, 4
  intentional, 1, 52–54
    assault and battery, 52
    defamation, 52–53
    invasion of privacy, 53–54
    medical abandonment, 54
  nonintentional, 43–51
    corporate negligence, 50–51
    failure to warn, 51
    negligence, 43–44
    res ipsa loquitur, 48–49
    vicarious liability, 49–50
Trademark, 4
Treatment program, 152
Trial,
  courts, 20
  defined, 22–23
  steps, 30–32
Trustworthiness requirement, 136–137

Unbundling, 239
United States
  constitution, 5, 119
  Supreme Court, 10, 24, 32, 119–120, 124
United States v. Sanders, 218
Upcoding, 239
U.S. ex rel. Cooper v. Blue Cross & Blue Shield of Florida, 240
U.S. ex rel. Kneepkins v. Gambro Healthcare, Inc., 241
U.S. ex rel. Merena v. SmithKline Beecham Clincial Laboratories, 240
U.S. ex rel. Stinson v. Prudential Ins., 240
U.S. ex rel. Thompson v. Columbia/HCA Healthcare Corp., 241
U.S. v. Geiger, 240
U.S. Postal Service, 241
  the Postal Dispection Service, 243
U.S. Public Health Service, 106
U.S. Sentencing Guidelines for Organizations, 246–247

Vann v. Harden, 62
Venereal disease, 106
Veterans Administration Hospitals, 100
Vicarious liability, 49–50
Voluntary testing (HIV/AIDS), 197–198

Warwick v. Bliss, 62
Whalen v. Roe, 119–120

Whistle-blowers, 240
Wilkinson v. Vesey, 132
Wright, Charles A., 147, 192

Ybarra v. Spangard, 48

Zaremski, Miles, 62